W9-AWW-577

ACP | MKSAP® 17
Medical Knowledge Self-Assessment Program®

Rheumatology

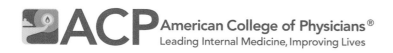

ACP American College of Physicians®
Leading Internal Medicine, Improving Lives

Welcome to the Rheumatology Section of MKSAP 17!

In these pages, you will find updated information on approaches to the patient with rheumatologic disease, principles of therapeutics, rheumatoid arthritis, osteoarthritis, systemic lupus erythematosus, infectious arthritis, idiopathic inflammatory myopathies, systemic vasculitis, systemic sclerosis, autoinflammatory diseases, true connective tissue diseases, and other clinical challenges. All of these topics are uniquely focused on the needs of generalists and subspecialists *outside* of rheumatology.

The publication of the 17th edition of Medical Knowledge Self-Assessment Program (MKSAP) represents nearly a half-century of serving as the gold-standard resource for internal medicine education. It also marks its evolution into an innovative learning system to better meet the changing educational needs and learning styles of all internists.

The core content of MKSAP has been developed as in previous editions—newly generated, essential information in 11 topic areas of internal medicine created by dozens of leading generalists and subspecialists and guided by certification and recertification requirements, emerging knowledge in the field, and user feedback. MKSAP 17 also contains 1200 all-new, psychometrically validated, and peer-reviewed multiple-choice questions (MCQs) for self-assessment and study, including 96 in Rheumatology. MKSAP 17 continues to include *High Value Care* (HVC) recommendations, based on the concept of balancing clinical benefit with costs and harms, with links to MCQs that illustrate these principles. In addition, HVC Key Points are highlighted in the text. Also highlighted, with blue text, are *Hospitalist*-focused content and MCQs that directly address the learning needs of internists who work in the hospital setting.

MKSAP 17 Digital provides access to additional tools allowing you to customize your learning experience, including regular text updates with practice-changing, new information and 200 new self-assessment questions; a board-style pretest to help direct your learning; and enhanced custom-quiz options. And, with MKSAP Complete, learners can access 1200 electronic flashcards for quick review of important concepts or review the updated and enhanced version of Virtual Dx, an image-based self-assessment tool.

As before, MKSAP 17 is optimized for use on your mobile devices, with iOS- and Android-based apps allowing you to sync your work between your apps and online account and submit for CME credits and MOC points online.

Please visit us at the MKSAP Resource Site (mksap.acponline.org) to find out how we can help you study, earn CME credit and MOC points, and stay up to date.

Whether you prefer to use the traditional print version or take advantage of the features available through the digital version, we hope you enjoy MKSAP 17 and that it meets and exceeds your personal learning needs.

On behalf of the many internists who have offered their time and expertise to create the content for MKSAP 17 and the editorial staff who work to bring this material to you in the best possible way, we are honored that you have chosen to use MKSAP 17 and appreciate any feedback about the program you may have. Please feel free to send us any comments to mksap_editors@acponline.org.

Sincerely,

Philip A. Masters, MD, FACP
Editor-in-Chief
Senior Physician Educator
Director, Content Development
Medical Education Division
American College of Physicians

Rheumatology

Committee

Michael H. Pillinger, MD, Section Editor[2]
Professor of Medicine, Biochemistry and Molecular
   Pharmacology
Department of Medicine
NYU School of Medicine
Section Chief, Rheumatology
VA New York Harbor Health Care System, New York
   Campus
New York, New York

Virginia U. Collier, MD, MACP, Associate Editor[2]
Hugh R. Sharp, Jr. Chair of Medicine
Christiana Care Health System
Newark, Delaware
Professor of Medicine
Sidney Kimmel Medical College at Thomas Jefferson
   University
Philadelphia, Pennsylvania

Daria B. Crittenden, MD[2]
Adjunct Assistant Professor of Medicine
New York University School of Medicine
Clinical Research Senior Medical Scientist
Bone Therapeutic Area
Amgen Inc.
Thousand Oaks, California

Gregory C. Gardner, MD, FACP[1]
Gilliland-Henderson Professor of Medicine
Fellowship Program Director
Division of Rheumatology
University of Washington
Seattle, Washington

Sharon L. Kolasinski, MD, FACP[2]
Professor of Clinical Medicine
Division of Rheumatology
Perelman School of Medicine at the University of
   Pennsylvania
Philadelphia, Pennsylvania

Bonita S. Libman, MD, FACP[2]
Professor of Medicine, Director of the Rheumatology
   Fellowship Training Program
Division of Rheumatology and Clinical Immunology
The University of Vermont Medical Center
Burlington, Vermont

Vikas Majithia, MD, MPH, FACP[2]
Professor of Medicine
Chief, Division of Rheumatology
Department of Medicine
University of Mississippi Medical Center
Jackson, Mississippi

Editor-in-Chief

Philip A. Masters, MD, FACP[1]
Director, Clinical Content Development
American College of Physicians
Philadelphia, Pennsylvania

Director, Clinical Program Development

Cynthia D. Smith, MD, FACP[2]
American College of Physicians
Philadelphia, Pennsylvania

Rheumatology Reviewers

Stewart F. Babbott, MD, FACP[1]
Pieter A. Cohen, MD[2]
Lia S. Logio, MD, FACP[2]
George F. Moxley, MD[2]

Rheumatology ACP Editorial Staff

Megan Zborowski[1], Senior Staff Editor
Margaret Wells[1], Director, Self-Assessment and Educational
   Programs
Becky Krumm[1], Managing Editor

ACP Principal Staff

Patrick C. Alguire, MD, FACP[2]
Senior Vice President, Medical Education

Sean McKinney[1]
Vice President, Medical Education

Margaret Wells[1]
Director, Self-Assessment and Educational Programs

Becky Krumm[1]
Managing Editor

Valerie A. Dangovetsky[1]
Administrator

Ellen McDonald, PhD[1]
Senior Staff Editor

Katie Idell[1]
Digital Content Associate/Editor

Megan Zborowski[1]
Senior Staff Editor

Randy Hendrickson[1]
Production Administrator/Editor

Linnea Donnarumma[1]
Staff Editor

Susan Galeone[1]
Staff Editor

Jackie Twomey[1]
Staff Editor

Kimberly Kerns[1]
Administrative Coordinator

---

1. Has no relationships with any entity producing, marketing, reselling, or distributing health care goods or services consumed by, or used on, patients.

2. Has disclosed relationship(s) with any entity producing, marketing, reselling, or distributing health care goods or services consumed by, or used on, patients.

Disclosure of Relationships with any entity producing, marketing, reselling, or distributing health care goods or services consumed by, or used on, patients:

Patrick C. Alguire, MD, FACP
Board Member
Teva Pharmaceuticals
Consultantship
National Board of Medical Examiners
Royalties
UpToDate
Stock Options/Holdings
Amgen Inc, Bristol-Myers Squibb, GlaxoSmithKline, Covidien, Stryker Corporation, Zimmer Orthopedics, Teva Pharmaceuticals, Express Scripts, Medtronic

Pieter A. Cohen, MD
Stock Options/Holdings (spouse)
Bio Reference Labs, Idexx Laboratories, Johnson & Johnson, Mettler Toledo International Inc., Stryker Corp., Biota Pharmaceuticals, Pfizer, ResMed Inc., Vertex Pharmaceuticals
Honoraria
Consumer Union, Wall Street Journal

Virginia U. Collier, MD, MACP
Stock Options/Holdings
Celgene, Pfizer, Merck, Abbott, Abbevie, Johnson and Johnson, Medtronic, McKesson, Amgen Inc., Wellpoint, Roche, Sanofi, Novartis, Covidien, Stryker, Amerisource Bergen, Schering Plough

Daria B. Crittenden, MD
Research Grants/Contracts
Savient Pharmaceuticals
Employment — Clinical Research Senior Medical Scientist
Amgen Inc.

Sharon L. Kolasinski, MD, FACP
Honoraria
Curatio CME, Georgetown University Rheumatology Division, American College of Rheumatology, Rush University Medical Center, New York University, Congress of Clinical Rheumatology, American College of Physicians Delaware Chapter
Consultantship
Vindico Medical Education
Research Grants/Contracts
Human Genome Sciences, UCB, Bristol-Myers Squibb, Amgen, Abbott

Bonita S. Libman, MD, FACP
Research Grants/Contracts
Human Genome Sciences, GlaxoSmithKline

Lia S. Logio, MD, FACP
Royalties
McGraw Hill

Vikas Majithia, MD, MPH, FACP
Speakers Bureau
GlaxoSmithKline
Research Grants/Contracts
GlaxoSmithKline

George F. Moxley, MD
Employment
Virginia Commonwealth University

Michael Pillinger, MD
Research Grants/Contracts
Takeda Incorporated, Savient Pharmaceuticals
Consultant
AstraZeneca, Crealta

Cynthia D. Smith, MD, FACP
Stock Options/Holdings
Merck and Co.; spousal employment at Merck

Acknowledgments

The American College of Physicians (ACP) gratefully acknowledges the special contributions to the development and production of the 17th edition of the Medical Knowledge Self-Assessment Program® (MKSAP® 17) made by the following people:

Graphic Design: Michael Ripca (Graphics Technical Administrator) and WFGD Studio (Graphic Designers).

Production/Systems: Dan Hoffmann (Director, Web Services & Systems Development), Neil Kohl (Senior

Architect), Chris Patterson (Senior Architect), and Scott Hurd (Manager, Web Projects & CMS Services).

MKSAP 17 Digital: Under the direction of Steven Spadt, Vice President, Digital Products & Services, the digital version of MKSAP 17 was developed within the ACP's Digital Product Development Department, led by Brian Sweigard (Director). Other members of the team included Dan Barron (Senior Web Application Developer/Architect), Chris Forrest (Senior Software Developer/Design Lead), Kara Kronenwetter (Senior Web Developer), Brad Lord (Senior Web Application Developer), John McKnight (Senior Web Developer), and Nate Pershall (Senior Web Developer).

The College also wishes to acknowledge that many other persons, too numerous to mention, have contributed to the production of this program. Without their dedicated efforts, this program would not have been possible.

MKSAP Resource Site (mksap.acponline.org)

The MKSAP Resource Site (mksap.acponline.org) is a continually updated site that provides links to MKSAP 17 online answer sheets for print subscribers; the latest details on Continuing Medical Education (CME) and Maintenance of Certification (MOC) in the United States, Canada, and Australia; errata; and other new information.

ABIM Maintenance of Certification

Check the MKSAP Resource Site (mksap.acponline.org) for the latest information on how MKSAP tests can be used to apply to the American Board of Internal Medicine for Maintenance of Certification (MOC) points.

Royal College Maintenance of Certification

In Canada, MKSAP 17 is an Accredited Self-Assessment Program (Section 3) as defined by the Maintenance of Certification (MOC) Program of The Royal College of Physicians and Surgeons of Canada and approved by the Canadian Society of Internal Medicine on December 9, 2014. Approval extends from July 31, 2015 until July 31, 2018 for the Part A sections. Approval extends from December 31, 2015 to December 31, 2018 for the Part B sections.

Fellows of the Royal College may earn three credits per hour for participating in MKSAP 17 under Section 3. MKSAP 17 also meets multiple CanMEDS Roles, including that of Medical Expert, Communicator, Collaborator, Manager, Health Advocate, Scholar, and Professional. For information on how to apply MKSAP 17 Continuing Medical Education (CME) credits to the Royal College MOC Program, visit the MKSAP Resource Site at mksap.acponline.org.

The Royal Australasian College of Physicians CPD Program

In Australia, MKSAP 17 is a Category 3 program that may be used by Fellows of The Royal Australasian College of Physicians (RACP) to meet mandatory Continuing Professional Development (CPD) points. Two CPD credits are awarded for each of the 200 *AMA PRA Category 1 Credits*™ available in MKSAP 17. More information about using MKSAP 17 for this purpose is available at the MKSAP Resource Site at mksap.acponline.org and at www.racp.edu.au. CPD credits earned through MKSAP 17 should be reported at the MyCPD site at www.racp.edu.au/mycpd.

Continuing Medical Education

The American College of Physicians (ACP) is accredited by the Accreditation Council for Continuing Medical Education (ACCME) to provide continuing medical education for physicians.

The ACP designates this enduring material, MKSAP 17, for a maximum of 200 *AMA PRA Category 1 Credits*™. Physicians should claim only the credit commensurate with the extent of their participation in the activity.

Up to 16 *AMA PRA Category 1 Credits*™ are available from July 31, 2015, to July 31, 2018, for the MKSAP 17 Rheumatology section.

Learning Objectives

The learning objectives of MKSAP 17 are to:
- Close gaps between actual care in your practice and preferred standards of care, based on best evidence
- Diagnose disease states that are less common and sometimes overlooked or confusing
- Improve management of comorbid conditions that can complicate patient care
- Determine when to refer patients for surgery or care by subspecialists
- Pass the ABIM Certification Examination
- Pass the ABIM Maintenance of Certification Examination

Target Audience

- General internists and primary care physicians
- Subspecialists who need to remain up-to-date in internal medicine and in areas outside of their own subspecialty area
- Residents preparing for the certification examination in internal medicine
- Physicians preparing for maintenance of certification in internal medicine (recertification)

Earn "Instantaneous" CME Credits Online

Print subscribers can enter their answers online to earn instantaneous Continuing Medical Education (CME) credits. You can submit your answers using online answer sheets that are provided at mksap.acponline.org, where a record of your MKSAP 17 credits will be available. To earn CME credits, you need to answer all of the questions in a test and earn a score of at least 50% correct (number of correct answers divided by the total number of questions). Take any of the following approaches:

1. Use the printed answer sheet at the back of this book to record your answers. Go to mksap.acponline.org, access the appropriate online answer sheet, transcribe your answers, and submit your test for instantaneous CME credits. There is no additional fee for this service.

2. Go to mksap.acponline.org, access the appropriate online answer sheet, directly enter your answers, and submit your test for instantaneous CME credits. There is no additional fee for this service.

3. Pay a $15 processing fee per answer sheet and submit the printed answer sheet at the back of this book by mail or fax, as instructed on the answer sheet. Make sure you calculate your score and fax the answer sheet to 215-351-2799 or mail the answer sheet to Member and Customer Service, American College of Physicians, 190 N. Independence Mall West, Philadelphia, PA 19106-1572, using the courtesy envelope provided in your MKSAP 17 slipcase. You will need your 10-digit order number and 8-digit ACP ID number, which are printed on your packing slip. Please allow 4 to 6 weeks for your score report to be emailed back to you. Be sure to include your email address for a response.

If you do not have a 10-digit order number and 8-digit ACP ID number or if you need help creating a user name and password to access the MKSAP 17 online answer sheets, go to mksap.acponline.org or email custserv@acponline.org.

Disclosure Policy

It is the policy of the American College of Physicians (ACP) to ensure balance, independence, objectivity, and scientific rigor in all of its educational activities. To this end, and consistent with the policies of the ACP and the Accreditation Council for Continuing Medical Education (ACCME), contributors to all ACP continuing medical education activities are required to disclose all relevant financial relationships with any entity producing, marketing, reselling, or distributing health care goods or services consumed by, or used on, patients. Contributors are required to use generic names in the discussion of therapeutic options and are required to identify any unapproved, off-label, or investigative use of commercial products or devices. Where a trade name is used, all available trade names for the same product type are also included. If trade-name products manufactured by companies with whom contributors have relationships are discussed, contributors are asked to provide evidence-based citations in support of the discussion. The information is reviewed by the committee responsible for producing this text. If necessary, adjustments to topics or contributors' roles in content development are made to balance the discussion. Further, all readers of this text are asked to evaluate the content for evidence of commercial bias and send any relevant comments to mksap_editors@acponline.org so that future decisions about content and contributors can be made in light of this information.

Resolution of Conflicts

To resolve all conflicts of interest and influences of vested interests, the American College of Physicians (ACP) precluded members of the content-creation committee from deciding on any content issues that involved generic or trade-name products associated with proprietary entities with which these committee members had relationships. In addition, content was based on best evidence and updated clinical care guidelines, when such evidence and guidelines were available. Contributors' disclosure information can be found with the list of contributors' names and those of ACP principal staff listed in the beginning of this book.

Hospital-Based Medicine

For the convenience of subscribers who provide care in hospital settings, content that is specific to the hospital setting has been highlighted in blue. Hospital icons (🄷) highlight where the hospital-based content begins, continues over more than one page, and ends.

High Value Care Key Points

Key Points in the text that relate to High Value Care concepts (that is, concepts that discuss balancing clinical benefit with costs and harms) are designated by the HVC icon (**HVC**).

Educational Disclaimer

The editors and publisher of MKSAP 17 recognize that the development of new material offers many opportunities for error. Despite our best efforts, some errors may persist in print. Drug dosage schedules are, we believe, accurate and in accordance with current standards. Readers are advised, however, to ensure that the recommended dosages in MKSAP 17 concur with the information provided in the product information material. This is especially important in cases of new, infrequently used, or highly toxic drugs. Application of the information in MKSAP 17 remains the professional responsibility of the practitioner.

The primary purpose of MKSAP 17 is educational. Information presented, as well as publications, technologies, products, and/or services discussed, is intended to inform subscribers about the knowledge, techniques, and experiences of the contributors. A diversity of professional opinion exists, and the views of the contributors are their own and not those of the American College of Physicians (ACP). Inclusion of any material in the program does not constitute endorsement or recommendation by the ACP. The ACP does not warrant the safety, reliability, accuracy, completeness, or usefulness of and disclaims any and all liability for damages and claims that may result from the use of information, publications, technologies, products, and/or services discussed in this program.

Publisher's Information

Copyright © 2015 American College of Physicians. All rights reserved.

This publication is protected by copyright. No part of this publication may be reproduced, stored in a retrieval system, or transmitted in any form or by any means, electronic or mechanical, including photocopy, without the express consent of the American College of Physicians. MKSAP 17 is for individual use only. Only one account per subscription will be permitted for the purpose of earning Continuing Medical Education (CME) credits and Maintenance of Certification (MOC) points/credits and for other authorized uses of MKSAP 17.

Unauthorized Use of This Book Is Against the Law

Unauthorized reproduction of this publication is unlawful. The American College of Physicians (ACP) prohibits reproduction of this publication or any of its parts in any form either for individual use or for distribution.

The ACP will consider granting an individual permission to reproduce only limited portions of this publication for his or her own exclusive use. Send requests in writing to MKSAP® Permissions, American College of Physicians, 190 N. Independence Mall West, Philadelphia, PA 19106-1572, or email your request to mksap_editors@acponline.org.

MKSAP 17 ISBN: 978-1-938245-18-3
(Rheumatology) ISBN: 978-1-938245-24-4

Printed in the United States of America.

For order information in the United States or Canada call 800-523-1546, extension 2600. All other countries call 215-351-2600, (M-F, 9 AM – 5 PM ET). Fax inquiries to 215-351-2799 or email to custserv@acponline.org.

Errata

Errata for MKSAP 17 will be available through the MKSAP Resource Site at mksap.acponline.org as new information becomes known to the editors.

Table of Contents

Rheumatology High Value Care Recommendations

The American College of Physicians, in collaboration with multiple other organizations, is engaged in a worldwide initiative to promote the practice of High Value Care (HVC). The goals of the HVC initiative are to improve health care outcomes by providing care of proven benefit and reducing costs by avoiding unnecessary and even harmful interventions. The initiative comprises several programs that integrate the important concept of health care value (balancing clinical benefit with costs and harms) for a given intervention into a broad range of educational materials to address the needs of trainees, practicing physicians, and patients.

HVC content has been integrated into MKSAP 17 in several important ways. MKSAP 17 now includes HVC-identified key points in the text, HVC-focused multiple choice questions, and, for subscribers to MKSAP Digital, an HVC custom quiz. From the text and questions, we have generated the following list of HVC recommendations that meet the definition below of high value care and bring us closer to our goal of improving patient outcomes while conserving finite resources.

High Value Care Recommendation: A recommendation to choose diagnostic and management strategies for patients in specific clinical situations that balance clinical benefit with cost and harms with the goal of improving patient outcomes.

Below are the High Value Care Recommendations for the Rheumatology section of MKSAP 17.

- A physical examination is essential when diagnosing musculoskeletal pain and can help to avoid unnecessary laboratory and radiographic testing.
- The most appropriate and cost-effective means of assessing the cause of acute monoarthritis is by aspiration and analysis of the synovial fluid for leukocytes, Gram stain with culture, and crystals.
- Laboratory studies such as erythrocyte sedimentation rate, rheumatoid factor, and antinuclear antibodies have low specificity for diagnosing rheumatologic disease in patients with low pretest probability, thus limiting their utility in this population.
- The dose of glucocorticoid therapy should not be prolonged or increased in patients with polymyalgia rheumatica who have clinically improved based on an elevated erythrocyte sedimentation rate, as this is a non-specific test (see Item 94).

- CT is useful in assessing bony abnormalities but is more expensive than plain radiography and exposes the patient to more radiation.
- MRI is useful in detecting soft-tissue abnormalities, inflammation, and fluid collections.
- Musculoskeletal ultrasonography is a low risk and relatively inexpensive way to detect soft-tissue abnormalities such as synovitis, tendinitis, bursitis, and joint fluid.
- Topical NSAIDs provide similar pain relief for inflammatory conditions as oral medications with fewer gastrointestinal effects and are preferred for patients 75 years or older; however, they are associated with more skin reactions and are significantly more expensive than oral NSAIDs.
- Rheumatoid factor, anti–cyclic citrullinated peptide antibodies, and inflammatory markers assist in confirming a diagnosis of rheumatoid arthritis; however, serologies should never be used as the sole criterion for diagnosis and should be avoided in patients with low pretest probability for disease due to the high rate of false-positive results.
- Plain radiography of the hands, wrists, and/or feet are indicated to aid in the diagnosis and to follow progression of rheumatoid arthritis; in contrast, MRI of peripheral joints should not be routinely performed to monitor disease progression.
- Methotrexate is the initial treatment of choice for patients with new-onset, rapidly progressive, or erosive rheumatoid arthritis (see Item 54).
- Leflunomide-induced liver chemistry elevation is common (seen in up to 20% of patients taking the medication) and is usually reversible with dose reduction or drug discontinuation; thus, further evaluation, including liver biopsy, is not necessary (see Item 75).
- Laboratory studies are indicated only when needed to rule out other diagnoses in patients with primary osteoarthritis (OA); the diagnostic role for MRI and ultrasonography in OA has not been established.
- In patients with suspected osteoarthritis, confirmatory plain radiographs with standing views are appropriate to solidify the diagnosis and rule out less common findings such as avascular necrosis, fractures, and malignancies (see Item 37).
- Additional testing such as autoantibody measurements or radiography is unnecessary in patients with clinically diagnosed hand osteoarthritis (see Item 43).

- In patients with osteoarthritis, initial treatment with acetaminophen for pain control is generally recommended (see Item 72).
- An NSAID should be initiated in patients with osteoarthritis if first-line therapy with acetaminophen does not provide adequate relief (see Item 89).
- Fibromyalgia is a clinical diagnosis characterized by chronic widespread pain, tenderness of the skin and muscles to pressure, fatigue, sleep disturbance, and exercise intolerance.
- Initial laboratory evaluation of fibromyalgia includes a complete blood count, chemistry panel, thyroid-stimulating hormone, and erythrocyte sedimentation rate or C-reactive protein; routine testing for antinuclear antibodies, rheumatoid factor, anti–cyclic citrullinated peptide antibodies, or muscle enzymes should be avoided.
- Nonpharmacologic therapy, including regular aerobic exercise, is the cornerstone of fibromyalgia treatment and should be initiated in all affected patients (see Item 67).
- Conventional radiography of the spine and sacroiliac joints is generally adequate to demonstrate synovitis, axial erosion, or new bone formation in patients with spondyloarthritis; CT should be reserved for identifying occult spine fractures and bony erosions in patients at high risk due to expense and higher level of radiation exposure.
- Patients with ankylosing spondylitis who are responding well to treatment should be monitored clinically and do not require periodic imaging studies less than every 2 years unless absolutely necessary (see Item 33).
- In patients with strongly suspected spondyloarthritis, MRI of the sacroiliac joints and/or spine should only be considered if conventional radiographs are negative.
- Age-appropriate cancer screening is recommended for patients with dermatomyositis or polymyositis, with consideration of additional testing for ovarian cancer; additional CT or PET scanning to look for underlying malignancy is not cost effective unless the patient has additional risk factors.
- Immediate treatment with prednisone, 60 mg/d (or 1 mg/kg/d), is indicated for patients with suspected giant cell arteritis to prevent visual complications (see Item 17).
- Sarcoidosis can manifest as Löfgren syndrome, which is characterized by acute arthritis, bilateral hilar lymphadenopathy, and erythema nodosum; when all three occur together, there is a 95% specificity for the diagnosis, and further diagnostic tests are unnecessary.
- Primary Raynaud phenomenon is common and carries a low risk for progression; thus, a serologic evaluation for underlying connective tissue disease is low yield and not cost effective unless severe and prolonged vasospastic episodes, asymmetric involvement of the digits, and abnormal nailfold capillary examination or digital pitting are present (see Item 73).

Rheumatology

Approach to the Patient with Rheumatologic Disease

Introduction

In the United States, the estimated prevalence of chronic arthritis among adults is 33%; older persons (>65 years of age) have a higher prevalence than younger persons (<44 years of age).

Inflammatory Versus Noninflammatory Pain

In patients with musculoskeletal pain, it is critical to distinguish between inflammatory and noninflammatory pain, which typically have different causes. Inflammatory pain involves classic signs and symptoms of redness, swelling, warmth, and tenderness. Inflammation is often associated with prolonged morning stiffness and, potentially, constitutional symptoms. Although noninflammatory pain may also manifest with tenderness, other signs of inflammation are generally mild or absent. **Table 1** compares the features of inflammatory and noninflammatory pain.

KEY POINT

- Inflammatory pain involves redness, swelling, warmth, and tenderness; prolonged morning stiffness and constitutional symptoms may also occur.

The Musculoskeletal Examination

A physical examination is essential when diagnosing musculoskeletal pain and can help to avoid unnecessary laboratory and radiographic testing. Pain may be articular (from the joint), periarticular (from soft-tissue structures around the joint such as tendons, bursae, or muscles), or referred (from structures proximal or distal to the joint, or neurogenic in origin). Inspection, palpation, and range of motion are generally sufficient to establish whether there is an articular or a periarticular condition. Peripheral joints are usually straightforward to examine, although adiposity or edema can make inspection and palpation difficult. Axial joints such as the spine, shoulders, and hips are more difficult to assess for warmth and swelling; tenderness, range of motion, and special maneuvers are often required to adequately assess these areas.

Differentiating between active (patient moves the joint using his/her own power) and passive (examiner moves the joint for the patient) range of motion is important because

TABLE 1.	Features of Inflammatory Versus Noninflammatory Pain	
Feature	**Inflammatory Pain**	**Noninflammatory Pain**
Physical examination findings	Erythema; warmth; soft-tissue swelling	No soft-tissue swelling; minimal or no warmth; bony enlargement and joint effusions may occur in osteoarthritis
Morning stiffness	>60 min	<30 min
Constitutional symptoms	Fever; fatigue; malaise	Generally absent
Synovial fluid	Leukocyte count >2000/µL (2.0 × 10⁹/L), predominantly neutrophils in acute inflammation and monocytes in chronic inflammation	Leukocyte count between 200/µL and 2000/µL (0.2 × 10⁹/L and 2.0 × 10⁹/L), predominantly monocytes
Other laboratory findings	Elevated inflammatory markers (ESR, CRP); anemia of chronic disease	Inflammatory markers usually normal or minimally elevated
Arthritis imaging studies	Symmetric/diffuse joint-space narrowing; periarticular osteopenia; erosions; bony proliferation in secondary osteoarthritis or spondyloarthritis; synovitis on MRI or ultrasound	Asymmetric/compartmental joint-space narrowing; osteophytes; subchondral sclerosis; limited or no synovitis on MRI or ultrasound

CRP = C-reactive protein; ESR = erythrocyte sedimentation rate.

pain with both passive and active range of motion implies an intrinsic joint condition, whereas pain with only active range of motion may be due to a periarticular condition.

See Musculoskeletal Pain in MKSAP 17 General Internal Medicine for more information.

KEY POINTS

HVC
- A physical examination is essential when diagnosing musculoskeletal pain and can help to avoid unnecessary laboratory and radiographic testing.
- Pain with both passive and active range of motion implies an intrinsic joint condition, whereas pain with only active range of motion may be due to a periarticular condition.

Arthritis

In addition to the presence or absence of inflammation, other features help to refine the differential diagnosis of musculoskeletal pain: pattern of joint involvement, number of joints involved, duration of symptoms, and presence or absence of symmetry.

Monoarticular Arthritis

Monoarticular arthritis (monoarthritis) involves a single joint. The differential diagnosis depends upon whether there is inflammation, the acuity of symptoms, and the patient's demographic and epidemiologic risk factors.

Inflammatory monoarthritis may be due to infection: bacterial in acute cases, and atypical organisms such as fungi, mycobacteria, or spirochetes (Lyme) in chronic cases. Noninfectious causes include crystal-related and autoimmune diseases. Crystal-related diseases typically present acutely but occasionally can be chronic, especially those caused by calcium pyrophosphate deposition. Noninflammatory monoarthritis is usually due to osteoarthritis or mechanical derangement (such as a torn meniscus or ligament). A history of trauma prior to onset of symptoms points toward noninflammatory arthritis.

The most appropriate and cost-effective means of assessing the cause of acute monoarthritis is by aspiration and analysis of the synovial fluid for leukocytes, Gram stain with culture, and crystals. If there is high suspicion for infection (especially atypical organisms) and synovial fluid cultures are unrevealing, synovial biopsy or other special tests may be needed. Blood in the synovial fluid (hemarthrosis) is typically associated with trauma except in patients with bleeding diatheses such as hemophilia.

Oligoarthritis

Oligoarthritis involves two to four joints, commonly in the lower extremities, and is often asymmetric. Although many diseases can manifest with oligoarthritis, the most common autoimmune inflammatory forms of oligoarthritis are the spondyloarthritis diseases (**Table 2**). Disseminated gonococcal infection, rheumatic fever, and Lyme disease may also present as inflammatory oligoarthritis. Osteoarthritis may cause a noninflammatory oligoarthritis, particularly if the involved joints share a history of trauma or overuse.

Polyarthritis

Polyarthritis involves five or more joints. The most common causes of chronic inflammatory polyarthritis include rheumatoid arthritis, systemic lupus erythematosus (SLE), and psoriatic arthritis (see Table 2). In contrast, acute onset of inflammatory polyarthritis is more commonly caused by viral infections such as hepatitis, parvovirus, rubella, herpes, HIV, adenovirus, mumps, or enterovirus. Polyarthritis may also be caused by a drug-induced serum sickness reaction, an immune complex reaction to bacterial infections such as endocarditis, or other forms of crystal or autoimmune diseases.

KEY POINT

- The most appropriate and cost-effective means of assessing the cause of acute monoarthritis is by aspiration and analysis of the synovial fluid for leukocytes, Gram stain with culture, and crystals.
HVC

Extra-Articular Manifestations of Rheumatologic Disease

Many rheumatologic diseases are systemic and therefore cause extra-articular manifestations in various sites and organs.

Constitutional Symptoms

Constitutional symptoms are common in systemic inflammatory diseases. Fever is especially typical of adult-onset Still disease and the autoinflammatory diseases (also known as the periodic fever syndromes) but may also occur in SLE, rheumatoid arthritis, and vasculitis, in which it is commonly low grade. Malaise and unintended weight loss also occur. In the absence of a clear cause, such symptoms may also suggest occult malignancy and/or infection.

Dermatologic Manifestations

Skin involvement is common in many rheumatologic diseases (**Table 3**, on page 4). Because of easy access by physical examination and/or biopsy, skin manifestations can be helpful in establishing a diagnosis, especially SLE, systemic sclerosis, and vasculitis. Some cutaneous findings may be subtle or unnoticed by the patient (for example, nail pitting); therefore, a high index of suspicion and a thorough physical examination may be required.

Inflammatory Eye Disease

Eye involvement is common in systemic rheumatologic diseases and provides direct visual access to both mucosal and central nervous system tissues. The location and type of ocular involvement may help narrow the differential diagnosis (**Table 4**, on page 4). Some diseases are particularly notable for ocular involvement, including rheumatoid arthritis (episcleritis and scleritis); spondyloarthritis and sarcoidosis (uveitis);

TABLE 2. Autoimmune Inflammatory Arthritis

Condition	Pattern of Joint Involvement	Extra-articular Features	Diagnostic Studies
Rheumatoid arthritis	Symmetric polyarthritis; involves small joints (wrist, MCP, PIP, MTP) but also can involve hips, knees, elbows, shoulders, and cervical spine; spares thoracic and lumbar spine and DIP joints	Rheumatoid nodules; dry eyes and mouth; interstitial lung disease; Felty syndrome (splenomegaly, leukopenia, leg ulcers)	Rheumatoid factor; anti-CCP; acute phase reactants; erosive changes on radiograph
Systemic lupus erythematosus	Symmetric polyarthritis with large and small joint involvement; minimal to no swelling	Constitutional (fever, fatigue); multi-organ involvement (rash, oral ulcers, alopecia, serositis, kidney disease, neurologic disease, cytopenias)	ANA; anti–double-stranded DNA; anti-Smith; anti-U1-RNP; anti-Ro/SSA; anti-La/SSB; no erosions on radiograph
Spondyloarthritis			
Ankylosing spondylitis	Sacroiliac and spinal involvement; symmetric; large joints (shoulders, hips); spares small joints	Uveitis	Calcification of anterior longitudinal ligament of spine on radiograph; sacroiliitis; usually HLA-B27 positive
Psoriatic arthritis	Asymmetric oligoarthritis or symmetric polyarthritis; DIP joint preference; dactylitis (sausage digits); enthesitis (insertion of tendon to bone); axial disease with sacroiliitis	Psoriasis; uveitis	"Pencil-in-cup" deformities; erosions and osteophytes on radiograph; sometimes HLA-B27 positive
Reactive arthritis (formerly known as Reiter syndrome)	Asymmetric oligoarthritis; knee and ankle involvement; enthesitis; Achilles tendinitis; plantar fasciitis; sacroiliitis	Uveitis; keratoderma blennorrhagicum; preceding infection (*Chlamydia*; enteropathic)	Sacroiliitis; sometimes HLA-B27 positive
Inflammatory bowel disease-associated arthritis	Asymmetric; sacroiliitis; knee and feet involvement	Crohn disease; ulcerative colitis	Sacroiliitis; sometimes HLA-B27 positive

ANA = antinuclear antibodies; CCP = cyclic citrullinated peptide; DIP = distal interphalangeal; MCP = metacarpophalangeal; MTP = metatarsophalangeal; PIP = proximal interphalangeal; RNP = ribonucleoprotein.

and vasculitis, especially granulomatosis with polyangiitis (formerly known as Wegener granulomatosis), which can affect all parts of the eye. Dry eyes (keratoconjunctivitis sicca) are a major feature of Sjögren syndrome, whether primary or in association with other rheumatologic diseases.

Scleritis can result in permanent loss of vision, especially if scleral perforation occurs. Severe uveitis can also cause permanent visual loss. Recognition and treatment of these entities are therefore an urgent matter.

Internal Organ Involvement

Internal organs are potential targets for rheumatologic diseases (**Table 5**, on page 5). Vasculitis may affect one or more internal organs and should be considered in the differential diagnosis of a multisystem disease. Certain patterns of involvement may be helpful in developing a differential diagnosis, such as pulmonary-renal syndrome (pulmonary vasculitis/hemorrhage and glomerulonephritis) that may occur with ANCA-associated vasculitis, SLE, or Goodpasture syndrome.

Rheumatologic and Musculoskeletal Manifestations in Systemic Disease

Nonrheumatologic systemic diseases may have rheumatologic or musculoskeletal manifestations (**Table 6**, on page 6).

KEY POINT

- Systemic rheumatologic diseases can cause constitutional symptoms and extra-articular manifestations in various sites, including the skin, eyes, and internal organs.

Laboratory Studies

In rheumatologic diseases, laboratory studies are used to aid in diagnosis, follow disease activity, assess the extent of disease-related internal organ involvement, and monitor patients taking chronic immunomodulatory medications. However, some

TABLE 3. Dermatologic Manifestations of Rheumatologic Disease

Disease	Manifestations
Systemic lupus erythematosus	Butterfly (malar) rash; photosensitive rash; discoid lupus erythematosus; subacute cutaneous lupus erythematosus; oral ulcerations (on the tongue or hard palate that are usually painless); alopecia; lupus panniculitis (painful, indurated subcutaneous swelling with overlying erythema of the skin)
Dermatomyositis	Gottron papules (erythematous plaques on extensor surfaces of MCP and PIP joints); photodistributed poikiloderma, including shawl sign (over the back and shoulders) and V sign (over the posterior neck/back or neck/upper chest); heliotrope rash (violaceous rash on the upper eyelid); mechanic's hands (hyperkeratotic, fissured skin on the palmar and lateral aspects of fingers); nailfold capillary abnormalities; holster sign (poikilodermic rash along lateral thigh)
Amyopathic dermatomyositis	Skin findings listed above under Dermatomyositis but without myositis findings
Systemic sclerosis	Skin thickening and hardening (limited disease involves face and skin distal to elbows/knees; diffuse disease involves skin proximal to distal forearms/knees); nailfold capillary changes
Vasculitis	Palpable purpura; cutaneous nodules; ulcers
Behçet syndrome	Painful oral and genital ulcers; erythema nodosum; acne/folliculitis; pathergy (skin inflammation/ulceration from minor trauma)
Sarcoidosis	Erythema nodosum
Psoriatic arthritis	Plaque psoriasis typically on extensor surfaces, umbilicus, gluteal fold, scalp, and behind ears; pustular psoriasis on palms and soles; arthritis may precede rash by up to 10 years; nail pitting; onycholysis
Reactive arthritis (formerly known as Reiter syndrome)	Keratoderma blennorrhagicum (psoriasiform rash on soles, toes, palms); circinate balanitis (psoriasiform rash on penis)
Adult-onset Still disease	Evanescent, salmon-colored rash on trunk and proximal extremities
Rheumatic fever (secondary to streptoccocal infection)	Erythema marginatum (annular pink to red nonpruritic rash with central clearing)
Lyme disease	Erythema chronicum migrans (slowly expanding, often annual lesion with central clearing)

MCP = metacarpophalangeal; PIP = proximal interphalangeal.

TABLE 4. Ocular Manifestations of Systemic Inflammatory Disease

Ocular Manifestation	Associated Systemic Inflammatory Disease
Uveitis	Spondyloarthritis (ankylosing spondylitis, reactive arthritis [formerly known as Reiter syndrome], inflammatory bowel disease) (anterior chamber); sarcoidosis (anterior and/or posterior chamber); Behçet syndrome (anterior and/or posterior chamber); granulomatosis with polyangiitis (formerly known as Wegener granulomatosis) (posterior chamber)
Episcleritis	Rheumatoid arthritis; spondyloarthritis; systemic vasculitis
Scleritis	Rheumatoid arthritis; relapsing polychondritis; inflammatory bowel disease; systemic vasculitis
Retinal disease	Systemic vasculitis; antiphospholipid antibody syndrome

commonly used laboratory studies have low specificity for diagnosing rheumatologic disease when the pretest probability of disease is low, and rigor must be applied when interpreting such results.

Tests That Measure Inflammation

Several tests may be abnormal when rheumatologic or other inflammation is present. These include erythrocyte sedimentation rate and acute phase reactants, particularly C-reactive protein but also fibrinogen and ferritin. Platelet counts also tend to rise with inflammation. Complement levels usually increase with inflammation but fall with immune complex formation.

Erythrocyte Sedimentation Rate

Erythrocyte sedimentation rate (ESR) measures the rate at which erythrocytes settle with gravity in an upright tube of anticoagulated whole blood. ESR is dictated by characteristics of the erythrocytes themselves (size, shape, surface charge) and by the presence of specific plasma proteins that alter the normal repulsive forces (that is, neutralize surface charge) between erythrocytes and promote their ability to aggregate and form rouleaux and sediment more quickly. Such plasma proteins include several acute phase reactants (especially fibrinogen) produced by the liver in response to proinflammatory cytokines arising in rheumatologic, infectious, or malignant conditions. The normal ESR rises with age and tends to be higher in women. An estimate of the maximal expected normal ESR based on age and gender is age in years/2 for men and (age in years + 10)/2 for women. Thus, a mildly elevated ESR in an older patient must be interpreted with caution.

TABLE 5. Internal Organ Involvement in Rheumatologic Disease

Organ	Disease	Type of Involvement
Heart		
	Kawasaki disease	Coronary artery vasculitis
	Systemic sclerosis	Arrhythmia; cardiomyopathy; pulmonary hypertension
	SLE	Pericarditis; valvular disease; cardiomyopathy
	RA	Pericarditis; cardiomyopathy
	Rheumatic fever; antiphospholipid antibody syndrome	Valvular disease
	GCA; Takayasu arteritis	Aortitis; heart failure; large-vessel vasculitis
Lung		
	RA	Serositis; ILD; rheumatoid nodules
	SLE; CTDs; HSP	Serositis; pneumonitis; pulmonary hemorrhage from vasculitis
	AAV; systemic vasculitis	Pulmonary hemorrhage; cavitary nodules
	Systemic sclerosis	ILD; pulmonary hypertension
	Antiphospholipid antibody syndrome	Pulmonary embolism
	Sarcoidosis	Hilar lymphadenopathy; ILD
	Goodpasture syndrome	Pulmonary hemorrhage
Kidney		
	SLE; CTDs; AAV; systemic vasculitis (except PAN)	Glomerulonephritis
	PAN	Renal artery vasculitis
	Antiphospholipid antibody syndrome	Renal infarct; renal vein thrombosis
	Sjögren syndrome	Acute interstitial nephritis/RTA
	Goodpasture syndrome	Glomerulonephritis
Gastrointestinal		
	PAN	Mesenteric vasculitis
	Spondyloarthritis	Inflammatory bowel disease
	HSP	Intestinal vasculitis; ulcerations
	Behçet syndrome	Ulcerations; inflammatory bowel disease
	FMF	Peritonitis
Neurologic		
	SLE; CTDs; AAV; systemic vasculitis	Mononeuritis multiplex; peripheral neuropathy
	PACNS	CNS vasculitis

AAV = ANCA-associated vasculitis; CNS = central nervous system; CTD = connective tissue disease; FMF = familial Mediterranean fever; GCA = giant cell arteritis; HSP = Henoch-Schönlein purpura; ILD = interstitial lung disease; PACNS = primary angiitis of the central nervous system; PAN = polyarteritis nodosa; RA = rheumatoid arthritis; RTA = renal tubular acidosis; SLE = systemic lupus erythematosus.

ESR elevations are used to identify and monitor disease activity in rheumatologic diseases, especially in polymyalgia rheumatica and giant cell arteritis; however, because the population with these diseases is older, ESR may be less reliable. ESR is an important component of several measures used to assess disease activity in rheumatoid arthritis and is included in the American College of Rheumatology's recommendations for use in clinical practice. Interpretation of an elevated ESR can be difficult in the presence of conditions independently causing elevated fibrinogen and/or other plasma proteins.

Although elevations in ESR most commonly indicate inflammation, some noninflammatory conditions (kidney disease, diabetes mellitus, pregnancy, and obesity) are also associated with elevated fibrinogen levels and can produce an elevated ESR. Some patients make paraproteins (for example, patients with multiple myeloma) that can also cause ESR elevations. Conditions associated with low ESR (due to

TABLE 6. Rheumatologic and Musculoskeletal Manifestations in Systemic Disease

Systemic Disease	Rheumatologic/Musculoskeletal Manifestations
Diabetes mellitus	Dupuytren contracture; adhesive capsulitis of the shoulder; diabetic amyotrophy (ischemic lumbosacral plexopathy); carpal tunnel syndrome; diffuse idiopathic skeletal hyperostosis; trigger finger; cheiroarthropathy (scleroderma-like thickening of hands); diabetic osteoarthropathy/Charcot foot
Hypothyroidism	Arthralgia/myalgia; myopathy (with elevated serum creatine kinase)
Hyperthyroidism	Osteoporosis; myopathy (serum creatine kinase not elevated)
Hyperparathyroidism	Calcium pyrophosphate deposition; osteoporosis
Acromegaly	Arthralgia/osteoarthritis; bone pain; calcium pyrophosphate deposition
Sickle cell disease	Sickle crisis; osteonecrosis; bone pain
Hemophilia	Hemarthroses
Carcinoma	Inflammatory polyarthritis or tendinitis; dermatomyositis; hypertrophic osteoarthropathy
Myeloma/lymphoma/leukemia	Cryoglobulinemia; amyloidosis; arthritis (particularly in children)
Hemochromatosis	Osteoarthritis (especially atypical joints such as metacarpophalangeal joints); calcium pyrophosphate deposition

reduced fibrinogen or abnormal erythrocyte shape and attraction) include heart and liver failure, sickle cell disease, polycythemia, and spherocytosis.

C-Reactive Protein

C-reactive protein (CRP) is an acute phase reactant synthesized by the liver during inflammation in response to proinflammatory cytokines. CRP can adhere to bacteria and activate complement, promoting phagocytosis. Values greater than 0.8 mg/dL (8.0 mg/L) are considered inflammatory, whereas levels between 0.2 mg/dL and 0.8 mg/dL (2.0 mg/L and 8.0 mg/L) are indeterminate.

CRP responds rapidly to inflammation, both rising and falling more quickly than ESR. CRP is more stable and less affected by other serum components compared with ESR. Like ESR, CRP is elevated with disease activity in most rheumatologic diseases and during other forms of inflammation (for example, infection or malignancy). However, in some patients with SLE, CRP will increase during infection but not during disease flare.

Complement

The complement system assists in bacterial opsonization and lysis during humoral immune responses; it also promotes inflammatory reactions. There are three complement cascades (classical, alternative, and mannose-binding lectin pathways); each is triggered differently, but all generate pro-opsonic and proinflammatory components.

Complement levels are generally increased in inflammatory states (that is, complement components are acute phase reactants). However, when immune complexes are present (for example, SLE or certain types of vasculitis), complement is consumed, leading to lower than normal levels. Rare genetic deficiencies of complement, particularly of the early complement components C1q, C2, and C4, paradoxically increase the risk of autoimmune disease, perhaps by impairing clearance of immune

complexes and apoptotic cells; genetic C4 deficiency may also be seen in lupus-like autoimmunity.

Reductions in C3 and C4 levels usually are measured to assess for immune complex–mediated consumption. CH50 tests measure the ability of serum complement to lyse immunoglobulin-coated erythrocytes. CH50 thus assesses overall activation of the classical complement pathway and is abnormal when any component of the classical system is depleted. However, CH50 is no longer routinely used because it is labor intensive, expensive, and usually no more useful in diagnosis and assessment than C3 and C4.

Autoantibody Tests

The presence of autoantibodies is characteristic of many rheumatologic diseases. Rheumatoid factor and antinuclear antibodies (ANA) are the most commonly ordered autoantibody tests. Rheumatoid factor is an immunoglobulin directed against the Fc portion of IgG, and ANA is directed against nuclear antigens. The specificity of these autoantibodies for a particular rheumatologic disease is relatively low because they may occur in other rheumatologic and nonrheumatologic diseases and even in healthy persons.

Rheumatoid factor presence is characteristic of rheumatoid arthritis, but a significant minority of patients with rheumatoid arthritis lack rheumatoid factor. Anti–cyclic citrullinated peptide antibodies are more specifically characteristic of RA and often appear earlier in the disease; using the two antibody tests together may be helpful. Rheumatoid factor is frequently present in healthy persons, especially at older ages, but usually in low titer.

The immunofluorescence assay is considered more reliable than the enzyme-linked immunosorbent assay (ELISA) for detecting ANA, but ELISA is less expensive and less labor intensive. About one third of the healthy population have a positive low-titer (1:40) ANA, and 3% to 5% have a titer of 1:160 or higher. Asymptomatic ANA positivity is more common in women and healthy first-degree relatives of patients with auto-immune disease. Higher ANA titers are more likely to be associated with rheumatologic disease. More than 95% of patients with SLE have a positive ANA; conversely, a negative ANA is rare in those with SLE. ANA occurs in other autoimmune diseases, including rheumatoid arthritis, other connective tissue diseases, infection, and malignancy. ANA can also be drug induced. ANA titer does not correlate with disease activity and should not be checked repeatedly during disease management.

A positive ANA in a patient with nonspecific symptoms is difficult to interpret. As with all tests, the positive predictive value of ANA rests upon the pretest probability of disease. The American College of Rheumatology's Choosing Wisely list currently recommends against testing ANA subserologies without the combination of a positive ANA and clinical suspicion of immune-mediated disease.

Table 7 provides details on these and other autoantibodies.

KEY POINTS

HVC
- Laboratory studies such as erythrocyte sedimentation rate, rheumatoid factor, and antinuclear antibodies have low specificity for diagnosing rheumatologic disease in patients with low pretest probability, thus limiting their utility in this population.

- Although elevations in erythrocyte sedimentation rate (ESR) most commonly reflect the presence of inflammation, increasing age and some noninflammatory conditions are also associated with elevated ESR.

- C-reactive protein responds rapidly to inflammation, both rising and falling more quickly than erythrocyte sedimentation rate (ESR) and is more stable and less affected by other serum components compared with ESR.

Imaging Studies

Imaging studies can be useful to diagnose and follow patients with rheumatologic diseases. For example, inflammatory arthritis can be evaluated with studies ranging from plain radiography to MRI, and medium- and large-vessel vasculitis can be detected using angiography. For all studies, it is important to consider whether the ordering of imaging tests will aid in the diagnosis or management of a suspected condition, and whether the benefits of such testing clearly outweigh the potential risks and costs.

Radiography

Plain radiography is used to assess inflammatory and degenerative arthritis (**Table 8**, on page 9). Autoimmune inflammatory arthritis may produce joint-space narrowing, erosions, and osteopenia, and in the case of spondyloarthritis, productive bony overgrowth. Crystal-related inflammatory diseases have characteristic radiographic findings, including punched-out bone lesions in gout or cartilage calcification (also known as chondrocalcinosis) in calcium pyrophosphate deposition.

Osteoarthritis causes compartmental joint-space narrowing and bony hypertrophy.

Plain radiography does not visualize soft tissues nearly as well as bone, and due to the two-dimensional nature of the images, not all bone findings are visible on every view (for example, visible on oblique but not anteroposterior imaging). Plain radiography may not detect early (within the first 6-12 months) or mild erosive arthritic changes. Despite these limitations, serial plain radiography can be useful for monitoring arthritis disease progression.

Plain radiography is relatively inexpensive and readily available. Despite low levels of ionizing radiation, plain radiography is considered safe except for pregnant women.

CT

In contrast to plain radiography, CT scanning permits multiple views and orientations from a single study. CT is more useful for bony abnormalities than for soft-tissue inflammation or fluid collections. Calcium pyrophosphate deposition is readily detected on CT, even when calcium deposits are overlooked on other modalities. CT is more sensitive in detecting bone erosions than plain radiographs or MRI.

CT is more expensive than plain radiography and exposes the patient to more radiation.

MRI

MRI is useful in detecting soft-tissue abnormalities, inflammation, and fluid collections, but is less effective than CT in demonstrating bony abnormalities and erosive changes. MRI is more sensitive than plain radiography in detecting early spine and sacroiliac joint inflammation.

MRI is more expensive than plain radiography and CT and is generally ordered when assessment of soft-tissue imaging is required. Although MRI does not expose the patient to radiation, MRI contrast (gadolinium) must be avoided in patients with kidney disease due to the risk of nephrogenic systemic fibrosis. Patient intolerance due to claustrophobia or inability of the patient to fit in the scanner due to large body habitus may limit the ability to obtain MRI data. Because data are currently inadequate to justify its use, the American College of Rheumatology Choosing Wisely list questions the utility of routinely ordering MRI of peripheral joints to monitor rheumatoid arthritis.

Ultrasonography

Musculoskeletal ultrasonography is increasingly utilized in rheumatologic disease. Ultrasonography can detect soft-tissue abnormalities such as synovitis, tendinitis, bursitis, and joint fluid, and Doppler can assess for increased tissue blood flow consistent with synovitis. Ultrasonography can diagnose and monitor disease, and can be used to guide arthrocentesis. Dynamic pathologies such as impingement can be visualized.

Unlike other modalities, ultrasonography is portable and can be used in the outpatient setting at the bedside for point-of-care evaluation and procedures. However, it is operator dependent, and training and practice are required

TABLE 7. Autoantibodies in Rheumatologic Disease

Autoantibody	Rheumatologic Condition	Sensitivity/Specificity	Comments
ANA	SLE; also SSc, Sjögren, and MCTD	SLE: 95% sensitivity; poor specificity	Does not correlate with disease activity
Anti–double-stranded DNA	SLE	SLE: 60% sensitivity, >95% specificity; *Crithidia* IFA or Farr assays more specific than ELISA	Found in more severe disease, especially kidney disease; antibody levels commonly follow disease activity and are useful to monitor
Anti-Smith	SLE	SLE: 30% sensitivity, 99% specificity	Most specific test for SLE; does not correlate with disease activity
Anti-U1-RNP	MCTD; SLE	100% sensitivity	High titer seen in MCTD (>1:10,000); does not correlate with disease activity
Anti-Ro/SSA; anti-La/SSB	Sjögren; SLE; RA; SSc	Sjögren: 70% sensitivity; SLE: 30% sensitivity	Sicca symptoms; in SLE, associated with photosensitive rash and neonatal lupus erythematosus (rash and conduction block)
Anti-Scl-70 (antitopoisomerase)	DcSSc	10%-30% sensitivity	Seen more often in patients with SSc who have pulmonary fibrosis
Anticentromere	LcSSc (CREST)	10%-30% sensitivity	Patients with SSc with this antibody are more likely to develop pulmonary hypertension
c-ANCA (antiproteinase-3)	GPA	90% sensitivity when disease is active; high specificity in classic presentations	Correlation with disease activity is unclear
p-ANCA (antimyeloperoxidase)	MPA; EGPA	MPA: 80% sensitivity; EGPA: 60% sensitivity; less specific than c-ANCA	Atypical p-ANCA (antimyeloperoxidase negative) can be seen in inflammatory bowel disease and with positive ANA
Anti–Jo-1	Myositis	20%-30% sensitivity	Associated with antisynthetase syndrome
Rheumatoid factor	RA; Sjögren; cryoglobulinemia	RA: 70% sensitivity; limited specificity, especially in patients without a classic disease presentation	RF is an antibody to Ig and hence many false positives (hepatitis C, SLE); 30% with RA are RF negative; may convert to positive later in RA course
Anti–cyclic citrullinated peptide	RA	RA: 70% sensitivity; more specific than RF for RA	Can be positive in RF-negative RA patients; often present before RF becomes positive; associated with erosions; predicts disease progression in undifferentiated arthritis
Antihistone	DILE	95% sensitivity; poor specificity	Also seen in patients with native lupus
Cryoglobulins	Vasculitis; hepatitis C; myeloma; SLE; RA	Type II or III cryoglobulins seen in patients with cryoglobulinemic vasculitis	May be present in connective tissue diseases in the absence of vasculitis

ANA = antinuclear antibodies; CREST = calcinosis, Raynaud phenomenon, esophageal dysmotility, sclerodactyly, and telangiectasia; DcSSc = diffuse cutaneous systemic sclerosis; DILE = drug-induced lupus erythematosus; EGPA = eosinophilic granulomatosis with polyangiitis (formerly known as Churg-Strauss syndrome); ELISA = enzyme-linked immunosorbent assay; GPA = granulomatosis with polyangiitis (formerly known as Wegener granulomatosis); IFA = immunofluorescent assay; LcSSc = limited cutaneous systemic sclerosis; MCTD = mixed connective tissue disease; MPA = microscopic polyangiitis; RA = rheumatoid arthritis; RF = rheumatoid factor; RNP = ribonucleoprotein; SLE = systemic lupus erythematosus; SSc = systemic sclerosis.

TABLE 8. Radiographic Findings of Common Rheumatologic Diseases

Rheumatologic Disease	Radiographic Findings
Rheumatoid arthritis	Bony erosions; periarticular osteopenia; subluxations; soft-tissue swelling; MCP and PIP involvement on hand radiograph
Osteoarthritis	Asymmetric joint-space narrowing; osteophytes; subchondral sclerosis and cystic changes; degenerative disk disease with collapse of disks; degenerative joint disease with facet joint osteophytes; these findings lead to spondylolisthesis (anterior/posterior misalignment of the spine) and kyphosis
Diffuse idiopathic skeletal hyperostosis	Calcification of the anterior longitudinal ligament; bridging horizontal syndesmophytes; usually more prominent on right side of spine than left
Ankylosing spondylitis	Sacroiliitis; squaring of the vertebral bodies; bridging vertical enthesophytes; shiny corners
Psoriatic arthritis	Destructive arthritis with erosions and osteophytes; DIP involvement; "pencil-in-cup" deformities on hand radiograph; arthritis mutilans
Gout	Punched-out erosions with sclerotic border and overhanging edge; periarticular soft-tissue swelling with calcifications in tophaceous deposits
Calcium pyrophosphate deposition	Chondrocalcinosis, most commonly of the knees, shoulders, wrists, pubic symphysis; leads to osteoarthritis

DIP = distal interphalangeal; MCP = metacarpophalangeal; PIP = proximal interphalangeal.

to achieve competency at performing and interpreting ultrasonography.

Ultrasonography is relatively inexpensive, and there is no ionizing radiation. **H**

KEY POINTS

HVC
- CT is useful in assessing bony abnormalities but is more expensive than plain radiography and exposes the patient to more radiation.

HVC
- MRI is useful in detecting soft-tissue abnormalities, inflammation, and fluid collections but should not be routinely used to monitor rheumatoid arthritis disease activity in peripheral joints.

HVC
- Musculoskeletal ultrasonography is a low risk and relatively inexpensive way to detect soft-tissue abnormalities such as synovitis, tendinitis, bursitis, and joint fluid.

Joint Aspiration

Synovial fluid aspiration is essential when evaluating for infection and crystal-related disease and can distinguish between inflammatory and noninflammatory conditions. The most useful tests of synovial fluid for infection are leukocyte count, stains, and cultures, as well as evaluation of synovial fluid for crystals under polarized light. Synovial fluid autoantibodies and protein and glucose levels are of limited utility and used primarily in research investigations. The gross appearance of synovial fluid can predict results in the laboratory. Normal fluid is clear and highly viscous. Inflammatory fluid is cloudy and watery. Infected fluid is cloudy to opaque and, while "thick" like pea soup, lacks the viscosity of normal fluid.

Synovial fluid leukocyte counts less than 200/µL (0.2 × 10^9/L) are considered normal, between 200/µL and 2000/µL (0.2 × 10^9/L and 2.0 × 10^9/L) are associated with

noninflammatory conditions, and greater than 2000/µL (2.0 × 10^9/L) are associated with inflammatory states. The higher the count is, the more inflammatory the fluid and the greater the suspicion for crystal-related or infectious disease.

There is no absolute cutoff value that distinguishes infection from crystal-related disease, because some infections may have lower counts than expected and crystal-related disease may have counts greater than 100,000/µL (100 × 10^9/L). Thus, the proper application of synovial fluid leukocyte counts requires conservative interpretation. Generally, counts greater than 50,000/µL (50 × 10^9/L) should be managed as infectious until explicitly proven otherwise; if there is clinical suspicion for infection, fluid should be sent for stains and cultures even in the setting of counts less than 50,000/µL (50 × 10^9/L).

See Crystal Arthropathies for a discussion on synovial fluid crystal evaluation. **H**

KEY POINT

- Synovial fluid leukocyte counts less than 200/µL (0.2 × 10^9/L) are considered normal, between 200/µL and 2000/µL (0.2 × 10^9/L and 2.0 × 10^9/L) are associated with noninflammatory conditions, and greater than 2000/µL (2.0 × 10^9/L) are associated with inflammatory states.

Principles of Therapeutics
Introduction

This section discusses the uses, mechanisms of action, targets, potential toxicities, and common monitoring parameters of medications used in rheumatologic disease. Specific applications of individual drugs are further discussed in the disease-specific sections.

Anti-Inflammatory Agents

Anti-inflammatory agents reduce pain and improve swelling, warmth, and redness but generally do not prevent disease progression.

NSAIDs

NSAIDs inhibit cyclooxygenase (COX) enzymes to block the generation of the lipid prostaglandin E_2 (PGE_2). PGE_2 stimulates inflammation, vasodilation, smooth muscle contraction, pain, and fever; NSAIDs therefore convey anti-inflammatory, analgesic, and antipyretic effects. However, PGE_2 also maintains gastric mucosa and promotes kidney sodium excretion and glomerular filtration. Other COX products include thromboxane A_2, a prothrombotic regulator of platelets, and prostacyclin, an antithrombotic and vasodilatory lipid. Because NSAIDs inhibit all of these, the consequences of COX inhibition are complex and accompanied by multiple potential side effects (**Table 9**). Side-effect risk is increased in older patients and those with preexisting comorbidities. Regular monitoring of blood pressure, kidney function, and blood counts during chronic NSAID use is recommended.

The identification of two distinct COX isoforms permitted the development of selective COX-2 inhibitors. Because the COX-1 isoform is responsible for platelet function and gastroprotection, COX-2 inhibitors cause less gastrotoxicity and bleeding than nonselective NSAIDs. However, COX-2 inhibitors are not less nephrotoxic and cause similar amounts of hypertension. The most selective COX-2 inhibitors also cause increased cardiovascular risk and have been removed from the market. However, nearly all NSAIDs may convey some cardiovascular risk.

In contrast to other NSAIDs, aspirin (acetylsalicylate) permanently inactivates COX enzymes. Platelets cannot generate replacement COX and are particularly vulnerable to this effect. Therefore, low-dose aspirin administration for cardiovascular disease permits a platelet-selective effect that reduces, but does not entirely alleviate, potential gastrointestinal toxicity. Higher doses promote more general COX inhibition and convey the same risks as other NSAIDs.

Oral NSAIDs vary in potency, kinetics, metabolism, cost, and selectivity for COX-1 versus COX-2. Selection of a particular NSAID depends mainly upon convenience of use and individual tolerance, including consideration of the patient's comorbidities. All NSAIDs should be used at the lowest effective dose for the shortest time; however, effective use of NSAIDs in rheumatologic disease often requires high and prolonged dosing. NSAIDs are not generally disease modifying; they improve arthritis symptoms but not long-term outcomes.

Topical NSAIDs such as diclofenac (available as a solution, spray, gel, or patch) provide similar pain relief for inflammatory conditions as oral medications with fewer gastrointestinal effects. The American College of Rheumatology currently recommends topical NSAIDs rather than oral NSAIDs for patients aged 75 years or older. However, they are associated with more skin reactions than placebo and are significantly more expensive than oral NSAIDs.

Glucocorticoids

Glucocorticoids are potent anti-inflammatories and are effective in many rheumatologic diseases; however, they are associated with multiple potential toxicities and should be used at the lowest effective dose for the shortest period possible. Intermediate to long-term use is associated with an increased risk of diabetes mellitus, osteoporosis, osteonecrosis, weight gain, fluid retention, hypertension, cardiovascular disease, striae and bruising, and glaucoma and cataracts; monitoring for adverse events can help limit morbidity. Virtually all patients receiving chronic glucocorticoids or frequent tapering doses should take calcium and vitamin D supplementation; patients receiving glucocorticoids for more than 4 weeks at doses greater than 5 mg of prednisone daily should be considered for bisphosphonate treatment.

Colchicine

Colchicine disrupts microtubules to interfere with leukocyte adhesion and migration. Other potential effects include inhibition of interleukin (IL)-1 generation. Colchicine is used to treat gout, familial Mediterranean fever, and hypersensitivity vasculitis. At low doses, colchicine is generally safe and well tolerated; higher doses routinely cause diarrhea. Acute colchicine overdose can be fatal; chronic low-level colchicine overdose can cause neuromyopathy. Colchicine is renally cleared; patients with kidney disease require dose adjustment. Colchicine is metabolized in the liver by the CYP3A4 cytochrome, and its absorption from the stomach is limited by the P-glycoprotein export pump; consequently, patients must reduce or avoid colchicine when also taking moderate/strong CYP3A4 inhibitors (for example, clarithromycin, most antiretroviral drugs) or P-glycoprotein inhibitors (for example, cyclosporine). When used in combination with statins (especially those metabolized by CYP3A4), colchicine may increase the risk of drug-induced myopathy.

TABLE 9.	Potential Toxicities of NSAID Use
Category	**Toxicity**
Cardiovascular	Hypertension; myocardial infarction; exacerbation of heart failure
Hemostatic	Bleeding diathesis
Gastrointestinal	Dyspepsia; reflux; peptic ulcer disease; gastrointestinal bleeding
Obstetric/ Gynecologic	Bleeding; delayed labor; premature ductus arteriosus closure
Pulmonary	Asthma exacerbation
Renal	Hypertension; decreased glomerular filtration; increased salt and water retention; increased renin production; uncommonly, allergic interstitial nephritis or acute tubular necrosis

HVC
- Topical NSAIDs provide similar pain relief for inflammatory conditions as oral medications with fewer gastrointestinal effects and are preferred for patients 75 years or older; however, they are associated with more skin reactions and are significantly more expensive than oral NSAIDs.
- Virtually all patients receiving chronic glucocorticoids or frequent tapering doses should take calcium and vitamin D supplementation; patients receiving glucocorticoids for more than 4 weeks at doses greater than 5 mg of prednisone daily should be considered for bisphosphonate treatment.

Analgesics

Simple analgesics are neither anti-inflammatory nor disease modifying but can help relieve pain in patients with arthritis.

Acetaminophen is generally well tolerated and has both analgesic and antipyretic effects; its mechanism of action is not well established. The maximum recommended daily dose by the FDA is 4 g/d, and doses greater than 4 g/d carry an increased risk for liver failure and even death. Because acetaminophen content in over-the-counter products (for example, for allergies, headaches, and colds) may not be taken into account by some patients when calculating the total daily dose, some guidelines limit maximum daily intake to 3 g/d in most patients and 2 g/d in patients with liver disease. In chronic acetaminophen use, periodic assessment of liver and kidney function may be prudent.

Opiates act on neurons to block pain signaling. Opiates are less effective for inflammatory than for malignancy pain, but milder opiates (for example, codeine or oxycodone) have an occasional role in treating patients with arthritis who cannot otherwise obtain relief. Opiates are potentially habit-forming, can cause constipation, and may cause respiratory depression at excessive doses. Tramadol is a centrally acting synthetic opioid analgesic that also weakly inhibits the reuptake of norepinephrine and serotonin; potential for addiction is lower than for traditional opioids.

Agents that modulate pain signals in the spinal cord (for example, pregabalin, gabapentin, tricyclic antidepressants such as amitriptyline, and dual serotonin-norepinephrine reuptake inhibitors such as duloxetine and milnacipran) are useful in patients with central chronic pain syndromes (for example, fibromyalgia) as well as musculoskeletal pain. Side effects include sedation and dry mouth. Concomitant use of serotonin reuptake inhibitors, tricyclic antidepressants, or monoamine oxidase inhibitors may lower seizure threshold and/or raise the risk of serotonin syndrome (mental status changes, autonomic instability, neuromuscular aberrations, and gastrointestinal symptoms).

Topical analgesics (such as capsaicin and lidocaine) may be useful and can limit systemic drug exposure when only a single area is painful.

- Simple analgesics are neither anti-inflammatory nor disease modifying but may help alleviate arthritis pain.
- Acetaminophen is generally well tolerated and beneficial, but excessive doses carry risk for liver failure and even death.

Disease-Modifying Antirheumatic Drugs

Disease-modifying antirheumatic drugs (DMARDs) are immunosuppressive agents used to achieve control and/or remission in rheumatologic disease. Most DMARDs increase the risk of infection, and each agent has its own specific potential toxicities.

Nonbiologic Disease-Modifying Antirheumatic Drugs

Table 10 summarizes the mechanisms of action, indications, and common monitoring parameters of various nonbiologic DMARDs. See Rheumatologic Medications and Pregnancy for information on these medications in women of childbearing potential.

Methotrexate

Methotrexate inhibits folic acid metabolism and increases extracellular adenosine levels. It is the recommended initial DMARD for most patients with rheumatoid arthritis and is useful in other disorders, including psoriatic arthritis, vasculitis, and sarcoidosis. Methotrexate is administered weekly along with daily folic acid supplementation, which limits toxicity without affecting efficacy. Potential toxicities include hepatitis and bone marrow suppression (leukopenia, anemia). Patients with liver disease should not receive methotrexate, and limitation of alcohol intake is strongly advised.

Hydroxychloroquine

Hydroxychloroquine is an antimalarial medication that appears to inhibit antigen processing. In systemic lupus erythematosus (SLE), hydroxychloroquine is used to control skin and joint disease, prevent systemic and organ-specific disease flare-ups, and reduce overall mortality. It is also used (alone or in combination with methotrexate and sulfasalazine) to treat undifferentiated connective tissue disease, rheumatoid arthritis, and other forms of inflammatory arthritis. Although its efficacy in arthritis is modest, its excellent side-effect profile makes it a useful adjunctive therapy.

Sulfasalazine

Sulfasalazine exerts systemic effects through its metabolite sulfapyridine and intracolonic effects via the salicylate moiety. Sulfasalazine is moderately effective in rheumatoid arthritis with or without methotrexate. It is also used to treat

TABLE 10. Nonbiologic Disease-Modifying Antirheumatic Drugs

Agent	Mechanism	Indications	Common Monitoring Parameters
Methotrexate	DHFR inhibition; extracellular adenosine level modification	RA; psoriasis; psoriatic arthritis; DM; PM; vasculitis	Baseline: chest radiography, hepatitis screening, CBC, LCTs, serum creatinine Thereafter: CBC, LCTs, serum creatinine every 3 months[a]
Hydroxychloroquine	Uncertain; appears to involve stabilization of lysosomal vacuoles, leading to inhibition of antigen processing and costimulatory activation	SLE; RA	Baseline: CBC, LCTs, serum creatinine Baseline/periodic ophthalmologic examinations approximately every 12 months to evaluate for hydroxychloroquine deposition, which rarely can lead to visual loss
Sulfasalazine	Antimetabolite; a pro-drug broken down into 5-amino salicylic acid (active metabolite in the gastrointestinal tract) and sulfapyridine (exerts systemic action)	RA; SpA; IBD	Baseline: CBC, LCTs, serum creatinine Thereafter: CBC, LCTs, serum creatinine every 3-6 months
Leflunomide	Blocks dihydroorotase, an enzyme involved in pyrimidine biosynthesis that targets replicating lymphocytes, which lack pyrimidine salvage pathways; antiproliferative	RA	Baseline: chest radiography, hepatitis screening, CBC, LCTs, serum creatinine Thereafter: CBC, serum creatinine every 3 months; LCTs every 8-12 weeks, and leflunomide temporarily or permanently discontinued for significant elevations >2 times normal and additional therapy with cholestyramine for elevations >3 times normal[a]
Azathioprine	Purine analogue; inhibits DNA synthesis essential for proliferating T- and B-lymphocytes	SLE; DM; PM; vasculitis; IBD	Baseline: CBC, LCTs, serum creatinine Thereafter: CBC, LCTs, serum creatinine every 3 months[a]
Cyclophosphamide	Alkylating agent; blocks DNA synthesis and causes cell death	Severe and life-threatening disease in SLE, DM, PM, and vasculitis	Close monitoring clinically and measuring CBC, chemistries, LCTs, urinalysis every 4-8 weeks
Mycophenolate mofetil	Inosine monophosphate inhibition; antiproliferative; mycophenolate is converted into the active metabolite, mycophenolic acid, which inhibits inosine monophosphate dehydrogenase (an enzyme in the purine synthetic pathway) and preferentially inhibits T- and B-lymphocytes	SLE (especially lupus nephritis); vasculitis; DM; PM	Baseline: CBC, LCTs, serum creatinine Thereafter: CBC, LCTs, serum creatinine every 3 months[a]
Cyclosporine	Inhibits calcineurin (a transcription activating factor); preferentially targets T cells	SLE; psoriasis; RA	Baseline: CBC, LCTs, serum creatinine Thereafter: CBC, LCTs, serum creatinine every 2-3 months[a]
Apremilast	Inhibits phosphodiesterase 4	Psoriasis; psoriatic arthritis	Baseline: weight Thereafter: weight, neuropsychiatric effects

CBC = complete blood count; DHFR = dihydrofolate reductase; DM = dermatomyositis; IBD = inflammatory bowel disease; LCTs = liver chemistry tests; PM = polymyositis; RA = rheumatoid arthritis; SLE = systemic lupus erythematosus; SpA = spondyloarthritis.

[a]Recommended monitoring interval is for a stable dose but may be shorter after initiation or in the case of abnormal results and must be individualized to the patient's risk of toxicity.

spondyloarthritis and inflammatory bowel disease. Toxicities include gastrointestinal upset, headache, agranulocytosis, hepatitis, and reversible oligospermia.

Leflunomide

Leflunomide inhibits lymphocyte activation by blocking the pyrimidine synthesis pathway. It is approved to treat rheumatoid arthritis, in which its efficacy is comparable to methotrexate. Toxicities include gastrointestinal upset, diarrhea, aminotransaminase elevations, cytopenias, infection, and teratogenesis.

Azathioprine

Azathioprine is a purine analogue that inhibits nucleotide synthesis. It is used to treat and/or maintain control of SLE, vasculitis, the inflammatory myopathies, and other autoimmune diseases. Toxicities include gastrointestinal intolerance, bone marrow suppression, hepatitis, and pancreatitis. Coadministration with allopurinol or febuxostat should be avoided because these three drugs compete for the same metabolic pathway, and toxic levels may ensue.

Cyclophosphamide

Cyclophosphamide is a DNA alkylating agent with potent immunosuppressive properties. It is used to treat severe and/or life-threatening manifestations of SLE (including nephritis), systemic sclerosis, the inflammatory myopathies, interstitial lung disease, and vasculitis. Toxicities include bone marrow suppression, leukopenia, anemia, infections, infertility, hemorrhagic cystitis and bladder cancer, and lymphoma and other malignancies. Evaluation of patients with painless hematuria and history of past cyclophosphamide treatment should include cystoscopy to evaluate for bladder cancer.

Mycophenolate Mofetil

Mycophenolate mofetil inhibits the purine pathway of nucleotide synthesis and may be at least as effective as cyclophosphamide for SLE (including nephritis) but with fewer, and milder, side effects. It is also used to treat autoimmune myositis and as a glucocorticoid-sparing agent in systemic vasculitis. Toxicities include diarrhea, cytopenias, and infection.

Cyclosporine

Cyclosporine is both a calcineurin and T-lymphocyte inhibitor that is efficacious in several autoimmune diseases, including rheumatoid arthritis, SLE, autoimmune myositis, psoriasis, and inflammatory bowel disease. Cyclosporine is mainly used as a third-line agent in rheumatologic disease because its potential toxicities (for example, nephrotoxicity, hypertension, tremors, and hirsutism) require close monitoring.

Apremilast

Apremilast was recently approved by the FDA for treatment of psoriasis and psoriatic arthritis. Apremilast inhibits phosphodiesterase 4, resulting in increases in cyclic adenosine monophosphate that inhibit inflammatory responses.

Although experience is limited, studies suggest that apremilast is well tolerated and of moderate efficacy.

KEY POINTS
- Methotrexate is the recommended initial disease-modifying antirheumatic drug for most patients with rheumatoid arthritis.
- Hydroxychloroquine is used in patients with systemic lupus erythematosus to control skin and joint disease, prevent systemic and organ-specific disease flare-ups, and reduce overall mortality.
- Cyclophosphamide is used to treat severe and/or life-threatening manifestations of systemic lupus erythematosus, systemic sclerosis, the inflammatory myopathies, interstitial lung disease, and vasculitis.
- Mycophenolate mofetil may be at least as effective as cyclophosphamide for systemic lupus erythematosus but with fewer, and milder, side effects.

Biologic Disease-Modifying Antirheumatic Drugs

Biologic DMARDs are protein-based products that alter the body's natural processes to block immune responses (**Figure 1**). Biologic DMARDs are more specific and typically more effective than nonbiologic DMARDs; however, they are significantly more expensive. Biologic DMARDS are generally administered parenterally; the suffixes of their names indicate their general structure (for example, "mab" for monoclonal antibody and "cept" for receptor derived).

Toxicities of biologic agents relate mainly to the pathways they block. Infection risk is elevated with most biologic agents; therapy should be temporarily interrupted during any significant infection. Biologic agents are frequently used in combination with a nonbiologic DMARD. However, concurrent use of two or more biologic agents is contraindicated because infection rates are increased with minimal, if any, added efficacy. See Vaccination and Screening in Immunosuppression for more details.

Table 11 on page 15 summarizes the structures, targets, indications, and common monitoring parameters of various biologic DMARDs. See Rheumatologic Medications and Pregnancy for information on these medications in women of childbearing potential.

Tumor Necrosis Factor α Inhibitors

Tumor necrosis factor (TNF)-α inhibitors are usually the treatment of first choice for patients with rheumatoid or psoriatic arthritis after inadequate response to nonbiologic DMARDs. TNF-α inhibitors also treat ankylosing spondylitis after failure of NSAIDs. TNF-α inhibitors are effective in 50% to 70% of patients with these diseases. Five TNF-α inhibitors (infliximab, adalimumab, etanercept, certolizumab pegol, and golimumab) are FDA approved to treat rheumatoid arthritis, psoriatic arthritis, and/or ankylosing spondylitis. These agents decrease disease activity and inhibit the progression of

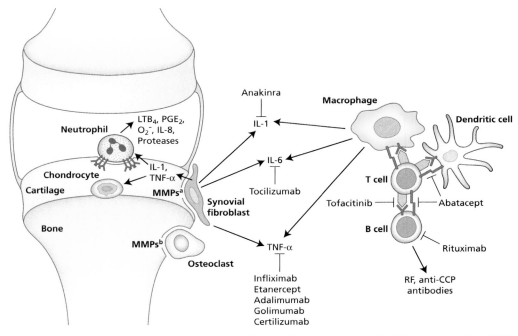

FIGURE 1. Biologic targets in rheumatoid arthritis. Various processes within the rheumatoid joint may be targeted by biologic (and nonbiologic) DMARDs. This figure illustrates the targets of specific biologic agents, described more fully in the text. CCP = cyclic citrullinated peptide; DMARD = disease-modifying antirheumatic drug; IL = interleukin; LTB_4 = leukotriene B_4; MMP = matrix metalloproteinase; O_2 = oxygen; PGE_2 = prostaglandin E_2; RF = rheumatoid factor; TNF = tumor necrosis factor.

[a]Activated synovial fibroblasts secrete MMPs and other enzymes that contribute to the degradation of articular cartilage.

[b]Activated osteoclasts secrete MMPs and other enzymes that contribute to marginal erosions of bone.

structural damage in rheumatoid arthritis, most effectively in combination with methotrexate. In psoriasis/psoriatic arthritis, they suppress both cutaneous and articular disease. In ankylosing spondylitis, TNF-α inhibitors improve both axial and peripheral joint symptoms, although radiographic progression of spinal disease may continue. They are also used off-label in uveitis, Behçet syndrome, sarcoidosis, inflammatory bowel disease, and pyoderma syndromes.

Common toxicities include risk of tuberculosis or hepatitis B reactivation as well as fungal (aspergillosis, histoplasmosis, coccidioidomycosis) and bacterial infections. Other potential toxicities include injection site and infusion reactions, leukopenia, induction of autoimmunity (such as drug-induced lupus erythematosus), and heart failure. Rarer toxicities include psoriasiform skin eruption and demyelinating syndromes. **H**

Despite early concerns, overall cancer incidence with use of TNF-α inhibitors does not appear to be increased, with the exception of skin cancer. Nonetheless, TNF-α inhibitors should usually be discontinued if the patient develops any malignancy. In patients with a remote history of malignancy, TNF-α inhibitors have been used cautiously without recurrence in a limited number of patients.

Other Biologic Disease-Modifying Antirheumatic Drugs
Other biologic agents are typically started after failure of one or two TNF-α inhibitors, although some are also approved as first-line therapies.

Abatacept
Abatacept interferes with antigen presentation to T cells and is indicated for moderate to severe rheumatoid arthritis in patients with inadequate response to methotrexate and/or TNF-α inhibition. Abatacept may be administered intravenously or as a subcutaneous injection. Abatacept is associated with increased risk of infection as well as COPD exacerbation. It may also be associated with an increased risk of lymphoma and lung cancer.

Rituximab
Rituximab depletes B cells and is used in combination with methotrexate to treat rheumatoid arthritis in patients who have not adequately responded to a TNF-α inhibitor. Rituximab has recently been shown to be effective in ANCA-associated vasculitis and has been used off-label for SLE and sarcoidosis. Rituximab is administered every 6 months in rheumatoid arthritis or as four weekly infusions for induction of remission in vasculitis. Toxicities include potentially severe infusion reactions; rare cases of progressive multifocal leukoencephalopathy have been reported. Despite depleting B-cell populations, rituximab has not been associated with significant increases in infections.

Tocilizumab
Tocilizumab blocks IL-6 receptors and is used to treat rheumatoid arthritis in patients who have experienced an inadequate response to TNF-α inhibitors. Tocilizumab may be associated

TABLE 11. Biologic Disease-Modifying Antirheumatic Drugs

Agent	Agent Structure	Target	Indications	Common Monitoring Parameters
Adalimumab	Fully humanized monoclonal antibody	TNF-α	RA; psoriatic arthritis; ankylosing spondylitis; IBD	TB, fungal, and other infections; CBC, serum creatinine, and LCTs at baseline; thereafter every 3-6 months
Etanercept	Soluble p75 TNF-α receptor/IgG Fc segment chimer	TNF-α	RA; psoriatic arthritis; ankylosing spondylitis	TB, fungal, and other infections; CBC, serum creatinine, and LCTs at baseline; thereafter every 3-6 months
Certolizumab pegol	Fab' segment of monoclonal antibody modified by polyethylene glycol strands to reduce immunogenicity	TNF-α	RA; psoriatic arthritis; ankylosing spondylitis	TB, fungal, and other infections; CBC, serum creatinine, and LCTs at baseline; thereafter every 3-6 months
Golimumab	Fully humanized monoclonal antibody	TNF-α	RA; psoriatic arthritis; ankylosing spondylitis	TB, fungal, and other infections; CBC, serum creatinine, and LCTs at baseline; thereafter every 3-6 months
Infliximab	Partially humanized mouse monoclonal antibody	TNF-α	RA; psoriatic arthritis; ankylosing spondylitis; IBD	TB, fungal, and other infections; CBC, serum creatinine, and LCTs at baseline; thereafter every 2-3 months
Abatacept	Soluble CTLA4 receptor/IgG Fc segment chimer	T-cell costimulation	RA	TB, fungal, and other infections; CBC, serum creatinine, and LCTs at baseline; thereafter every 3-6 months
Rituximab	Chimeric (mouse + human) monoclonal antibody	CD20+ B cells	RA; ANCA-associated vasculitis	Infections; IgG levels; CBC, chemistries, and LCTs at baseline and at 2 weeks; thereafter every 3-6 months
Tocilizumab	Humanized monoclonal antibody	IL-6 receptor	RA; JIA; Castleman disease	TB and other infections; CBC, chemistries, and LCTs at baseline and with each infusion or every 2-3 months; lipid profile every 3-6 months
Belimumab	Human monoclonal antibody	BLyS/BAFF	SLE	IgG levels; CBC, chemistries, and LCTs at baseline and 2 weeks; thereafter every 3 months
Tofacitinib	Orally available small molecule agent	JAK	RA	TB and other infections; CBC, chemistries, and LCTs at baseline and every 3 months
Ustekinumab	Human monoclonal antibody	IL-12/IL-23	Psoriasis; psoriatic arthritis	Close monitoring for TB and other infections; CBC, chemistries, and LCTs at baseline and every 3 months
Anakinra	Recombinant receptor antagonist	IL-1β receptor	RA; AOSD; cryopyrin-associated syndromes	CBC at baseline and every 3 months
Rilonacept	Dual IL-1β receptors chimerically attached to IgG Fc segment	IL-1	Cryopyrin-associated syndromes; refractory gout	CBC at baseline and every 3 months
Canakinumab	Fully humanized antibody	IL-1β	Cryopyrin-associated syndromes	CBC at baseline and every 3 months

AOSD = adult-onset Still disease; BAFF = B-cell-activating factor; BLyS = B-lymphocyte stimulator; CBC = complete blood count; IBD = inflammatory bowel disease; IL = interleukin; JAK = Janus kinase; JIA = juvenile idiopathic arthritis; LCTs = liver chemistry tests; RA = rheumatoid arthritis; SLE = systemic lupus erythematosus; TB = tuberculosis; TNF = tumor necrosis factor.

with elevated liver chemistries, leukopenia, thrombocytopenia, and elevated serum lipid levels. Reactivation of tuberculosis and invasive fungal infections can occur, and rare cases of colon or small bowel perforation have been reported in patients with a history of diverticulitis.

Tofacitinib

Tofacitinib is an oral agent that is FDA approved to treat moderate to severe rheumatoid arthritis in patients who have experienced an inadequate response to methotrexate. In contrast to protein-based biologics, tofacitinib is the first small molecule, specific signal transduction inhibitor to be used in rheumatologic disease and works by inhibiting Janus kinase (JAK) pathway signaling. Tofacitinib may be associated with bone marrow suppression and elevated liver chemistries. Tuberculosis, invasive fungal infections, and bacterial and viral infections can occur. Like tocilizumab, tofacitinib can induce lipid abnormalities and carries a risk of intestinal perforation.

Ustekinumab

Ustekinumab is an anti–IL-12/IL-23 antibody that is FDA approved to treat active psoriatic arthritis and moderate to severe plaque psoriasis. Ustekinumab is administered subcutaneously every 12 weeks. Serious infections are uncommon but have been reported.

Interleukin-1β Inhibitors

Anakinra is FDA approved to treat rheumatoid arthritis but is infrequently used due to limited efficacy. However, anakinra is approved for a cryopyrin-associated periodic fever syndrome (neonatal-onset multisystem inflammatory disease) and is used off-label in similar autoinflammatory syndromes such as Muckle-Wells syndrome, familial cold autoinflammatory syndrome, and adult-onset Still disease. Rilonacept and canakinumab are also beneficial in the treatment of cryopyrin-associated periodic fever syndromes. Anakinra and canakinumab may also be considered for off-label use in severe cases of gout refractory to other therapies.

Belimumab

Belimumab is an anti-BLyS (B lymphocyte stimulator) antibody that is FDA approved to treat active SLE in patients on standard therapy. Belimumab is generally well tolerated, but cytopenias and infection may occur. In one trial, belimumab failed to demonstrate efficacy among black patients with SLE. **H**

KEY POINTS

- Infection risk is elevated with most biologic agents; therapy should be temporarily interrupted during any significant infection.
- Tumor necrosis factor α inhibitors are usually the treatment of first choice for patients with rheumatoid or psoriatic arthritis after inadequate response to non-biologic disease-modifying antirheumatic drugs.

(Continued)

KEY POINTS *(continued)*

- Other biologic agents are typically started after failure of one or two tumor necrosis factor α inhibitors, although some are also approved as first-line therapies.

Vaccination and Screening in Immunosuppression

Patients with autoimmune diseases are at increased risk for infection, and risk may be significantly increased with the institution of immunosuppressive therapies. Accordingly, patients with rheumatologic disease should be fully vaccinated according to general guidelines; specific recommendations for immunocompromised patients may also apply. Whenever possible, patients should be brought up to date on vaccinations prior to starting immunosuppressive agents because vaccine responses may be diminished when on treatment. Nonetheless, immunosuppressed patients do respond immunologically to vaccines and should not generally be deprived of the opportunity to be vaccinated.

Patients on nonbiologic DMARDs can receive vaccines of all types. Because of a theoretical risk of infection in a higher state of immunosuppression, the use of live attenuated vaccines (for example, herpes zoster vaccine, yellow fever vaccine) is currently contraindicated for patients on biologic therapies. However, such patients may be administered live attenuated vaccines approximately 4 weeks before starting biologic therapy.

Prior to initiating aggressive immunosuppressive therapy, the following recommendations for screening have been suggested:

- Tuberculosis screening with tuberculin skin testing or interferon-γ release assay, particularly for patients initiating most biologic therapies
- Hepatitis B and C serologies, particularly for patients initiating potentially hepatotoxic agents (methotrexate, leflunomide) or TNF-α inhibitor therapy
- HIV screening
- Strongyloidiasis screening if patient is from an endemic area

Patients with latent or active tuberculosis, active hepatitis B, or untreated HIV infection require initiation of infection therapy prior to initiating immunosuppressive therapy. Repeat screening for tuberculosis should be performed annually, with similar repeat screening for hepatitis, HIV, and strongyloidiasis in the presence of ongoing risk.

KEY POINTS

- Whenever possible, patients should be brought up to date on vaccinations prior to starting immunosuppressive therapy.
- Live attenuated vaccines are currently contraindicated for patients on biologic therapies; however, live attenuated vaccines may be administered approximately 4 weeks before starting biologic therapy. *(Continued)*

KEY POINTS *(continued)*

- Prior to initiating aggressive immunosuppressive therapy, screening for infections (tuberculosis, hepatitis B and C, HIV) is indicated; if needed, infection therapy must be started before initiating immunosuppressive therapy.

Urate-Lowering Therapy

The American College of Rheumatology guidelines currently indicate that urate-lowering therapy (ULT) should be initiated in patients with gout who have had two or more attacks within a 1-year period, one attack in the setting of chronic kidney disease of stage 2 or worse, one attack with the presence of tophi visible on examination or imaging, or one attack with a history of urolithiasis. ULT reduces total body uric acid burden; the treatment target is a serum urate level of 6.0 mg/dL (0.35 mmol/L) or less. Over time, urate lowering reduces risk of future gout attacks and promotes regression of tophi. Treatment with ULT is usually life-long.

Anti-inflammatory prophylaxis to prevent gout attacks is recommended when ULT is initiated because of the paradoxical increased risk of acute gout attacks when serum urate levels are rapidly decreased by medication. See Crystal Arthropathies for more information on gout prophylaxis.

Allopurinol

Allopurinol is a first-line agent for serum urate reduction in patients with gout. Allopurinol is a purine analogue that inhibits xanthine oxidase, the final enzyme in the pathway of urate synthesis from purine precursors. Allopurinol is metabolized by the liver and renally excreted; its active metabolite oxypurinol has a half-life of 12 to 17 hours, or longer in patients with kidney disease.

Allopurinol is generally well tolerated and should be initial treatment for patients requiring ULT due to its extensive use history and cost-benefit profile. However, it can very rarely provoke a severe hypersensitivity reaction with fever, lymphadenopathy, widespread erythema, purpura, and skin necrosis and should therefore be discontinued at the first sign of a rash. Allopurinol should be avoided in patients taking other purine analogues such as azathioprine or 6-mercaptopurine because toxic levels of either or both drug may ensue. Patients should be periodically monitored for liver function, kidney function, and complete blood count levels during allopurinol treatment.

Allopurinol is FDA approved for dosing up to 800 mg/d. However, the dose most commonly used in routine practice is 300 mg/d, a dose that is sufficient to achieve the serum urate target in only half the patients treated. Although concern was expressed regarding allopurinol dosing and the risk of hypersensitivity, it appears that gradual dose escalation with careful monitoring is a safe approach, even in patients with kidney disease. The American College of Rheumatology recommends a starting dose of 100 mg/d (50 mg/d in patients with stage 4 or 5 chronic kidney disease) with a urate check and titration upward every 2 to 5 weeks, until a target level of 6.0 mg/dL (0.35 mmol/L) or less is achieved.

Febuxostat

Febuxostat is an alternative first-line therapy for urate lowering. In contrast to the purine analogue allopurinol, febuxostat is a non-purine, non-competitive xanthine oxidase inhibitor that is more specific than allopurinol. Febuxostat is newer and more expensive than allopurinol. It is less likely to cause hypersensitivity reactions and may be used in patients who have had adverse reactions to allopurinol. Febuxostat is excreted via the gastrointestinal tract and kidneys and needs no dose adjustment for patients with mild to moderate chronic kidney disease. Febuxostat should be avoided in patients taking other purine analogues such as azathioprine or 6-mercaptopurine because toxic levels of either or both drug may ensue.

Febuxostat is approved at doses of 40 mg/d or 80 mg/d in the United States and 120 mg/d in Europe. The 40-mg dose is roughly equivalent to 300-mg allopurinol in efficacy, whereas the 80-mg dose is superior to 300-mg allopurinol. To date, studies comparing the efficacy of febuxostat versus higher doses of allopurinol are lacking. Patients should be monitored for liver function during therapy with this agent.

Probenecid

Probenecid is a second-line agent that promotes kidney uric acid excretion (uricosuric effect). Probenecid may also be used in conjunction with a xanthine oxidase inhibitor for synergistic effect. Probenecid has limited efficacy in patients with a creatinine clearance less than 50 mL/min and is relatively contraindicated in patients with kidney stones or hyperuricosuria (indicating uric acid overproduction). Probenecid requires frequent daily dosing and adequate hydration, and it has multiple drug-drug interactions. Kidney function and complete blood count levels should be monitored.

Pegloticase

Humans lack the gene for uricase, which converts uric acid to the more soluble allantoin; therefore, repletion of uricase is a potential strategy for lowering uric acid. Pegloticase is a recombinant pegylated uricase that dramatically lowers serum urate. Pegloticase is indicated for patients with persistent moderate to severe gout who have failed standard ULT. Pegloticase is administered intravenously every 2 weeks; gout flares are common, and infusion reactions may occur. Patients on pegloticase must eschew other ULTs and should have serum urate levels checked before each infusion. Increase of serum urate to greater than 6.0 mg/dL (0.35 mmol/L) suggests failure of the drug due to immunogenicity, which indicates that the patient is at risk for infusion reactions, and requires discontinuation.

KEY POINTS

- Urate-lowering therapy is indicated for patients with gout who have had two or more attacks within a 1-year period, one attack in the setting of chronic kidney disease of stage 2 or worse, one attack with the presence of tophi visible on examination or imaging, or one attack with a history of urolithiasis.
- Allopurinol and febuxostat are first-line agents for serum urate reduction; allopurinol is less expensive but can rarely cause a severe hypersensitivity reaction and should be discontinued at the first sign of a rash.

Rheumatologic Medications and Pregnancy

Some rheumatologic medications have potentially adverse effects on pregnancy. **Table 12** discusses these agents and their relative risks.

KEY POINTS

- Methotrexate is highly teratogenic and abortifacient and must be discontinued at least 3 months prior to conception.
- Hydroxychloroquine is relatively safe in pregnancy and should not be discontinued.
- Leflunomide is extremely teratogenic and must not be used before/during pregnancy; if leflunomide is inadvertently administered, cholestyramine treatment is required to remove the drug from the body before pregnancy.

Nonpharmacologic and Nontraditional Management

Physical and Occupational Therapy

Physical and occupational therapy are integral to the comprehensive management of many types of arthritis. Physical therapy can help manage pain and functional deficits in arthritis. Overuse injuries related to occupational or recreational activities or loss of strength and flexibility after surgical intervention also respond well to graded exercise. Modalities such as local heat or cold, electrical stimulation, and massage can provide analgesia and may enhance the ability of the patient to exercise.

Occupational therapy refers not only to rehabilitative efforts for enhancing workplace functioning but also to therapy for the hands and upper extremities, including splinting, range of motion exercises, and instruction in joint-sparing techniques.

Complementary and Alternative Medicine

Complementary and alternative medicine (CAM) refers to a diverse group of interventions outside the mainstream of medicine taught in U.S. medical schools. Nearly 40% of Americans use CAM, usually as an adjunct to traditional medical care. Patients with rheumatologic diseases and chronic pain syndromes are more likely to use CAM.

Natural Products

Vitamins, minerals, herbal preparations, and probiotics are labeled as dietary supplements, which permits sale without proof of specific effects or content verification. Although labels on these products commonly make broad statements about particular health benefits, most have not been studied in well-controlled trials.

Glucosamine sulfate and chondroitin sulfate are the most commonly used dietary supplements for arthritis. Earlier trials suggested analgesic benefit, but recent studies have shown little effect on symptoms and/or radiographic disease progression in osteoarthritis, and current guidelines do not recommend their use.

Omega-3 fatty acids present in fish oil inhibit prostaglandin and leukotriene production and reduce inflammation. Clinical trials in rheumatoid arthritis show modest benefit.

Numerous herbal products for arthritis are available over the counter, including ginger, curcumin, bromelain, evening primrose and borage oils, feverfew, willow bark, cat's claw, and *Boswellia*. Although many of these have been shown to have in vitro anti-inflammatory effects, clinical trials are lacking.

Mind-Body Practices

Mind-body practices include tai chi, yoga, acupuncture, meditation, deep-breathing exercises, guided imagery, hypnotherapy, progressive relaxation, and qi gong. Randomized controlled trials support the use of tai chi for reducing pain and enhancing function in patients with osteoarthritis. Some data suggest that yoga may also be beneficial. Acupuncture has been the subject of numerous studies in osteoarthritis, and modest, short-term reductions in pain and improved function have been demonstrated. Few studies have assessed the other modalities.

Role of Surgery

When medications fail to adequately control pain or prevent disability, surgery can be considered. Surgery may be needed acutely or planned electively in chronic circumstances. Osteoarthritis is the most frequent reason for total joint arthroplasty. The knee, hip, and, occasionally, the shoulder are replaced when end-stage joints cause pain at rest or at night or when function is compromised to an unacceptable level. Joint replacements in other locations have less predictable benefit. Arthroscopy is performed primarily for specific indications such as the removal of a loose body or repair of a torn meniscus. Arthroscopy in routine degenerative disease has not been shown to be superior to sham surgery in controlled trials. Arthroscopic synovectomy may be helpful in rheumatoid arthritis when excessive pannus accumulates and does not respond to medical management.

TABLE 12. Rheumatologic Medications and Pregnancy

Medication/Class	FDA Pregnancy Category[a]	Comments
Anti-Inflammatory Agents		
NSAIDs	Various	May impede implantation and may be associated with a small increased risk of miscarriage when used before 20 weeks' gestation. Use of NSAIDs after 30 weeks' gestation can lead to premature closure of the ductus arteriosus.
Glucocorticoids	Various	In the first trimester, they can increase the risk of cleft palate in the fetus and of gestational diabetes in the mother throughout pregnancy. Nonetheless, they can be useful in the management of active autoimmune disease in pregnancy. Non-fluorinated glucocorticoids (e.g., prednisone, prednisolone, methylprednisolone) have limited ability to cross the placenta and may be preferred, except when treating the fetus (e.g., neonatal lupus erythematosus).
Colchicine	C	Should be used only if the potential benefit justifies the potential risk to the fetus.
Analgesics		
Acetaminophen	B	Generally considered safe at standard dosing, but does cross the placenta.
Opiates	Various	Some opiates/opioids cross the placenta; may cause fetal opioid withdrawal at birth.
Tramadol	C	Should be used only if the potential benefit justifies the potential risk to the fetus; post-marketing reports suggest the possibility of neonatal seizures, withdrawal syndrome, and still birth.
Topical agents	Varies by agent, concentration, and vehicle	Topical use may limit serum levels; individual agents should be reviewed for pregnancy impact prior to use.
Nonbiologic DMARDs		
Methotrexate	X	Highly teratogenic and abortifacient; must be discontinued at least 3 months before pregnancy.
Hydroxychloroquine	C	Despite a C rating, relatively safe in pregnancy and should not be discontinued.
Sulfasalazine	B	Relatively safe during pregnancy.
Leflunomide	X	Extremely teratogenic; must not be used before/during pregnancy; cholestyramine administration is required to remove the drug from the body in all women of childbearing potential upon discontinuation and specifically in those wishing to become pregnant; should be followed up with measurement of leflunomide and its metabolite levels to ensure removal of the drug.
Azathioprine	D	Routine use in pregnancy is not recommended; however, despite a D rating, azathioprine may be safer than some other DMARDs and may be used if an immunosuppressive agent is imperatively needed.
Cyclophosphamide	D	Not used in pregnancy unless absolutely necessary.
Mycophenolate mofetil	D	Teratogenic; should not be used in pregnancy; discontinue for 3 months before attempting pregnancy.
Cyclosporine	C	May be used in pregnancy only if benefits outweigh the risks.
Biologic DMARDs		
TNF-α inhibitors	B	Accumulating retrospective data suggest low risk in pregnancy, but evidence is limited; can be continued if absolutely needed; different agents may have different considerations regarding crossing the placenta.
Ustekinumab, anakinra	B	Should be used only if the potential benefit justifies the undefined risk to the fetus.
Abatacept, rituximab, tocilizumab, belimumab, tofacitinib, rilonacept, canakinumab	C	Should be used only if the potential benefit justifies the potential risk to the fetus; tofacitinib may be teratogenic at high doses.
Urate-Lowering Therapy		
Allopurinol	C	Should be used only if the potential benefit justifies the potential risk to the fetus.
Febuxostat	C	Should be used only if the potential benefit justifies the potential risk to the fetus.
Probenecid	B	No current evidence for adverse impact on pregnancy.
Pegloticase	C	Should be used only if the potential benefit justifies the potential risk to the fetus.

DMARD = disease-modifying antirheumatic drug; TNF = tumor necrosis factor.

[a]See MKSAP 17 General Internal Medicine for information on the FDA pregnancy categories.

KEY POINTS
- Physical and occupational therapy are integral components of a comprehensive management plan for many types of arthritis.
- When medications fail to adequately control pain or prevent disability, surgery can be considered.

Rheumatoid Arthritis

Introduction

Rheumatoid arthritis (RA) is a systemic autoimmune disorder of unknown cause that typically presents as a symmetric inflammatory polyarthritis. Characteristically affected joints include the proximal interphalangeal and metacarpophalangeal joints of the hands and feet and the wrists, but other joints can also be involved. Prolonged morning stiffness is common. RA is also associated with extra-articular manifestations, including inflammation of the skin, eyes, pleura, and pericardium. Early diagnosis and immunomodulation offer the best opportunity to avoid permanent joint damage and multisystem complications.

Epidemiology

RA affects approximately 1% of the population worldwide. Women are affected two to three times more often than men. Onset can occur at any age, with peak incidence between ages 30 and 60 years.

Pathophysiology and Risk Factors

Genetic Factors

The risk of RA is increased in relatives of affected persons, primarily as a result of shared genetic factors. Siblings of those with RA have at least twice the risk of developing RA as unrelated individuals, and offspring of affected persons have about three times the risk. Based on twin studies, the heritability of RA is estimated at 60%, suggesting that genetic factors account for the majority of disease susceptibility within the population.

More than 20 risk alleles have been identified, with the largest contribution coming from genes in the major histocompatibility complex (MHC) region. Alleles encoding the "shared epitope" of the HLA-DRB1 molecule have the strongest association with RA (especially severe articular disease, multisystem disease, and rheumatoid vasculitis). The shared epitope corresponds to a specific amino acid sequence in the antigen-binding site of the MHC molecule, suggesting a possible (but unproven) role in facilitating the presentation of specific but currently unidentified antigens. This association of RA with a gene determining a specific antigen response capacity underscores the relationship of disease to immune dysregulation.

Autoantibodies

Autoantibodies, including rheumatoid factor and anti–cyclic citrullinated peptide (CCP) antibodies, are often present in the peripheral blood and synovial fluid of patients with RA. These autoantibodies typically precede clinical disease by years; their possible role in pathogenesis remains an area of investigation. Although they aid in diagnosis, autoantibodies are neither necessary nor sufficient for diagnosing RA.

Rheumatoid factor, an immunoglobulin directed against the Fc portion of IgG, is associated with increased risk of RA diagnosis as well as erosive and/or more widespread joint disease. However, some patients with RA lack rheumatoid factor, and it is also found in other diseases as well as in healthy persons, limiting its diagnostic specificity.

Anti-CCP antibodies occur less frequently than rheumatoid factor but have more diagnostic specificity. Anti-CCP antibodies are directed against citrullinated proteins, including proteins present in inflamed joint tissues, suggesting that anti-CCP antibodies may play a pathogenic role. Clinically, the presence of anti-CCP antibodies predicts a greater risk of erosive disease and radiographic progression.

Environmental Factors

Several environmental exposures increase the risk of RA in genetically susceptible persons. For individuals carrying the shared epitope, smoking conveys up to a fivefold increase in RA risk (more in the presence of rheumatoid factor or anti-CCP antibodies). Smoking risk may be mediated, in part, by the ability of cigarette smoke to induce protein citrullination in the lungs, which may serve as antigens to drive anti-CCP antibody production.

Occupational exposure to silica or asbestos, as well as occupations involving electrical or carpentry work, has also been associated with increased RA risk.

Infection

Although it has long been hypothesized that infection could trigger RA, no definitive proof of the role of any individual organism exists. Nonetheless, observations about *Porphyromonas gingivalis*, the pathogenic agent in periodontitis, continue to stimulate investigations. The presence of periodontal disease is epidemiologically linked to RA. Furthermore, *P. gingivalis* has the ability to generate citrullinated peptides, suggesting a possible antigenic effect.

More recent studies have focused on a possible role for the intestinal microbiome in promoting immune responses leading to RA.

Hormones

The increased incidence of RA in women is most evident prior to menopause, suggesting a role for sex hormones in the modulation of disease. However, the relationship between RA and hormones is complex. Estrogen levels alone cannot adequately explain the link between gender and RA risk because oral contraceptives and postmenopausal hormone replacement have no predictable effect on disease risk.

KEY POINTS

- Rheumatoid arthritis typically presents as a symmetric inflammatory polyarthritis affecting small joints and is associated with prolonged morning stiffness and extra-articular manifestations.
- Possible risk factors for rheumatoid arthritis include genetic and environmental factors, autoantibodies, infection, and hormones.

Diagnosis

A careful history, physical examination, and assessment of clinical manifestations are the first steps in the evaluation of a patient with suspected RA. Laboratory and imaging studies are indicated to properly establish the diagnosis. Differential diagnoses, including infection, should be excluded. The American College of Rheumatology classification criteria provide guidelines for identifying patients with RA, with the goal of permitting early diagnosis and management (**Table 13**).

Clinical Manifestations

Patients with RA characteristically present with pain and swelling in multiple (>3) small joints of the hands and/or feet, along with morning stiffness lasting at least 1 hour. Distal interphalangeal joint involvement is distinctly rare. Many patients have 12 or more affected joints. Rarely, only a single joint may be initially involved.

Initial symptoms often worsen gradually over weeks to months; fewer than 10% of patients have an abrupt onset of disease. RA frequently interferes with activities of daily living, including occupational and recreational activities. Constitutional symptoms such as increased fatigue and malaise are common. Depression and myalgia may occur and, less often, fever, anorexia, and weight loss. Musculoskeletal manifestations are listed in **Table 14**.

Physical examination reveals tenderness and swelling of the joints, sometimes with warmth and erythema; symmetric joint involvement is common. Joint symmetry refers to involvement of the same rank of joints on both sides (for example, hand metacarpophalangeal joints), rather than exact

TABLE 13. The 2010 American College of Rheumatology/European League Against Rheumatism Classification Criteria for Rheumatoid Arthritis

Target Population: newly presenting patients

1) who have at least 1 joint with definite clinical synovitis (swelling)

2) with synovitis not better explained by another disease (rheumatology consult may be indicated)

Classification Criteria for RA (score-based algorithm: add score of categories A-D; a score of ≥6/10 is needed for classification of a patient as having definite RA; score may change over time)

	Score
A) Joint Involvement (swollen or tender)	
1 large joint (shoulders, elbows, hips, knees, ankles)	0
2-10 large joints	1
1-3 small joints (with or without involvement of large joints)[a]	2
4-10 small joints (with or without involvement of large joints)	3
>10 joints (at least 1 small joint)	5
B) Serology (at least 1 test result is needed for classification)	
Negative RF and negative anti-CCP antibodies	0
Low-positive RF or low-positive anti-CCP antibodies (>ULN but ≤3 times ULN)	2
High-positive RF or high-positive anti-CCP antibodies (>3 times ULN)	3
C) Acute Phase Reactants (at least 1 test result is needed for classification)	
Normal CRP and normal ESR	0
Abnormal CRP or abnormal ESR	1
D) Duration of Joint Symptoms (by patient self-report)	
<6 weeks	0
≥6 weeks	1

CCP = cyclic citrullinated peptide; CRP = C-reactive protein; ESR = erythrocyte sedimentation rate; RA = rheumatoid arthritis; RF = rheumatoid factor; ULN = upper limit of normal for the laboratory and assay.

[a]"Small joints" refers to the metacarpophalangeal joints, proximal interphalangeal joints, second through fifth metatarsophalangeal joints, thumb interphalangeal joints, and wrists.

Adapted with permission from John Wiley & Sons, from Aletaha D, Neogi T, Silman AJ, et al. 2010 Rheumatoid arthritis classification criteria: an American College of Rheumatology/European League Against Rheumatism collaborative initiative. Arthritis Rheum. 2010 Sep;62(9):2569-81. [PMID: 20872595] Copyright 2010 American College of Rheumatology.

TABLE 14. Musculoskeletal Manifestations of Rheumatoid Arthritis

Feature	Findings	Comments
Joint inflammation	Morning stiffness; joint tenderness; soft-tissue swelling; palpable joint effusion; local warmth; pain on active and passive range of motion	Assess duration of morning stiffness by asking "How long does it take from when you wake up in the morning until you feel as good as you are going to feel for the rest of the day?"
Distribution of joint involvement	Symmetric; initially small joints; progresses proximally to larger joints; commonly involves MCP, PIP, MTP, and wrist joints	DIP joint involvement is uncommon (seen in psoriatic arthritis, osteoarthritis).
Joint damage	Decreased range of motion; contractures; ulnar deviation; subluxation; cervical instability; basilar invagination	Marginal erosions may be evident earliest at the 5th MTP joint. Cartilage degradation causes joint-space narrowing. Ankylosis can occur in long-standing disease.
Periarticular involvement	Bursitis; tenosynovitis; tendinopathy; swan neck and boutonnière deformities; flexion contractures; popliteal (Baker) and ganglion cysts	Olecranon bursitis and rotator cuff tendinopathy are common. Tenosynovitis can cause trigger finger but is less prominent than in spondyloarthritis. Popliteal (Baker) cysts are contiguous with the knee joint.
Muscular weakness	Disuse atrophy; drug-induced myopathy (glucocorticoids and other drugs)	Interosseous and quadriceps muscles are common sites of atrophy from disuse.
Decreased bone quality	Periarticular osteopenia; generalized loss of bone mineral density; increased risk of fracture	Risk of fracture may be underestimated by bone mineral density alone.

DIP = distal interphalangeal; MCP= metacarpophalangeal; MTP = metatarsophalangeal; PIP = proximal interphalangeal.

mirroring of involved digits. See **Figure 2** for examples of involvement of the hands in RA.

Because viral and other infections can cause transient symmetric arthritis of small joints, active signs of inflammation for at least 6 weeks should be documented before diagnosis of RA is established.

Laboratory Studies

Laboratory studies, including rheumatoid factor, anti-CCP antibodies, and inflammatory markers, can assist in confirming a diagnosis of RA; however, serologies should never be used as the sole criterion for diagnosis because of limitations in sensitivity and specificity.

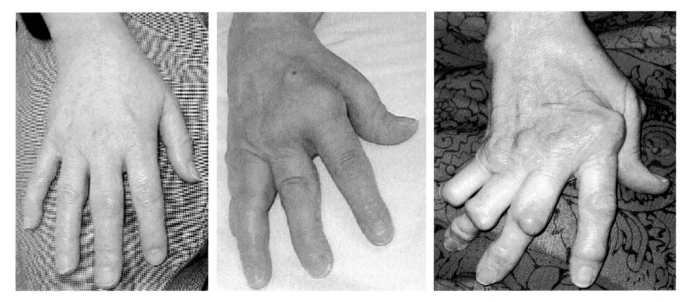

FIGURE 2. Involvement of the hands in rheumatoid arthritis. Early rheumatoid arthritis with mild fusiform soft-tissue swelling of the proximal interphalangeal joints (*left panel*). Moderate to severe rheumatoid arthritis with synovitis of the metacarpophalangeal joints and swan neck deformities of the second and third digits (*center panel*). Severe deforming rheumatoid arthritis with ulnar deviation, multiple rheumatoid nodules, and proximal interphalangeal joint subluxations (*right panel*).

Rheumatoid factor is approximately 70% sensitive for the diagnosis of RA. Approximately 50% of patients with RA have detectable rheumatoid factor at onset, increasing to 60% to 80% in established disease. Conversely, up to 20% of patients with RA lack rheumatoid factor. Moreover, rheumatoid factor occurs in other rheumatologic diseases (Sjögren syndrome, systemic lupus erythematosus, polymyositis, dermatomyositis); cryoglobulinemia due to hepatitis B or C virus infection; primary biliary cirrhosis; subacute bacterial endocarditis; and certain lung diseases (sarcoidosis, B-cell lymphomas). Rheumatoid factor can also be present in healthy persons. Thus, the positive predictive value of rheumatoid factor is poor in populations with a low pretest probability of RA. Testing patients with fibromyalgia, osteoarthritis, or nonspecific aches and pains is therefore not recommended because a positive result is more likely to represent a false positive. Higher titers of rheumatoid factor are more likely to be associated with RA as well as with more severe RA disease, multisystem manifestations, and involvement of more joints. However, fluctuations in rheumatoid factor do not mirror disease activity, and serial testing lacks clinical utility in established disease.

Anti-CCP antibody testing has similar sensitivity but superior specificity compared with rheumatoid factor. Although anti-CCP antibody specificity is reported to be around 95%, anti-CCP antibodies occasionally occur in other rheumatologic diseases, active tuberculosis, and chronic lung disease. The dual presence of rheumatoid factor and anti-CCP antibodies makes a diagnosis of RA substantially more likely. Seronegative RA has an identical clinical appearance as seropositive RA but is more likely to occur in men.

Elevation of inflammatory markers such as erythrocyte sedimentation rate (ESR) or C-reactive protein (CRP) suggests RA disease activity; however, normal levels do not absolutely rule out RA activity.

A normochromic, normocytic anemia and/or thrombocytosis may reflect chronic inflammatory RA disease.

Imaging Studies

More than half of inadequately treated patients with RA develop bone erosions within the first 2 years of disease; therefore, baseline and subsequent radiographs are indicated to aid in the diagnosis and to follow disease progression. Plain radiographs of the hands, wrists, and/or feet may show characteristic findings of periarticular osteopenia and marginal (near the edges of the joint) erosions (**Figure 3**); however, erosive changes may not be evident early in the disease course. The earliest site of RA erosion of the foot is classically at the fifth metatarsophalangeal joint (**Figure 4**). In the presence of long-standing inflammation, relatively uniform joint-space narrowing may occur across the entire affected joint.

Musculoskeletal ultrasonography is increasingly utilized for RA diagnosis and management. It requires specialized training and is operator dependent but is more sensitive

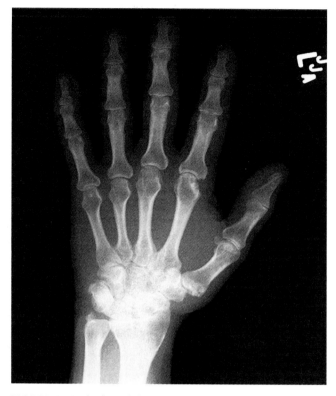

FIGURE 3. Hand radiograph showing rheumatoid arthritis. Periarticular osteopenia is present at the metacarpophalangeal joints. Marginal erosions are present at the second proximal interphalangeal and metacarpophalangeal joints, as well as the ulnar styloid. Both are characteristic of rheumatoid arthritis and findings that can aid in diagnosis. Joint-space narrowing (a nonspecific finding) is seen at the second and fifth proximal interphalangeal joints.

than radiography for identifying synovitis and erosions. However, it may not be more specific for RA diagnosis than the standard approach.

MRI is sensitive for identifying erosions, synovitis, and tenosynovitis, but its value in RA diagnosis and management is not established. The American College of Rheumatology Choosing Wisely list questions the utility of routinely ordering MRI of peripheral joints to monitor rheumatoid arthritis. However, MRI can be used in the evaluation of cervical spine involvement if subluxation or myelopathy is suspected.

KEY POINTS

- Patients with rheumatoid arthritis characteristically present with pain and swelling in multiple (>3) small joints of the hands and/or feet and prolonged morning stiffness.
- Rheumatoid factor, anti–cyclic citrullinated peptide antibodies, and inflammatory markers assist in confirming a diagnosis of rheumatoid arthritis; however, serologies should never be used as the sole criterion for diagnosis and should be avoided in patients with low pretest probability for disease due to the high rate of false-positive results. *(Continued)*

HVC

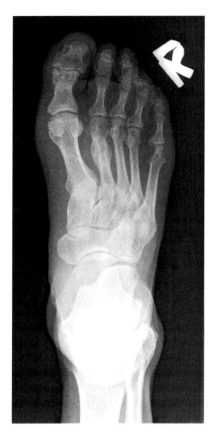

FIGURE 4. Foot radiograph showing rheumatoid arthritis. Characteristic changes of rheumatoid arthritis are frequently seen in the small joints of the feet, as seen here with severe erosive change at the fifth metatarsophalangeal joint and marginal erosions at the first and second metatarsophalangeal joints and the first interphalangeal joint. Nonspecific cystic changes in bone may be seen in many different forms of arthritis.

KEY POINTS *(continued)*

HVC
- Plain radiography of the hands, wrists, and/or feet is indicated to aid in the diagnosis and to follow progression of rheumatoid arthritis; in contrast, MRI of peripheral joints should not be routinely performed to monitor disease progression.

Complications and Extra-Articular Manifestations

Joints

In the absence of appropriate immunosuppressive therapy, patients can develop increasing numbers of swollen and tender joints, subluxation and malalignment, tenosynovitis and ligamentous laxity, reduced grip strength, loss of range of motion, and loss of function. Permanent joint damage and radiographic abnormalities can occur within the first year.

Skin

RA may affect various organs in addition to joints. The skin is most commonly affected, with rheumatoid nodules being the most frequent manifestation. These firm, subcutaneous masses measure from a few millimeters to several centimeters and may be mobile or adhere to the underlying periosteum. Rheumatoid nodules occur alone or in clusters, often on pressure areas such as the elbows, finger joints, ischial and sacral prominences, occiput, and Achilles tendons (see Figure 2). Although usually in periarticular locations on extensor surfaces, they may appear in any location, including the lungs, heart, and muscle.

Pyoderma gangrenosum is also seen in RA. It usually occurs as a single painful lesion on the lower extremities, beginning as a tender erythematous or violaceous papule and rapidly expanding into a purulent, necrotic, nonhealing ulcer (see MKSAP 17 Dermatology, Cutaneous Manifestations of Internal Disease).

Rheumatoid vasculitis is a late complication of RA that affects small and medium vessels and may involve the skin and other organs. It is most common in seropositive male patients with long-standing disease. Small-vessel involvement presents as purpura, petechiae, splinter hemorrhages, nailfold infarctions, and peripheral neuropathy. In medium-vessel disease, nodules, ulcerations, livedo reticularis, and digital infarcts can occur.

Eyes

The most common eye manifestation of RA is keratoconjunctivitis sicca, as is also seen in Sjögren syndrome and systemic lupus erythematosus. Episcleritis occurs with more severe RA disease activity, appears acutely, and causes eye redness and pain; changes in vision rarely occur. Scleritis, uveitis, ulcerative keratitis, and corneal filamentary keratitis also occur during more severe disease and may lead to visual impairment. See Eye Disorders in MKSAP 17 General Internal Medicine for more information.

Pulmonary Involvement

Pleuritis is the most common RA pulmonary manifestation but is frequently asymptomatic. Exudative pleural effusions may occur. Rheumatoid nodules in the lungs can be difficult to diagnose because they are often peripheral in location and usually measure less than 1 cm in diameter. Interstitial lung disease occurs in up to 10% of patients, particularly in male smokers with long-standing, seropositive disease.

Cardiac Involvement

RA is an independent risk factor for both coronary artery disease and heart failure; patients with severe extra-articular disease are at particularly increased risk of cardiovascular death. Pericarditis is common but is often asymptomatic. Rarely, pericarditis is severe, unresponsive to glucocorticoids, and may be restrictive. Successful treatment with disease-modifying agents appears to reduce cardiac comorbidity.

Other Complications

Felty syndrome is a rare complication occurring in patients with severe, erosive, seropositive, long-standing RA. Felty syndrome is characterized by neutropenia (absolute neutrophil count <2000/μL [2.0×10^9/L]) and splenomegaly, often accompanied by fever, anemia, thrombocytopenia, and/or vasculitis, and can predispose to recurrent bacterial infections. Felty syndrome has limited responsiveness to disease-modifying drugs and may require use of granulocyte colony-stimulating factor.

Unusual complications of long-standing, severe RA include mesangioproliferative glomerulonephritis, amyloidosis, atlantoaxial subluxation due to erosion of the odontoid process, and peripheral neuropathy.

KEY POINTS

- Extra-articular manifestations of rheumatoid arthritis include rheumatoid nodules, rheumatoid vasculitis, keratoconjunctivitis sicca, pleuritis, and pericarditis.

- Rheumatoid arthritis is an independent risk factor for coronary artery disease and heart failure; patients with severe extra-articular disease are at particularly increased risk of cardiovascular death.

Management

General Considerations

RA management often requires a team approach to comprehensively provide optimal care of the joints and other organs and to address psychosocial needs. The American College of Rheumatology treatment recommendations for early and established RA are presented in **Figure 5** and **Figure 6**, respectively.

Once a diagnosis of RA is established, management with disease-modifying antirheumatic drugs (DMARDs) is mandated to minimize damage and reduce disability. The initial goal of treatment is to rapidly reduce disease activity, but the ultimate goal is remission (absence of signs and symptoms of significant inflammatory activity). This "treat-to-target" approach requires treatment protocols and regular follow-up visits to reassess clinical status and response to changes in medication. Therapy is advanced at each follow-up visit until the therapeutic target is reached. The usual interval of follow-up is every 2 to 3 months to reassess whether goals are being met and toxicity is present. Patients may be seen by rheumatologists more frequently if disease activity is high or less often (for example, every 6 to 12 months) if remission has been achieved. In long-standing refractory disease, low disease activity may be an acceptable alternative target, and response-limiting factors such as the presence of structural damage, functional impairment, medical comorbidities, drug side-effect risks, and other individual patient-related factors must be taken into account.

Disease activity is assessed based on history, physical examination, and the use of composite disease activity scores that incorporate findings such as the number of tender or swollen joints and laboratory studies such as ESR or CRP. Composite scores provide a more comprehensive and standardized assessment that can account for variability between patients and within the course of disease for a single patient. Furthermore, treatment targets can be expressed as a single number facilitating comparisons over time. In clinical trials, the most

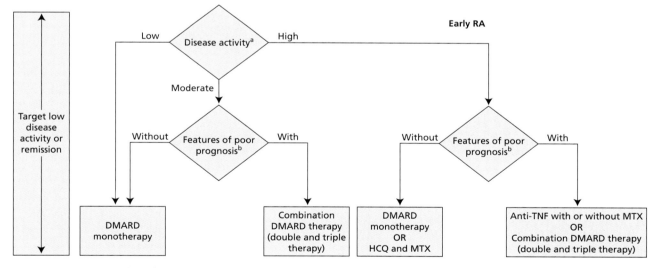

FIGURE 5. 2012 American College of Rheumatology recommendations update for the treatment of early rheumatoid arthritis, defined as a disease duration <6 months. DMARDs include hydroxychloroquine, leflunomide, methotrexate, minocycline, and sulfasalazine. DMARD = disease-modifying antirheumatic drug; HCQ = hydroxychloroquine; MTX = methotrexate; RA = rheumatoid arthritis; TNF = tumor necrosis factor.

[a]Definitions of disease activity are available at http://onlinelibrary.wiley.com/journal/10.1002/(ISSN)2151-4658) and were categorized as low, moderate, or high.

[b]Patients were categorized based on the presence or absence of 1 or more of the following poor prognostic features: functional limitation (e.g., Health Assessment Questionnaire score or similar valid tools), extra-articular disease (e.g., presence of rheumatoid nodules, RA vasculitis, Felty syndrome), positive rheumatoid factor or anti-cyclic citrullinated peptide antibodies, and bony erosions by radiograph.

Adapted with permission from John Wiley & Sons, from Singh JA, Furst DE, Bharat A, et al. 2012 update of the 2008 American College of Rheumatology recommendations for the use of disease-modifying antirheumatic drugs and biologic agents in the treatment of rheumatoid arthritis. Arthritis Care Res (Hoboken). 2012;64(5):625-639. [PMID: 22473917] Copyright 2012 American College of Rheumatology.

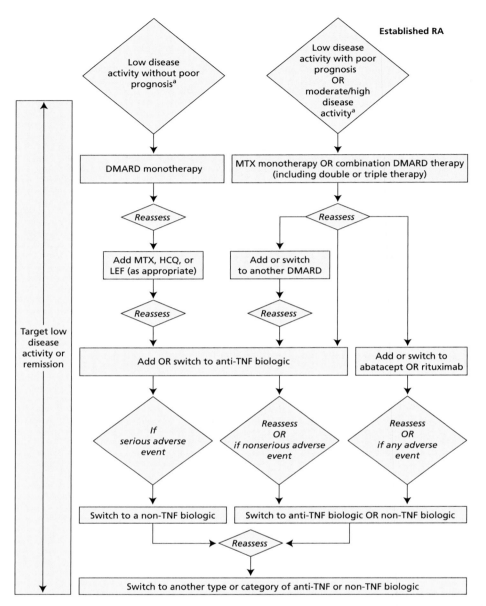

FIGURE 6. 2012 American College of Rheumatology (ACR) recommendations update for the treatment of established rheumatoid arthritis (RA), defined as a disease duration >6 months or meeting the 1987 ACR classification criteria. Depending on a patient's current medication regimen, the management algorithm may begin at an appropriate rectangle in the figure, rather than only at the top of the figure. DMARDs include HCQ, LEF, MTX, minocycline, and sulfasalazine (therapies are listed alphabetically; azathioprine and cyclosporine were considered but not included). DMARD monotherapy refers to treatment in most instances with HCQ, LEF, MTX, or sulfasalazine; in few instances, where appropriate, minocycline may also be used. Anti-TNF biologics include adalimumab, certolizumab pegol, etanercept, infliximab, and golimumab. Non-TNF biologics include abatacept, rituximab, or tocilizumab (therapies are listed alphabetically). DMARD = disease-modifying antirheumatic drug; HCQ = hydroxychloroquine; LEF = leflunomide; MTX = methotrexate; RA = rheumatoid arthritis; TNF = tumor necrosis factor.

[a]Definitions of disease activity are available at http://onlinelibrary.wiley.com/journal/10.1002/(ISSN)2151-4658) and were categorized as low, moderate, or high. Features of poor prognosis included the presence of 1 or more of the following: functional limitation (e.g., Health Assessment Questionnaire score or similar valid tools), extra-articular disease (e.g., presence of rheumatoid nodules, RA vasculitis, Felty syndrome), positive rheumatoid factor or anti–cyclic citrullinated peptide antibodies, and bony erosions by radiograph.

Adapted with permission from John Wiley & Sons, from Singh JA, Furst DE, Bharat A, et al. 2012 update of the 2008 American College of Rheumatology recommendations for the use of disease-modifying antirheumatic drugs and biologic agents in the treatment of rheumatoid arthritis. Arthritis Care Res (Hoboken). 2012;64(5):625-639. [PMID: 22473917] Copyright 2012 American College of Rheumatology.

frequently used disease assessment instrument has been the Disease Activity Score 28 (DAS28), which incorporates the number of tender and swollen joints out of a predetermined set of 28 joints, a weighted ESR or CRP, and a global health assessment. An example of low disease activity based on DAS is ≥2.6

to <3.2 (see Figure 5), and high disease activity based on DAS is >5.1 (see Figure 6). Other disease activity scales to determine the appropriate level of treatment are available.

Patient education is fundamental to managing RA and includes discussing medications and side effects, advising on lifestyle choices (diet, weight loss, exercise), and assessing psychosocial needs. Physical and occupational therapy may be appropriate throughout the course of RA. Appropriate exercise can strengthen and protect joints and is an important adjunct in combating fatigue and optimizing function. Smoking cessation is important not only because of its link to disease risk, but also because continued smoking may impair the response to therapy and exacerbate rheumatoid lung disease.

Disease-Modifying Antirheumatic Drugs

Principles, toxicities, baseline evaluation and monitoring, use of vaccinations, and pregnancy issues associated with medications used in RA are discussed in Principles of Therapeutics.

Nonbiologic Disease-Modifying Antirheumatic Drugs

Methotrexate is the recommended initial DMARD for most patients with RA and is appropriate at disease onset as well as in patients whose disease is well established. It is generally continued indefinitely and can be used alone or in combination with biologic DMARDs. Methotrexate is usually well tolerated and has good efficacy, high long-term compliance rates, and relatively low cost but requires regular monitoring. Methotrexate or another nonbiologic DMARD should be tried before initiating therapy with a considerably more expensive biologic DMARD. Generally, the dose of methotrexate is titrated up until the treatment target is achieved. If the response is below target at an oral dose of 25 mg weekly, clinicians may switch to parenteral administration since absorption and efficacy may improve. However, if toxicity or lack of efficacy is encountered at this dose, the use of a biologic agent is indicated.

Hydroxychloroquine and sulfasalazine have long-acting effects and may be used alone, together, or in combination with methotrexate. Triple therapy with these three agents has a reasonable side-effect profile and can be highly efficacious in symptom control and in reducing the risk of structural damage.

Leflunomide may be used with or as a substitute for methotrexate. It is appropriate as a first choice in the treatment of RA or as an alternative to methotrexate if side effects or other considerations limit methotrexate use.

Biologic Disease-Modifying Antirheumatic Drugs

The decision to add a biologic agent should be made based on inadequate response to a nonbiologic DMARD (especially methotrexate) while balancing the patient-specific risks of biologic therapy. Biologic agents are commonly added to methotrexate but are not used in combination with other biologics because of an unacceptable increase in infection without added efficacy.

Tumor necrosis factor (TNF)-α inhibitors are the most widely used biologic agents for RA and are available in both intravenous and subcutaneously administered injections. All TNF-α inhibitors interfere with the actions of TNF-α, a major proinflammatory cytokine in RA pathogenesis. TNF-α stimulates synovial cell proliferation and synthesis of collagenase,

leading to cartilage degradation. In addition, TNF-α increases bone resorption, inhibits proteoglycan synthesis, and increases expression of adhesion molecules, thus enhancing inflammatory cell recruitment as well as production of additional proinflammatory cytokines and arachidonic acid metabolites.

TNF-α inhibitors are highly effective for treating RA, leading to rapid (weeks), significant improvement in signs and symptoms for most patients. Their use is associated with increased likelihood of achieving remission in both new-onset and established disease, reduction in radiographic progression, normalization of acute phase reactants, and reduced cardiovascular risk. Their efficacy is enhanced when used in combination with methotrexate.

Other biologic agents target other proinflammatory cytokines and pathways. Tocilzumab is a monoclonal antibody that neutralizes IL-6, a cytokine that activates T cells, B cells, macrophages, osteoclasts, and the hepatic acute phase response. Abatacept blocks necessary second signals between antigen-presenting cells and T cells during antigen presentation, thereby blocking T-cell activation. Rituximab is a monoclonal antibody that depletes B-cell populations, leading to a reduction in B-cell cytokine production, B-cell help for T-cell activation, and the production of a number of autoantibodies, including rheumatoid factor and anti-CCP antibodies. All of these agents have efficacy similar to TNF-α inhibitors.

Tofacitinib is a new oral agent and the first small molecule therapy for RA that specifically targets an intracellular signaling molecule in immune/inflammatory pathways. Tofacitinib inhibits Janus-associated kinases, which signal in response to membrane cytokine receptors to activate STATs (signal transducers and activators of transcription). Tofacitinib appears to have efficacy similar to biologic agents.

Glucocorticoids

Oral or intra-articular glucocorticoids are used as adjunctive therapy in RA. Glucocorticoids act rapidly to control inflammation and joint symptoms and can be useful until slower-acting DMARDs achieve full effect. Glucocorticoids are also used to manage intermittent flares in patients already taking other agents. Regular, frequent use of glucocorticoids should signal the need for increasing the DMARD dose or adding/switching DMARDs. Given their many side effects, glucocorticoids should be employed at the lowest dose and shortest period possible and should never be used as standing monotherapy.

NSAIDs

NSAIDs can ameliorate RA joint symptoms. However, NSAIDs lack disease-modifying activity, do not alter the destructive course of untreated RA, and should never be used as monotherapy.

Surgical Therapy

Surgical interventions are available to patients with RA complications or advanced disease unresponsive to pharmacologic therapy. Large joint (hip, knee) replacement is an option for

H
CONT.

intractable disease unresponsive to medical management. Patients with pain at rest or night pain are particularly appropriate for total joint replacement. Patients with RA have a higher risk of prosthetic joint infection than patients having total joint arthroplasty for other indications. Repair procedures for tendon ruptures and rotator cuff disease are occasionally needed. Degenerative disk disease may be accelerated in the presence of RA, and spinal procedures such as laminectomy may be indicated. Improvements in pharmacologic management have made surgical approaches to RA increasingly uncommon.

Patients with RA undergoing general anesthesia for any kind of surgery should have cervical spine radiography with flexion and extension views to assess for atlantoaxial subluxation, which rarely can lead to neurologic compromise when the neck is extended during intubation. H

KEY POINTS

- Methotrexate is the recommended initial disease-modifying antirheumatic drug for most patients with rheumatoid arthritis.
- The use of tumor necrosis factor α inhibitors or other biologic agents in patients with rheumatoid arthritis can achieve remission in new-onset and established disease, reduce risk of radiographic progression, normalize acute phase reactants, and reduce cardiovascular risk.

Pregnancy and Rheumatoid Arthritis

Nulliparity has been suggested as a risk factor for RA, but data are conflicting. During pregnancy, patients with RA may experience relative disease quiescence, but disease may flare postpartum. There is also evidence that the incidence of RA is increased in the year after delivery, particularly after the first pregnancy. Breastfeeding may decrease the risk.

Methotrexate and leflunomide are absolutely contraindicated in pregnancy and must be discontinued prior to conception. Limited case studies suggest that use of TNF-α inhibitors during pregnancy may be safe, but a relationship to rare birth defects has been raised by a single report. Decisions regarding the use of any biologic agent in pregnancy should incorporate risk-benefit analysis. Both hydroxychloroquine and sulfasalazine are considered relatively safe in pregnancy. Non-fluorinated glucocorticoids such as prednisone, prednisolone, or methylprednisolone have limited ability to cross the placenta and may be preferred. NSAIDs may impede implantation and may be associated with a small increased risk of miscarriage when used prior to 20 weeks' gestation. Use of NSAIDs after 30 weeks' gestation can lead to premature closure of the ductus arteriosus.

See Rheumatologic Disease and Pregnancy in Principles of Therapeutics for more information on these and other medications and their role in pregnancy.

KEY POINTS

- Methotrexate and leflunomide are absolutely contraindicated in pregnancy and must be discontinued prior to conception.
- Both hydroxychloroquine and sulfasalazine are considered relatively safe in pregnancy.

Osteoarthritis
Introduction

Osteoarthritis (OA) is characterized by loss of cartilage accompanied by reactive bony changes, including osteophyte formation, subchondral bony sclerosis, and subchondral cysts. OA typically affects the knees, hips, hands, spine, and feet. Pain and loss of function are the hallmark features; however, OA is variable in its clinical presentation, which can range from asymptomatic radiographic changes to severe and disabling pain and permanent impairment and deformity.

Epidemiology

OA is the most common form of arthritis, affecting at least 30 million persons in the United States. Prevalence increases with age; OA among younger populations is frequently related to a history of recreational or occupational injury in a specific joint or to a strong genetic predisposition. Whereas early OA is slightly more common in men, at older ages women are slightly more frequently affected. Overall, radiographic knee OA is present in about 35% of adults over the age of 60, and radiographic hand OA is present in 55% to 65%. OA is the most common cause of disability in patients over age 65.

Pathophysiology

OA is the consequence of biomechanical and biochemical processes involving the cartilage, synovium, bone, and soft tissues surrounding the joint. These processes can be initiated by a single traumatic event, repeated microtrauma, or genetic, metabolic, or systemic factors affecting the integrity of cartilage. During OA progression, matrix metalloproteinases (MMPs), including collagenase, stromelysin, and gelatinase, are secreted by chondrocytes and degrade cartilage collagen. Inappropriately low levels of tissue inhibitors of metalloproteinases (TIMPs) may reduce the ability of cartilage to resist MMPs.

Inflammatory cytokines such as interleukin (IL)-1β may induce MMP production and suppress collagen production. Ineffective repair responses within the joint may be mediated by insulin-like growth factor and transforming growth factor β, leading to abnormal bone growth, including osteophyte formation and subchondral sclerosis.

Risk Factors

Risk factors for OA include advanced age, female gender, obesity, and joint injury caused by repetitive use, trauma, or certain occupations. Joint malalignment, ligamentous laxity, meniscal injury, or surgical meniscectomy can accelerate the onset of OA, as can quadriceps weakness and defects in proprioception, all resulting in abnormal joint forces. Family history may indicate risk; a multitude of genetic variants has been associated with various OA subsets, but no single gene has emerged as definitively predicting onset or severity.

OA risk varies depending on the joint involved. The lifetime risk for symptomatic knee OA is approximately 45%, with a higher risk after job- or sports-related injury or overuse or among those who are obese. Lifetime risk of symptomatic hip OA is approximately 27%, is higher in women, and is less strongly related to obesity and trauma compared with knee OA. Hand OA risk is increased on the basis of genetic predisposition and is more common in women. Manual labor and obesity confer additional risk for hand OA.

KEY POINTS

- Osteoarthritis is characterized by loss of cartilage and the presence of osteophytes, subchondral bony sclerosis, and subchondral cysts.
- Risk factors for osteoarthritis include advanced age, female gender, obesity, and acute or chronic joint injury.

Classification
Primary Osteoarthritis

Primary (idiopathic) OA constitutes most cases of OA, which are designated as such when no specific antecedent event or predisposing disease is present. The designation of primary OA does not exclude the impact of routine factors such as obesity, aging, or a chronic history of significant but non-injurious joint use. Primary OA typically affects the knees, hips, hands, spine, and feet and may be localized (a single or few joints) or generalized (multiple joints). It typically becomes clinically evident around the age of 55 years.

Erosive Osteoarthritis

Erosive OA is a subset of primary OA in which radiographic erosions are seen. Erosive OA typically involves the interphalangeal joints of the fingers and is associated with intermittent flares of swelling and redness of the affected joints. Diagnosis is radiographic, based on the presence of central erosions (contrasting with the marginal erosions of rheumatoid and psoriatic arthritis) and collapse of the subchondral

bone in the affected joints. Patients with erosive OA are more likely to have pain and disability than those without erosive features. In contrast to rheumatoid arthritis, erosive OA is common in the distal interphalangeal joints, does not typically affect the wrists or elbows, and is not associated with rheumatoid factor, anti-cyclic citrullinated peptide antibodies, or an elevated erythrocyte sedimentation rate or C-reactive protein level.

Prevalence of erosive OA is approximately 3% in the general population over the age of 55 years and 10% among those with any symptomatic hand OA. Men and women are equally affected.

Secondary Osteoarthritis

Secondary OA indicates joint degeneration in the setting of preexisting joint abnormality. It may occur in the setting of trauma or congenital anatomic abnormalities (such as hip dysplasia). Secondary OA may follow inflammatory arthritis (such as rheumatoid or gouty arthritis or calcium pyrophosphate deposition), avascular necrosis, infectious arthritis, Paget disease, osteopetrosis (congenitally increased bone mass and skeletal fragility), or osteochondritis dissecans (in which a portion of bone and cartilage separates from the surrounding bone). Finally, secondary OA may occur in the setting of metabolic or systemic diseases such as hemochromatosis (iron overload, which is associated with a characteristic OA pattern involving the second and third metacarpophalangeal joints and is diagnosed with the aid of transferrin saturation measurement), ochronosis (excessive accumulation of homogentisic acid), Gaucher disease, hemoglobinopathy, or Ehlers-Danlos syndrome.

Diffuse Idiopathic Skeletal Hyperostosis

Diffuse idiopathic skeletal hyperostosis (DISH) is often considered in the same context as OA by virtue of its lack of systemic inflammation, the presence of characteristic bony remodeling changes, a similar epidemiology, and its frequent coexpression with OA. DISH is diagnosed on plain radiograph by the presence of flowing osteophytes involving the anterolateral aspect of four or more contiguous vertebrae most easily detected in the thoracic spine (**Figure 7**). Intervertebral disk spaces are typically preserved; apophyseal or sacroiliac joint inflammatory changes are absent. Peripheral enthesitis and ossification of ligaments in nonvertebral locations may occur. DISH is distinguished from primary OA of the spine (with which it may co-occur) by the manner in which the flowing osteophytes bridge the vertebrae, by its anatomic location, and by the relative preservation of the disk spaces when OA is absent. Complications include dysphagia, unstable spinal fractures, spinal stenosis, postsurgical heterotropic ossifications, difficult intubation, difficult gastroscopy, aspiration pneumonia, and myelopathy. Radiographically, DISH may be difficult to differentiate from ankylosing spondylitis (see Spondyloarthritis).

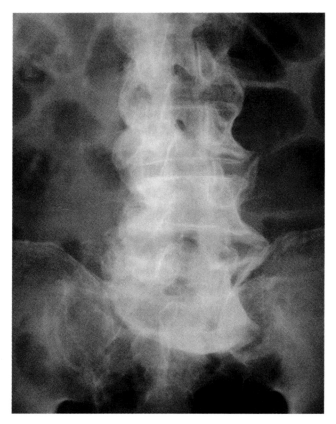

FIGURE 7. Diffuse idiopathic skeletal hyperostosis. This disorder is characterized by calcification of the enthesis regions (where the tendons or ligaments insert into bone) and the spinal ligaments. The diagnosis is confirmed on radiograph by the presence of flowing osteophytes along the anterolateral aspect of at least four contiguous vertebral bodies (most easily detected in the thoracic spine), preserved vertebral height, and absent findings typical for ankylosing spondylitis.

The prevalence of DISH increases with age and is approximately 15% in patients over 50 years of age. In contrast to OA, DISH is twice as common in men than in women.

KEY POINTS

- Primary osteoarthritis (OA) constitutes most cases of OA, which are designated as such when no clear antecedent event or predisposing disease is present.

- Erosive hand osteoarthritis is associated with intermittent flares of swelling and redness of the affected joints as well as the presence of central erosions and collapse of subchondral bone in the interphalangeal joints as seen on plain radiographs.

- Secondary osteoarthritis can occur in settings of trauma and metabolic or systemic disease or following joint damage from inflammatory or infectious arthritis.

- Diffuse idiopathic skeletal hyperostosis is characterized by flowing osteophytes involving the anterolateral aspect of four or more contiguous vertebrae most easily detected in the thoracic spine.

Diagnosis
Clinical Manifestations

A thorough history and physical examination are warranted in the initial evaluation of the patient with suspected OA. Patients with symptomatic OA describe pain and stiffness in the affected joint(s). Pain may occur intermittently and be associated with joint use. Patients often report a decline in function associated with the pain. Stiffness may worsen with rest and improve with activity, but typically lasts for only brief periods (less than 30 minutes).

On physical examination, affected joints may be tender, or the patient may report discomfort only when the joint is put through a range of motion (often reduced due to pain and/or deformity). Joint effusions may occur; erythema and warmth are less common than in inflammatory arthritis. More advanced disease may be accompanied by change in the physical appearance of the joints, manifesting as bony enlargement and/or changes in alignment. The most commonly affected joints are the first carpometacarpal and distal and proximal interphalangeal joints of the hands, knees, hips, and apophyseal joints of the spine.

Hand OA typically presents with pain, aching, or stiffness for most days of the prior month. Bony enlargement of a distal interphalangeal joint is termed a Heberden node (**Figure 8**); similar enlargement in a proximal interphalangeal joint is termed a Bouchard node. Occasionally, an individual joint in the hand may be swollen or erythematous (inflammatory or erosive OA), but the presence of multiple swollen joints, particularly proximal joints, should lead to consideration of concomitant calcium pyrophosphate deposition or rheumatoid or psoriatic arthritis.

Diagnosis of knee or hip OA is established in the presence of knee or groin pain for most days of the prior month. Hip involvement can occasionally result in referred pain that is perceived by the patient as knee pain. Crepitus on active joint

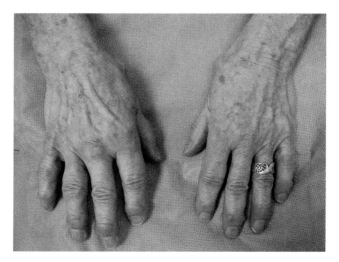

FIGURE 8. Heberden nodes in osteoarthritis are bony spurs at the dorsolateral and medial aspects of the distal interphalangeal joints.

motion, limited range of motion, and morning stiffness lasting less than 30 minutes are typical. Bony enlargement of the knee is common. Knee effusions, which are usually cool, are also common. Chronic effusions may be associated with the formation of popliteal fossa fluid collections (Baker cysts). Knee malalignment is common and may result in a "knocked knee" or "bow-legged" appearance. Long-standing knee OA is associated with quadriceps muscle atrophy.

OA of the spine is a common source of back pain and is often seen in association with degenerative disk disease. Physical examination may demonstrate reduced range of motion and associated muscle spasm; spinal tenderness is rarely present.

Laboratory and Imaging Studies

No specific laboratory abnormalities are associated with primary OA. In most cases, laboratory studies are indicated only when needed to rule out other diagnoses. If NSAID use is contemplated, it is appropriate to first evaluate kidney function. Although arthrocentesis is not mandatory for diagnosing OA, synovial fluid examination should be considered if needed to help rule out inflammatory arthritis (rheumatoid arthritis, crystal-induced disease), hemarthrosis, or infection. Noninflammatory synovial fluid (leukocyte count <2000/μL [2.0×10^9/L]) is typical of OA.

Joint-space narrowing (articular cartilage loss), subchondral sclerosis, and marginal osteophyte formation are the radiographic hallmarks of OA (**Figure 9**); periarticular osteopenia and marginal erosions (as seen in rheumatoid arthritis) are absent. In OA of the knee and hip, joint-space narrowing characteristically occurs mainly on the weight-bearing areas of the joint, distinguishing it from inflammatory arthritis (**Figure 10**). Subchondral sclerosis is seen on plain

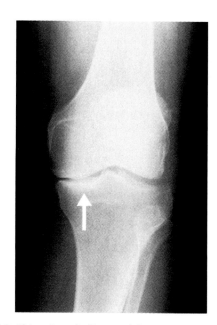

FIGURE 10. Plain radiograph of knee medial compartment osteoarthritis showing joint-space narrowing and subchondral sclerosis (*arrow*).

radiographs as increased bone density subjacent to joint-space narrowing. Both subchondral sclerosis and osteophytes reflect reaction of bone to growth factors stimulated by the mechanical changes driving OA. In erosive hand OA, central erosions are visible on radiograph. However, plain radiography is insensitive for the detection of early OA, and OA severity on plain radiographs is inconsistently associated with pain and other symptoms.

MRI and ultrasonography are currently being investigated as potential tools in OA diagnosis and management.

Differential Diagnosis

Polyarthritis of the proximal hand digits may warrant exclusion of rheumatoid arthritis because both OA and rheumatoid arthritis can affect these joints. Whereas rheumatoid arthritis rarely, if ever, affects the distal interphalangeal joints, psoriatic arthritis may affect both proximal and distal joints, but tends to affect these joints more globally than OA. The presence of extensive inflammation and/or morning stiffness, a positive rheumatoid factor, anti-cyclic citrullinated peptide antibodies, elevated erythrocyte sedimentation rate or C-reactive protein, anemia of chronic disease or thrombocytosis without other explanation, or inflammatory synovial fluid also favor the diagnosis of rheumatoid arthritis.

Calcium pyrophosphate deposition can co-occur with OA, may be related to severe presentations of OA, and can promote inflammation that is difficult to distinguish from rheumatoid arthritis when metacarpophalangeal joint and wrist involvement is present. It can be a cause of acute monoarticular or oligoarticular arthritis, particularly in the knee. Joints may be chronically painful or abruptly warm and swollen, and large knee effusions can result.

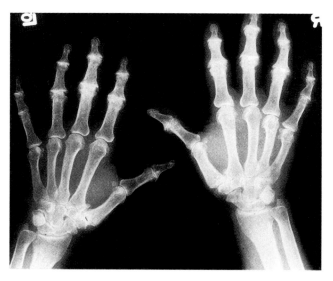

FIGURE 9. Plain radiograph of hand osteoarthritis showing joint-space narrowing, subchondral sclerosis, and osteophyte formation involving the distal interphalangeal and proximal interphalangeal joints.

KEY POINTS

- Laboratory studies are indicated only when needed to rule out other diagnoses in patients with primary osteoarthritis (OA); the diagnostic role for MRI and ultrasonography in OA has not been established.

- Joint-space narrowing, subchondral sclerosis, and marginal osteophyte formation are the radiographic hallmarks of osteoarthritis; periarticular osteopenia and marginal erosions (as seen in rheumatoid arthritis) are absent.

- Polyarthritis of the proximal hand digits may warrant exclusion of rheumatoid arthritis because both osteoarthritis and rheumatoid arthritis can affect these joints.

Management

OA management requires a comprehensive, individualized evaluation of symptoms, level of functioning, and patient expectations. Because no single intervention addresses all of the ways in which OA can impact quality of life, a multidisciplinary perspective promotes the best patient outcomes.

Nonpharmacologic Therapy

Exercise (aquatic or land based) is among the most important nonpharmacologic treatments for most patients with OA. Exercise prescriptions should first address acutely symptomatic joints, targeting rehabilitation within the physical capabilities of the patient. Exercise should be repeated regularly and should not overuse the joints or exacerbate symptoms. Exercise should be advanced as the patient improves and can include strengthening, stretching, range of motion, and aerobic activity. Although a physical or occupational therapist is often useful initially and can also provide thermal agents and manual therapy, the goal is to assist patients in incorporating exercise into their daily self-management routine.

Evidence for the efficacy of exercise is most convincing for knee OA. Because excessive weight contributes to both knee OA risk and symptomatology, measures to promote weight loss (exercise, food diaries, support groups, meal planning, nutritional counseling, portion size regulation, evaluation of psychosocial factors and coping strategies) are usually appropriate for overweight patients with knee OA. Obese patients undergoing bariatric surgery may experience reduction in knee OA symptoms.

Properly fitting footwear and/or orthotics can improve ambulation among patients with OA of the feet, ankles, knees, hips, and/or spine. Assistive devices such as canes and walkers can reduce lower extremity symptoms and may permit delay or deferral of surgical intervention. Canes should be held on the side opposite from the affected joint. Short-term use of splints (for example, thumb spica), cushions, and ergonomic supports (for example, in vehicles and at desks and workstations), as well as the use of grab bars and other specialized equipment in bathrooms, can relieve symptoms and enhance functioning. Chronic bracing can be used for severely affected joints that may be unstable, particularly when patients are poor candidates for surgery.

Pharmacologic Therapy

Because no disease-modifying agents are currently available for the treatment of OA, pharmacologic options address the symptoms of OA rather than its underlying cause. Most treatment guidelines suggest the initial use of acetaminophen for pain control, with recognition of potential hepatotoxicity leading to some recommendations limiting the total daily dose to approximately ≤3 g/d. If acetaminophen proves inadequate, an over-the-counter or prescription NSAID should be used. NSAIDs are available in oral, topical, and intravenous forms. Oral preparations are usually first-line NSAID therapy in patients without a contraindication to treatment due to efficacy and cost-effectiveness. Topical NSAIDs are considered to provide similar pain relief OA as oral medications with fewer gastrointestinal effects. Furthermore, the American College of Rheumatology currently recommends topical NSAIDs rather than oral NSAIDs for patients aged 75 years or older. However, they are associated with more skin reactions and are significantly more expensive than oral NSAIDs. NSAIDs can be also be used in combination with acetaminophen. Treatment guidelines suggest using the lowest effective NSAID dose for the shortest time period in order to reduce risk of side effects. However, many patients with OA require years of NSAID use given the prolonged timeframe over which the disease is symptomatic and the limited number of pharmacologic alternatives.

Tramadol is a centrally acting opioid analgesic that weakly inhibits norepinephrine-serotonin reuptake; potential for addiction is lower than for traditional opioids. Tramadol may be useful for managing OA pain when acetaminophen or NSAIDs are ineffective or contraindicated (for example, patients with a history of bleeding peptic ulcer, heart failure, or chronic kidney disease).

Duloxetine is a dual serotonin-norepinephrine reuptake inhibitor indicated for chronic musculoskeletal pain, including pain due to OA. Duloxetine may be used as an adjunct to more rapidly acting analgesics or as a single agent in patients with chronic OA pain.

Traditional opiates may rarely be warranted to control pain in patients with OA who have not responded to other agents or are poor candidates for other interventions to treat painful joints, such as surgery. Patient selection, informed consent, and monitoring of response and for side effects should proceed according to treatment guidelines established for opiate treatment of any chronic pain.

Although early trials suggested an analgesic benefit from glucosamine sulfate and chondroitin sulfate, subsequent studies have shown a minimal effect on symptoms and no moderation in the progression of disease. Therefore, guidelines do not recommend their use.

See Principles of Therapeutics for a discussion on medication toxicities and side effects.

Intra-articular Injection

When a single symptomatic joint is present, injection directly into the joint may deliver medication to the affected site while minimizing the potential for systemic effects. Intra-articular injections may be used along with or in place of oral or topical analgesics.

Glucocorticoid Injection

Numerous glucocorticoid preparations are available for intra-articular injection, including triamcinolone acetonide, triamcinolone hexacetonide, and methylprednisolone. Glucocorticoids can reduce OA knee pain within days to weeks. When a joint effusion is present, glucocorticoid injections can be particularly helpful after drainage of the excessive joint fluid. Intra-articular facet joint injections may provide pain relief from cervical or lumbar spinal OA, although studies are limited. Local side effects include skin hypopigmentation, subcutaneous tissue atrophy, and joint infection. The frequency of glucocorticoid injections is usually limited to every 3 months due to theoretical concerns about adverse effects on the joint.

Hyaluronic Acid Injection

Although multiple individual trials of hyaluronic acid injection have suggested analgesic benefit for knee OA, recent meta-analyses suggest that any such benefit may be clinically trivial. Functional benefit has also not been demonstrated. However, the possibility that specific patient subsets may obtain benefit from hyaluronic acid injection is not yet determined. Side effects are uncommon but include transient postinjection joint inflammation. The risk of joint infection after hyaluronic acid injection is not currently known.

Surgical Therapy

When pain or functional impairment cannot be controlled by other means, orthopedic intervention for OA deserves consideration. The decision to proceed with surgery should take into consideration the patient's medical comorbidities and level of preoperative strength and mobility. Radiographic severity alone is an imperfect predictor of symptoms and an inadequate gauge of the need for surgery; decision making should incorporate an appreciation for the likely benefit in terms of quality of life and patient expectations, particularly regarding employment and recreational activities. Pain at rest or that awakens the patient in the middle of the night despite analgesic use is often present in those considering surgery. Preoperative anxiety and depression are associated with worse postoperative outcomes. Morbidly obese patients may experience earlier failure of prostheses and are often advised to lose weight prior to surgery.

For knee and hip OA, the most effective surgical intervention is total joint arthroplasty (removal of the affected articular surfaces followed by replacement with metal and polyethylene prosthetic components). In properly selected patients, arthroplasty can reduce pain, improve function, and enhance quality of life. Patients are transiently anticoagulated to reduce the rate of postoperative deep venous thrombosis to about 1%. Prosthetic joint infection occurs in 1% to 2% of patients undergoing total joint arthroplasty; patients with diabetes mellitus are at increased risk. After 10 years, 85% to 90% of total joint replacements for OA remain functional. However, about 20% of total knee and 10% of total hip arthroplasty patients continue to have some level of persistent pain.

Arthroscopy may be helpful in knee OA when retrieval of a loose body is required to prevent locking of the joint. However, the routine use of arthroscopic lavage and debridement for OA has fallen out of favor because several studies have demonstrated no benefit of this procedure compared with blinded sham surgery.

KEY POINTS

- A regular exercise program, physical therapy, nutritional counseling, and appropriate footwear, splints, canes, or other assistive devices can benefit patients with osteoarthritis.
- Acetaminophen is the initial choice for osteoarthritis pain control in most instances; if acetaminophen provides inadequate relief, NSAIDs should usually be tried.
- Intra-articular glucocorticoids reduce osteoarthritis knee pain within days to weeks.
- The most effective surgical intervention for knee or hip osteoarthritis is total joint arthroplasty, which can reduce pain, improve function, and enhance quality of life.

Fibromyalgia

Introduction

Fibromyalgia is characterized by chronic widespread pain, tenderness of skin and muscles to pressure, fatigue, sleep disturbance, and exercise intolerance. Patients with fibromyalgia often have coexisting somatic conditions such as pelvic pain, headaches, and temporal mandibular joint pain. Effective treatment addresses both the biologic and psychologic aspects of chronic pain.

Epidemiology

Using the 1990 American College of Rheumatology fibromyalgia classification criteria (widespread body pain, tender points), prevalence in the general population ranges from 0.06% to 10%. Fibromyalgia increases with age up to the sixth decade and declines thereafter. The female-male ratio is 9:1, but this may change with use of newer diagnostic criteria.

Fibromyalgia may co-occur in patients with inflammatory diseases such as rheumatoid arthritis (25%), systemic lupus erythematosus (30%), and primary Sjögren syndrome (50%). Psychologic distress, mood disorder, victimization, and disordered sleep have also been reported to play contributory roles. The role of physical trauma as an initiator of fibromyalgia is controversial. Importantly, not all patients with fibromyalgia have evidence of psychologic distress or physical trauma, underlining that such factors may contribute to, but do not define, fibromyalgia.

Pathophysiology

Studies suggest that the pain state of fibromyalgia is mediated by aberrant chronic pain reflex arcs centered on the dorsal ganglia of the spine. These arcs function independently but may be exacerbated by acute or chronic pain input such as that seen in arthritis or by the input contributed by psychologic distress. Functional MRI brain studies indicate that pain perception among patients with fibromyalgia is indistinguishable from, but more readily triggered than, pain perception in unaffected individuals. Patients with fibromyalgia demonstrate elevation in pain-facilitating neurotransmitters (glutamate and substance P) and reduction of neurotransmitters that down-regulate pain (norepinephrine, serotonin, and γ-aminobutyric acid). Endogenous opioid levels are paradoxically elevated along with decreased opioid receptor availability, perhaps accounting for the poor response to narcotics seen in those with fibromyalgia.

Diagnosis

The 2010 American College of Rheumatology fibromyalgia diagnostic criteria eliminated the tender point examination, owing to sensitivity biases that resulted in overdiagnosis among women. Current criteria include documentation of self-reported pain for at least 3 months at 19 different body locations (Widespread Pain Index [WPI]) along with a severity score (scale of 0-3) for three reported symptoms: fatigue, waking unrefreshed, and cognitive symptoms (Symptoms Severity Scale [SSS]). The combination of a WPI of ≥7 plus an SSS of ≥5, or a WPI between 3 and 6 plus an SSS of ≥9, establishes a diagnosis of fibromyalgia for the purposes of study enrollment.

In routine clinical practice, the combination of widespread pain ("hurt all over"), waking unrefreshed ("always tired and fatigued"), cognitive fatigue (forgets words or loses track of conversations in mid-sentence), and exercise intolerance ("if I overdo it, I pay for it for several days") are clues to the diagnosis. Previous lack of response to multiple medications, including NSAIDs, is also a diagnostic clue. Cross-sectional data suggest that obstructive sleep apnea may be common. Examination is generally unremarkable except for diffuse tenderness to palpation. The association of fibromyalgia with some inflammatory diseases requires that these disorders be considered when performing a history and physical examination.

Initial laboratory studies include a complete blood count, chemistry panel, thyroid-stimulating hormone, and erythrocyte sedimentation rate (ESR) or C-reactive protein (CRP). ESR and CRP should be normal; elevated levels should prompt additional evaluation. Antinuclear antibodies, rheumatoid factor, or anti–cyclic citrullinated peptide antibodies should not be obtained unless examination or initial laboratory testing suggests that these are indicated. Muscle enzymes are frequently checked but are useful only in patients who are actually weak on examination.

Management

Patients with fibromyalgia typically benefit from validation of their symptoms by a physician because many patients have previously had their complaints disregarded by caregivers or family. These patients should be reassured that the condition is not an indication of a more serious problem and that additional diagnostic testing is generally unhelpful. Discussing the current understanding of fibromyalgia ("a problem of central pain processing") can be useful when the treatment program is described. The goal is to have the patient actively involved in a program that improves pain processing centrally and increases pain thresholds. Four issues need to be addressed: psychologic distress and/or mood disorder, sleep disturbance (may be tied to the distress), pain, and deactivation. Although patients often avoid aerobic exercise, it is critical for functional improvement. A physical therapist can be useful to discuss daily stretching and a slowly progressive home aerobic exercise program. Sleep hygiene should be reviewed. When another rheumatologic disease or significant psychologic distress is present, referral to a specialist is suggested.

Three drugs are FDA approved for fibromyalgia: the anticonvulsant pregabalin and the dual serotonin-norepinephrine reuptake inhibitors duloxetine and milnacipran. Each provides a modest benefit over placebo, with 30% to 50% of patients experiencing more than 30% reduction in pain. The latter two agents can also address coexisting mood disorder. Off-label therapies that have provided benefit include the tricyclic antidepressants (which have some demonstrated sleep utility), and, to a lesser extent, the selective serotonin reuptake inhibitors, particularly when administered in conjunction with a tricyclic agent.

The combination of medications, reactivation, and a productive lifestyle offers the best chance for significant improvement. Patients should be reassured that the chances of further deterioration are low but should also be aware that there currently is no medical cure for this condition.

KEY POINTS

HVC

- Fibromyalgia is a clinical diagnosis characterized by chronic widespread pain, tenderness of the skin and muscles to pressure, fatigue, sleep disturbance, and exercise intolerance. *(Continued)*

KEY POINTS *(continued)*

- Initial laboratory evaluation of fibromyalgia includes a complete blood count, chemistry panel, thyroid-stimulating hormone, and erythrocyte sedimentation rate or C-reactive protein; routine testing for antinuclear antibodies, rheumatoid factor, anti–cyclic citrullinated peptide antibodies, or muscle enzymes should be avoided.

- Management of fibromyalgia addresses psychologic distress and/or mood disorder, sleep disturbance, pain, and deactivation.

- For patients with fibromyalgia, aerobic exercise is critical for functional improvement.

- Pregabalin, duloxetine, and milnacipran are FDA approved and modestly effective for fibromyalgia.

Spondyloarthritis

Introduction

Spondyloarthritis refers to a group of disorders that share an overlapping set of features, including inflammation of the axial skeleton, tendons, and entheses (insertion of tendon to bone); tendon and enthesis calcification; an association with HLA-B27; and mucocutaneous, gastrointestinal, and ocular inflammation.

The four disorders of spondyloarthritis are ankylosing spondylitis, psoriatic arthritis, inflammatory bowel disease (IBD)–associated arthritis, and reactive arthritis (formerly known as Reiter syndrome). Patients who have some of these features but do not meet criteria for one of the four disorders may be designated as having undifferentiated spondyloarthritis.

KEY POINT

- Spondyloarthritis refers to a group of disorders that share an overlapping set of features, including inflammation of the axial skeleton, tendons, and entheses; tendon and enthesis calcification; an association with HLA-B27; and mucocutaneous, gastrointestinal, and ocular inflammation.

Pathophysiology

Genetic Factors

The gene most strongly associated with spondyloarthritis is the class I major histocompatibility complex molecule HLA-B27, which is present in approximately 90% of patients with ankylosing spondylitis. Among first-degree relatives of patients with ankylosing spondylitis, the presence of HLA-B27 confers an increased risk (approximately 10%-30%) of developing the disease. Moreover, ankylosing spondylitis is rare in low HLA-B27 prevalence populations. However, HLA-B27 alone is insufficient to produce spondyloarthritis because most individuals who are positive for HLA-B27 never develop the disease.

Although less strongly associated with other forms of spondyloarthritis, HLA-B27 is present in up to 70% of patients with reactive and/or IBD-associated arthritis. HLA-B27 is also present in 60% to 70% of patients with axial psoriatic arthritis and in 25% of those with peripheral psoriatic arthritis without axial involvement.

Environmental Factors

The strongest evidence that infectious triggers can play a role in spondyloarthritis is found in reactive arthritis, which typically develops after specific gastrointestinal or genitourinary infections. However, the immunobiology underlying infectious triggers remains uncertain, and infectious agents have not been shown to trigger ankylosing spondylitis. A disrupted mucosal barrier between the gut and bloodstream, potentially fostering unopposed interaction of microorganisms with immune tissues, has been hypothesized to promote IBD-associated arthritis.

Reactive arthritis and psoriatic arthritis may be more severe among patients with HIV infection, particularly when HLA-B27 is present. Unexpectedly severe presentations of either disease may warrant evaluation for underlying HIV infection in appropriate cases.

KEY POINTS

- The gene most strongly associated with spondyloarthritis is HLA-B27, which is present in approximately 90% of patients with ankylosing spondylitis.

- The strongest evidence that infectious triggers can play a role in spondyloarthritis is found in reactive arthritis, which typically develops after specific gastrointestinal or genitourinary infections.

- Reactive arthritis and psoriatic arthritis may be more severe among patients with HIV infection, particularly when HLA-B27 is present; unexpectedly severe presentations of either disease may warrant evaluation for underlying HIV infection in appropriate cases.

Classification

Although the disorders comprising spondyloarthritis share common clinical features, each disorder has a greater or lesser tendency to manifest specific features (**Table 15**). However, the features can overlap and the phenotype of each syndrome also varies from patient to patient, making the distinction sometimes challenging.

Ankylosing Spondylitis

Ankylosing spondylitis characteristically affects the axial skeleton and also has extra-articular manifestations (see Table 15). Ankylosing spondylitis is more common in men than women (3:1 ratio), although some studies suggest it is underrecognized in the female population. Peak age of onset is in the second to third decade of life.

TABLE 15. Clinical Features of Spondyloarthritis

	Ankylosing Spondylitis	Psoriatic Arthritis	IBD-Associated Arthritis	Reactive Arthritis
Musculoskeletal				
Axial involvement	Axial involvement predominates; initially symmetrically involves the SI joints and lower spine, progressing cranially; does not skip regions	May occur at any level; may start in the cervical spine; may skip regions; may be asymmetric	May be asymptomatic but can follow a course similar to ankylosing spondylitis; SI involvement often asymmetric; arthritis does not parallel IBD activity	Less common than in other forms of spondyloarthritis
Peripheral involvement	Enthesitis (e.g., Achilles tendinitis) with or without asymmetric large-joint oligoarthritis; hip involvement can cause significant functional limitation; shoulders can be involved	Various patterns, most commonly polyarticular; DIP involvement is associated with nail involvement; dactylitis; enthesitis; tenosynovitis; arthritis mutilans	Two patterns: mono/oligoarticular large joint lower extremity (parallels IBD activity), and polyarticular small joint upper extremity (does not parallel IBD activity); dactylitis and enthesitis may occur	Enthesitis and asymmetric large-joint oligoarthritis; usually self-limited; nonerosive; some patients experience recurrent or persistent arthritis; may develop features of other forms of spondyloarthritis
Dermatologic	Psoriasis may coexist	Psoriasis typically precedes joint involvement; nail pitting; onycholysis	Pyoderma gangrenosum; erythema nodosum	Keratoderma blennorrhagicum; circinate balanitis
Ophthalmologic	Uveitis (typically anterior, unilateral, recurrent)	Conjunctivitis more common than uveitis (anterior; can be bilateral, insidious, or chronic)	Uveitis (anterior; can be bilateral, insidious, or chronic); conjunctivitis, keratitis, and episcleritis are rare	Conjunctivitis is more common than uveitis
Gastrointestinal	Asymptomatic intestinal ulcerations	—	Crohn disease; ulcerative colitis	Prior GI infection in some patients
Genitourinary	Urethritis (rare)	—	Nephrolithiasis	Prior GU infection in some patients; sterile urethritis; prostatitis; cervicitis; salpingitis
Cardiovascular	Aortic valve disease; aortitis; conduction abnormalities; CAD	Association with traditional CAD risk factors	Thromboembolism	—
Pulmonary	Restrictive lung disease from costovertebral rigidity; apical fibrosis (rare)	—	—	—
Bone quality	Falsely elevated bone mineral density from syndesmophytes; increased risk of spine fracture	Increased risk of fracture; multifactorial	High risk for vitamin D deficiency, low bone density, and fracture	Localized osteopenia

CAD = coronary artery disease; DIP = distal interphalangeal; GI = gastrointestinal; GU = genitourinary; IBD = inflammatory bowel disease; SI = sacroiliac.

Inflammatory low back pain of insidious onset is the hallmark of ankylosing spondylitis, manifesting as pain and stiffness that are worse after immobility and are better with use. Symptoms are prominent in the morning (>1 hour); night pain is characteristic and may awaken the patient. Buttock pain is common and bilateral, and it correlates with sacroiliitis. Early in its course, ankylosing spondylitis almost always affects the lumbar spine; longer and more severe disease may involve the thoracic and cervical regions as well. *Ankylosis* refers to the bony bridging of the vertebrae resulting from chronic inflammation; the calcified ligaments and disk capsules in such cases are read on radiographs as *syndesmophytes*. Fusion of the spine may occur over time, leading to rigidity and kyphosis.

Risk factors for poor prognosis include male gender, early age of onset, tobacco use, and the presence of hip or peripheral arthritis, psoriasis, IBD, iritis, or elevated erythrocyte sedimentation rate (ESR). Mortality is increased, primarily relating to increased rates of cardiovascular disease (coronary artery disease, aortic valve regurgitation, aortic aneurysm, conduction disturbance), cancer, and infection.

Psoriatic Arthritis

Psoriatic arthritis is an inflammatory arthritis that is associated with psoriasis (see Table 15). Peak age of onset is between 40 and 60 years; men and women are equally affected. Prevalence of psoriatic arthritis is approximately 1% in the general population. Although estimates of the prevalence of psoriatic arthritis in patients with psoriasis vary, more recent studies using standardized diagnostic criteria indicate that psoriatic arthritis is present in approximately 15% to 20% of those with psoriasis. Psoriasis most commonly precedes the onset of arthritis but may occur with or after arthritis onset.

The most common patterns of joint involvement are an asymmetric lower extremity oligoarthritis (resembling reactive arthritis) or a symmetric polyarthritis involving the distal interphalangeal (DIP), proximal interphalangeal (PIP), and/or metacarpophalangeal (MCP) and metatarsophalangeal (MTP) joints (distribution similar to rheumatoid arthritis but includes the DIPs). Less common presentations include DIP involvement only as well as a chronic resorptive arthritis (arthritis mutilans) causing digital shortening and a "telescoping" appearance. Spondylitis (spine or sacroiliac arthritis) may occur; in contrast to ankylosing spondylitis, it is usually asymmetric and may skip regions.

Dactylitis (diffuse swelling of joints, tendons, and/or ligaments of a digit, creating a sausage-like appearance) occurs in approximately 50% of patients with psoriatic arthritis (**Figure 11**). Nail involvement such as pitting or onycholysis (**Figure 12**) is commonly observed concurrent with DIP joint involvement.

The recently developed Classification Criteria for Psoriatic Arthritis (CASPAR) convey a sensitivity and specificity of more than 90% (**Table 16**). Patients with a characteristic pattern of

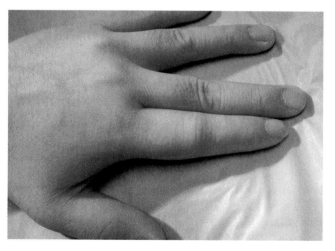

FIGURE 11. Dactylitis ("sausage digit") associated with psoriatic arthritis. Dactylitis manifests as swelling of the entire digit and arises from inflammation of the flexor tendon and adjacent soft tissue.

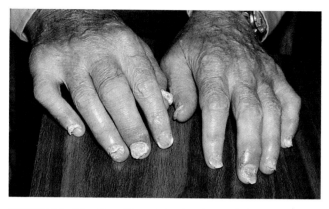

FIGURE 12. This patient with psoriatic arthritis has onycholysis and onychodystrophy (malformation of a fingernail or toenail).

TABLE 16. Classification Criteria for Psoriatic Arthritis (CASPAR)
Inflammatory articular disease (joint, spine, entheseal)
Plus three or more of the following:
Psoriasis (current, personal history of, family history of)
Psoriatic nail dystrophy
Negative rheumatoid factor[a]
Dactylitis/swelling of entire digit (current, personal history of)
Radiologic evidence of juxta-articular new bone formation (joint of hand or foot)
[a]Five to ten percent of patients may have a positive rheumatoid factor or anti–cyclic citrullinated peptide antibodies; this would not exclude the diagnosis as long as the patient meets sufficient other criteria.

psoriatic joint involvement (especially DIP arthritis and/or dactylitis), but without apparent psoriasis, should undergo a thorough examination for occult psoriatic skin or nail changes. Although patients with psoriatic arthritis are characteristically seronegative, 5% to 10% may demonstrate rheumatoid factor or anti–cyclic citrullinated peptide (CCP) antibodies, possibly owing to overlapping genetic proclivities. Typical radiographic changes of psoriatic arthritis include a combination of marginal joint erosions and new bone formation; classic findings include pencil-in-cup changes (**Figure 13**).

Prognosis of psoriatic arthritis is variable, with studies suggesting a relationship between disease severity and mortality. Severity of skin disease neither predicts nor correlates with severity of arthritis. Elevated ESR and the presence of radiologic joint damage at presentation predict both arthritis progression and mortality; the presence of nail lesions may be protective. Cardiovascular disease is the most common cause of mortality.

Inflammatory Bowel Disease-Associated Arthritis

Inflammatory arthritis is present in 20% to 30% of patients with ulcerative colitis or Crohn disease. IBD-associated arthritis may be axial or peripheral. Peripheral joint involvement

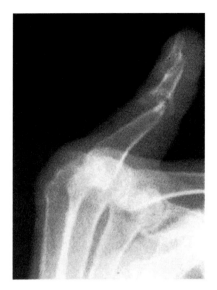

FIGURE 13. Pencil-in-cup deformity in psoriatic arthritis. Note the erosion and remodeling of the index proximal interphalangeal joint with a cup-like appearance of the distal bone on the ulnar aspect of the joint; the bone proximal to the joint becomes so eroded as to look like a pencil point within the cup.

may be oligoarticular (type 1) or polyarticular (type 2). Only the oligoarticular peripheral arthritis parallels IBD activity. See Table 15 for more information.

Reactive Arthritis

Reactive arthritis is a noninfectious inflammatory arthritis that can occur after specific gastrointestinal or genitourinary infections. Asymmetric monoarthritis or oligoarthritis in the lower extremities is the most common presentation, but up to 20% of patients have polyarthritis. Enthesopathy (including at the Achilles tendon insertion to the calcaneus), dactylitis, and sacroiliitis may occur. Erosive disease is uncommon. See Table 15 for clinical features.

Despite the preceding infection, reactive arthritis is an autoimmune, rather than infectious, arthritis. It is hypothesized that exposure of a susceptible patient to a defined infectious antigen may induce a cross-reaction to a similarly structured, previously tolerated self-antigen (molecular mimicry), resulting in autoimmunity and self-perpetuating inflammation. Therefore, use of antibiotics specifically to treat reactive arthritis has failed to demonstrate benefit.

Gastrointestinal pathogens associated with reactive arthritis include *Yersinia*, *Salmonella*, *Shigella*, *Campylobacter*, and, rarely, *Escherichia coli* and *Clostridium difficile*. The most common genitourinary pathogen is *Chlamydia trachomatis*; cases due to *Ureaplasma urealyticum* have been reported.

Reactive arthritis typically occurs approximately 3 to 6 weeks after the infectious trigger, with a latency range of 2 weeks to 6 months. In a significant minority of cases, the triggering infection may go unrecognized. The presence of HLA-B27

and severity of initial infection may increase the risk of developing reactive arthritis.

Up to 50% of reactive arthritis cases resolve by 6 months, but 20% of patients progress to chronic disease. Recurrent infectious episodes may convey an increased risk of recurrent reactive arthritis.

KEY POINTS

- Inflammatory low back pain of insidious onset is the hallmark of ankylosing spondylitis, manifesting as pain and stiffness that are worse after immobility and are better with use.
- Psoriatic arthritis typically presents as an asymmetric lower extremity oligoarthritis or a symmetric polyarthritis involving the distal interphalangeal, proximal interphalangeal, and/or metacarpophalangeal and metatarsophalangeal joints, often with dactylitis.
- Arthritis of varying patterns may occur in patients with inflammatory bowel disease (IBD); however, only oligoarticular peripheral arthritis parallels IBD activity.
- Reactive arthritis is a noninfectious, autoimmune inflammatory arthritis that can occur after specific gastrointestinal or genitourinary infections and typically presents as asymmetric monoarthritis or oligoarthritis in the lower extremities; enthesopathy, dactylitis, and sacroiliitis may also occur.

Diagnosis

Diagnosis of a specific spondyloarthritis disorder is based on the characteristic history and physical examination, as well as radiographic findings such as sacroiliitis and enthesitis (**Table 17**). The clinical setting may provide a clue to diagnosis. For example, ankylosing spondylitis should be considered in patients with chronic inflammatory back pain who are younger than 45 years old. Peripheral arthritis or tendinitis is less likely to occur in ankylosing spondylitis and should raise suspicion for a different form of spondyloarthritis. Psoriatic arthritis should be considered if there is a prior or current diagnosis of psoriasis, especially along with the characteristic arthritis patterns previously described. IBD-associated arthritis should be considered if there is a prior diagnosis of IBD or current symptoms and signs of possible IBD. Reactive arthritis should be considered if there is a history of preceding infection, especially gastrointestinal or genitourinary infection. Considerable overlap exists between these diseases; for example, a patient with ankylosing spondylitis may also have psoriasis and/or IBD.

Diagnosis may be supported by the presence of HLA-B27 and/or elevated inflammatory markers. Patients lacking laboratory and radiographic evidence of disease may nonetheless have sufficient historical and physical manifestations (characteristic inflammatory arthritis, along with dactylitis, enthesitis, inflammatory eye disease, or psoriasis) to support a

TABLE 17. Evaluation of Patients with Suspected Spondyloarthritis

History
Inflammatory back and/or joint pain[a]
Family history of SpA or psoriasis
Positive response to NSAIDs
Symptoms consistent with, or existing diagnosis of, psoriasis, IBD, and/or ocular inflammation (iritis, uveitis, conjunctivitis)
Preceding infection
Urethritis symptoms in the absence of ongoing infection

Physical Examination Findings
Spine/SI joint tenderness; limited ROM of spine[b]; tenderness and/or swelling of joints, tendons (dactylitis), and/or tendon insertions to bone (enthesitis, especially Achilles tendon insertion)
Rash and/or nail changes indicative of psoriasis
Ocular inflammation (iritis, uveitis, conjunctivitis)

Laboratory Studies
Positive HLA-B27
Elevated C-reactive protein and/or erythrocyte sedimentation rate

Radiography
Plain radiography of SI joints and/or symptomatic area of spine (lumbar, thoracic, cervical) showing characteristic changes; if plain radiograph is negative, consider MRI of SI joints +/− spine
Plain radiograph of symptomatic peripheral joints to look for erosions and new bone formation suggestive of inflammatory arthritis/enthesitis

IBD = inflammatory bowel disease; ROM = range of motion; SI = sacroiliac; SpA = spondyloarthritis.

[a]Inflammatory joint pain is worse overnight, in the morning, and after immobility; improves with joint use; and is associated with morning stiffness lasting longer than 1 hour.

[b]Schober test, chest expansion, and occiput-wall distance measurements can be useful.

diagnosis. Classification criteria for psoriatic arthritis (CASPAR) and for peripheral and axial spondyloarthritis (Assessment of SpondyloArthritis international Society) have been developed; although these are primarily intended for research purposes, they provide informative paradigms for clinicians diagnosing these disorders.

See **Figure 14** and **Figure 15** for more information on diagnosing spondyloarthritis.

Laboratory Studies

No specific serologic tests are available to diagnose spondyloarthritis. Rheumatoid factor, anti-CCP antibodies, and antinuclear antibodies are usually negative, although low-titer positivity may occasionally be present. Elevated inflammatory markers such as ESR, C-reactive protein, and serum amyloid A protein often correlate with disease activity but may also be normal, especially in patients with ankylosing spondylitis. HLA-B27 testing can define a probability for spondyloarthritis but cannot independently confirm or exclude any specific diagnosis. Although infection has usually resolved by the time of arthritis onset in patients with reactive arthritis, DNA amplification urine testing for *Chlamydia trachomatis* should be performed because some individuals may have asymptomatic persistent infection or carriage of this organism.

Imaging Studies

Conventional radiography of the spine and sacroiliac joints is inexpensive and generally adequate to demonstrate synovitis, axial erosion, or new bone formation in patients with spondyloarthritis, although results may be normal in early disease. With peripheral spondyloarthritis, conventional radiography may detect erosive changes with bony proliferation at the entheses.

Sacroiliitis is usually bilateral and symmetric in ankylosing spondylitis but may be unilateral or absent in other forms of spondyloarthritis. On plain radiographic imaging, sacroiliac erosion initially appears as irregular widening of the joint space, accompanied by sclerotic changes. Later, the joint space narrows, and eventually the sacroiliac joint may fuse. Vertebral plain radiographic findings in ankylosing spondylitis include sclerosis at the attachment of annulus fibrosis to the anterior corner of the vertebral endplate ("shiny corner"), and erosion at the point of contact between the disk and the vertebra. In later disease, vertebrae may lose their normal anterior concavity due to periosteal bone proliferation, resulting in squaring of the vertebral bodies. Calcification of the anterior longitudinal ligament and bridging syndesmophyte formation are late features, leading to ankylosis and a "bamboo" spine appearance (**Figure 16**, on page 41). This may be difficult to differentiate

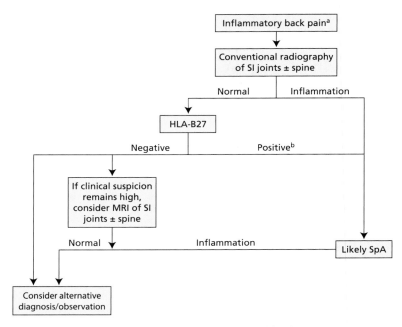

FIGURE 14. Diagnostic evaluation for suspected axial spondyloarthritis. SI = sacroiliac; SpA = spondyloarthritis.

[a]Characterized by pain and stiffness in the spine that is worse after immobility and better with use; prominent morning pain lasting >1 hour; buttock pain is common and typically bilateral.

[b]Particularly if at least one other feature typical of SpA is present: uveitis, enthesitis, dactylitis, psoriasis, inflammatory bowel disease, positive family history of SpA, or elevated inflammatory markers.

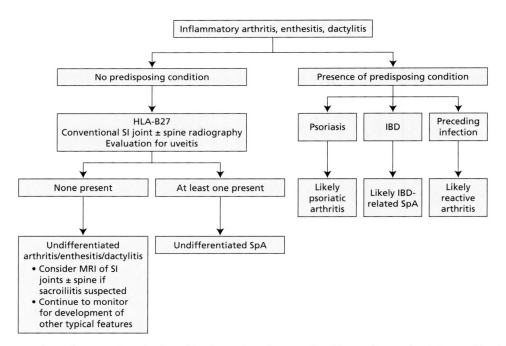

FIGURE 15. Diagnostic evaluation for suspected peripheral spondyloarthritis. IBD = inflammatory bowel disease; SI = sacroiliac; SpA = spondyloarthritis.

from diffuse idiopathic skeletal hyperostosis (DISH); however, the changes in ankylosing spondylitis are usually on both sides of the spine, whereas in DISH they are characteristically right sided. Furthermore, DISH is most commonly thoracic, whereas ankylosing spondylitis starts with sacroiliitis and lumbar arthritis and usually does not skip regions as it ascends.

CT is more sensitive than conventional radiography for detecting bony erosions and may be helpful when disease is suspected but plain radiographs are negative. CT is also useful for detecting subtle vertebral body fractures in patients with ankylosing spondylitis who are at increased risk of spine fractures. However, CT is expensive and conveys increased levels of

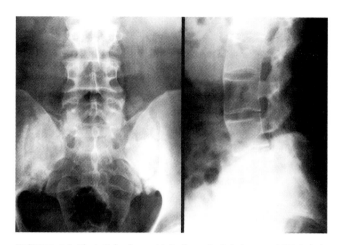

FIGURE 16. The initial radiographic findings of ankylosing spondylitis include irregularities along the margins of the sacroiliac joints leading to eventual ankylosis and fusion. Inflammation of the ligamentous attachments erodes the corners of the vertebral bodies, which produces a squared-off appearance. Over time, ossification of these ligaments leads to the development of a rigid "bamboo spine," named because the shape of the vertebrae resemble bamboo on radiograph.

ionizing radiation exposure. Accordingly, CT is not routinely used to monitor spondyloarthritis disease progression.

MRI can detect early inflammation in the spine and sacroiliac joints, even before bony changes are detected on radiograph or CT. MRI of the sacroiliac joints and/or spine should be obtained if there is high suspicion for spondyloarthritis and conventional radiographs are negative. However, MRI is more expensive and less generally available.

Musculoskeletal ultrasonography can detect peripheral enthesitis and arthritis but has no current role in detecting sacroiliitis or axial involvement.

KEY POINTS

- In patients with spondyloarthritis, rheumatoid factor, anti–cyclic citrullinated peptide antibodies, and antinuclear antibodies are usually negative.
- HLA-B27 testing can support, but cannot independently confirm or exclude, a diagnosis of spondyloarthritis.
- **HVC** Conventional radiography of the spine and sacroiliac joints is generally adequate to demonstrate synovitis, axial erosion, or new bone formation in patients with spondyloarthritis; CT should be reserved for identifying occult spine fractures and bony erosions in patients at high risk due to expense and higher level of radiation exposure.
- **HVC** In patients with strongly suspected spondyloarthritis, MRI of the sacroiliac joints and/or spine should only be considered if conventional radiographs are negative.

Management

General Considerations

Management of spondyloarthritis should include exercise to preserve spine and peripheral joint strength and range of motion. Glucocorticoid injections may be helpful in providing symptomatic relief, particularly if there are one or two active isolated joints in which a local injection may reduce the need for systemic medication. Pharmacologic therapy is needed for control of symptoms in most forms of spondyloarthritis, although the most effective medication regimen may vary by type of spondyloarthritis present.

A mainstay of pharmacologic therapy is NSAIDs. The various NSAIDs studied are equally effective, but differences exist in individual response to, and tolerance of, a given NSAID; thus, it can be helpful to try a second NSAID if the first has produced an inadequate response. Maximal daily NSAID dosing is generally required to produce a positive response in spondyloarthritis, but the dose may subsequently be reduced depending on patient response and tolerance.

For patients with more serious disease not adequately controlled with NSAIDs or who cannot tolerate NSAIDs, nonbiologic and biologic disease-modifying antirheumatic drugs (DMARDs) can be helpful. However, these agents may increase the risk of infection, and certain drugs are extremely expensive or may require parenteral administration.

Patients with severe end-stage joint or soft-tissue damage may need surgery such as tendon repair or joint replacement. Surgery to correct severe spine flexion deformities in ankylosing spondylitis may be considered but can be challenging and risky due to difficulties with intubation for anesthesia, spine fragility, and stabilization.

Ankylosing Spondylitis

Exercise is a particularly important component of ankylosing spondylitis therapy and can help preserve mobility and prevent kyphosis. A physical therapist can assist patients in developing a home exercise routine that can be maintained over time. Glucocorticoid injections to the sacroiliac joints can relieve symptoms and facilitate exercise.

NSAIDs are considered first-line therapy for ankylosing spondylitis. Studies of full-dose NSAIDs demonstrate symptomatic relief as well as reduced sacroiliac and spine inflammation as seen on MRI in some patients. In contrast to their limited effects in modifying the course of almost all other rheumatologic diseases, some studies suggest that daily NSAID use may reduce progression of spine damage caused by ankylosing spondylitis.

Tumor necrosis factor (TNF)-α inhibitors are indicated for patients who have had inadequate responses to NSAIDs. If the first TNF-α inhibitor produces an inadequate response, a different TNF-α inhibitor may be more successful. TNF-α inhibitors demonstrably improve pain and mobility as well as reduce inflammation in axial joints. Although recent reports suggest that they may help slow radiographic disease progression, more studies are needed for confirmation.

Nonbiologic DMARDs such as methotrexate and sulfasalazine are not helpful in treating axial disease but may be helpful in treating accompanying peripheral arthritis.

Monitoring of patients with ankylosing spondylitis for response to therapy or progression of disease can include patient history, physical examination, and laboratory testing (such as erythrocyte sedimentation rate and C-reactive protein). Serial imaging can also be used to help monitor patients with ankylosing spondylitis, but the 2010 Assessment of SpondyloArthritis international Society/European League Against Rheumatism (ASAS/EULAR) guidelines recommend against repeating spinal radiography more frequently than every 2 years unless absolutely necessary in specific cases.

Psoriatic Arthritis

NSAIDs can improve symptoms of inflammation and are therefore commonly used for pain control but have not been shown to prevent progression of erosions in psoriatic arthritis. Glucocorticoids (systemically or by intra-articular injection) can provide short-term relief, although flare-ups of psoriasis may occur after discontinuation of systemic glucocorticoids.

Nonbiologic DMARDs can treat peripheral arthritis and enthesitis but are unlikely to improve axial disease. Methotrexate has demonstrated efficacy in psoriatic arthritis and also helps psoriasis. Sulfasalazine and hydroxychloroquine can be useful for the arthritis, although there are reports of hydroxychloroquine-induced exacerbation of psoriasis in some patients.

Several biologic agents are highly efficacious in psoriatic arthritis and should be considered for more severe disease, when nonbiologic DMARDs have provided inadequate benefit, and/or in the presence of radiographic evidence of bony damage. TNF-α inhibitors can prevent progression of joint damage and are also effective for treating the accompanying psoriasis. Combination therapy with methotrexate and a TNF-α inhibitor may be more helpful than monotherapy for some patients. Paradoxical worsening of psoriasis has been reported in some patients receiving TNF-α inhibitors. Ustekinumab, a biologic agent that targets interleukin (IL)-12 and IL-23, is FDA approved for use in both severe psoriasis and psoriatic arthritis. Ustekinumab can slow progression of radiographic disease and can be used in combination with methotrexate.

Inflammatory Bowel Disease-Associated Arthritis

NSAIDs may be contraindicated in patients with IBD due to risk of bowel flare-up, limiting their usefulness in IBD-associated arthritis. Glucocorticoids, systemically or by local injection, may provide short-term relief.

Methotrexate may ameliorate IBD-associated arthritis and can also treat the underlying bowel disease, especially Crohn disease. Similarly, sulfasalazine may also be effective for both IBD and IBD-related arthritis.

With the exception of etanercept (a receptor-based rather than antibody-based biologic agent), TNF-α inhibitors are effective treatments for IBD-associated arthritis that can be used when nonbiologic agents fail. However, paradoxical worsening of IBD has been reported in some patients receiving these agents.

Reactive Arthritis

Reactive arthritis is usually self-limited, with symptoms resolving within 6 months; in most cases, symptom-based treatment is sufficient. NSAIDs provide symptomatic relief, and intra-articular glucocorticoid injections may provide local benefit. In patients who progress to severe and/or chronic disease, DMARDs such as sulfasalazine, methotrexate, or leflunomide should be tried, although data for this indication are limited. A few case reports of benefit from TNF-α inhibitors have been published, but more studies are needed.

Antibiotic therapy has not been shown to be effective in reactive arthritis except in rare cases of demonstrated persistent infection.

KEY POINTS

- Management of spondyloarthritis generally includes exercise to preserve strength and range of motion, glucocorticoid injections for symptomatic relief, and pharmacologic therapy.

- NSAIDs are first-line therapy for ankylosing spondylitis; tumor necrosis factor α inhibitors are used when patients have had inadequate response to NSAIDs.

- In patients with psoriatic arthritis, NSAIDs are typically used to control inflammatory symptoms; nonbiologic disease-modifying antirheumatic drugs can treat peripheral arthritis and enthesitis, and biologic agents should be considered for more severe disease.

- Methotrexate or sulfasalazine can be used to treat both the arthritis and bowel disease associated with inflammatory bowel disease–associated arthritis; tumor necrosis factor α inhibitors other than etanercept can be tried when nonbiologic agents fail.

- Antibiotic therapy has not been shown to be effective in reactive arthritis except in rare cases of demonstrated persistent infection.

Systemic Lupus Erythematosus

Introduction

Systemic lupus erythematosus (SLE) is characterized by multiorgan involvement and the presence of autoantibodies, including antibodies directed at intranuclear antigens.

Pathophysiology

SLE demonstrates a polygenic inheritance pattern. Clinical disease results from the interaction of genes, environment, and random effects, resulting in loss of tolerance to self-antigens and active autoimmunity.

Patients with SLE have abnormalities in how dying cells are handled by the immune system. The nuclear material of dying cells may be inadequately cleared, engendering an immune response, and promoting up-regulation of autoreactive T and B cells and autoantibodies directed against nuclear and other antigens. Recent studies suggest a role for type 1 interferons in SLE induction. Single gene mutations causing deficiencies of the complement components C1q, C2, or C4 can promote SLE, possibly by impairing clearance of immune complexes and/or apoptotic cell debris.

Epidemiology

Approximately 90% of patients with SLE are women, with disease risk dramatically increasing with the appearance of female sex hormones; the female-to-male ratio is 1:1 in childhood versus 9:1 in adulthood. The disease is more common, and often more severe, among women of African American, Chinese, and Hispanic backgrounds.

KEY POINTS

- Systemic lupus erythematosus is characterized by multiorgan involvement and the presence of autoantibodies, many directed at intranuclear antigens.

- Approximately 90% of patients with systemic lupus erythematosus are women, with disease risk dramatically increasing with the appearance of female sex hormones.

Clinical Manifestations

Mucocutaneous Involvement

Skin and/or mucous membranes are affected in 80% to 90% of patients with SLE; skin manifestations are classified as acute, subacute, or chronic.

The characteristic SLE skin manifestation is acute cutaneous lupus erythematosus (ACLE), also known as malar or butterfly rash, which affects 40% to 50% of patients (**Figure 17**). ACLE consists of erythema and edema over the cheeks and

bridge of the nose and potentially the forehead and chin; it characteristically spares the nasolabial folds. A more generalized form of ACLE can also involve the dorsum of the arms and hands, including the areas between the fingers but sparing the knuckle pads. Skin sequelae such as atrophy are not seen.

Subacute cutaneous lupus erythematosus (SCLE) is a photosensitive rash that occurs over the arms, neck, and face (**Figure 18**). It consists of erythematous, annular, or polycyclic lesions, often with a fine scale. SCLE may leave postinflammatory changes (hypo- or hyperpigmentation) but does not cause atrophy. Anti-Ro/SSA autoantibodies are present in 70% of patients with SCLE.

The most common chronic cutaneous manifestation is discoid lupus erythematosus (DLE) (**Figure 19**). DLE occurs in

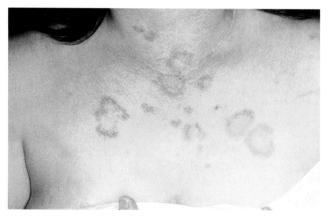

FIGURE 18. Rash in subacute cutaneous lupus erythematosus. This patient has an annular polycyclic rash characterized by scaly erythematous circular plaques with central hypopigmentation.

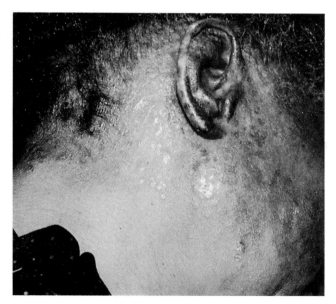

FIGURE 19. Chronic cutaneous lupus erythematosus consists of chronic, slowly progressive, scaly, infiltrative papules and plaques or atrophic red plaques on sun-exposed skin surfaces, most commonly the face, neck, and scalp. Healed lesions result in depressed scars, atrophy, telangiectasias, and hyperpigmentation or hypopigmentation.

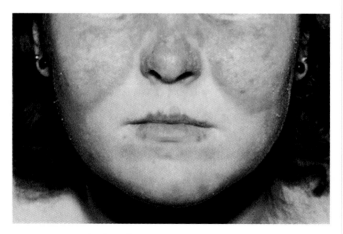

FIGURE 17. Malar (butterfly) rash. This patient has a classic acute cutaneous lupus erythematosus rash in a butterfly distribution that spares the nasolabial folds. It is erythematous and raised, with a very slight scale. This rash will resolve completely with treatment without leaving any skin atrophy.

20% of patients with SLE but more commonly occurs as an isolated, nonsystemic finding; patients with isolated DLE usually do not go on to develop SLE. DLE usually affects the scalp and face and presents as hypo- or hyperpigmented, possibly erythematous, patches or thin plaques that may be variably atrophic or hyperkeratotic. In contrast to ACLE and SCLE, DLE can cause scarring, atrophy, and permanent alopecia.

Painless oral or nasopharyngeal ulceration occurs in 5% of patients with SLE. Nonscarring alopecia is a common feature of active SLE, with hair regrowth a sign of disease control. Raynaud phenomenon occurs in 60%, reflecting arterial vasospasm of the digits.

Musculoskeletal Involvement

Joint involvement occurs in 90% of patients with SLE, with inflammatory polyarthralgia the most common presentation. Frank arthritis occurs in 40% of patients with SLE. Both small and large peripheral joints can be affected; the synovial fluid is only mildly inflammatory. SLE arthritis is nonerosive. However, persistent periarticular inflammation can damage joints supporting soft-tissue structures, resulting in reducible subluxation of the digits, swan neck deformities, and ulnar deviation (Jaccoud arthropathy).

Pain or limitation of motion of the large joints, especially the hips, should raise concern for possible osteonecrosis. Up to 37% of patients with SLE develop osteonecrosis by serial MRI scan of the hips, but less than 10% become symptomatic. Large necrotic areas (for example, >20% of the femoral head) may progress to bony collapse, whereas smaller lesions often resolve without structural perturbation. The occurrence of osteonecrosis is attributable to glucocorticoid use and other factors, including Raynaud phenomenon and lupus vasculitis, which may disrupt the blood supply to vulnerable bone volumes. Prednisone doses greater than 20 mg/d and cushingoid facial features are markers of risk. Patients with osteonecrosis have night pain and use pain. Early diagnosis is by MRI, with more advanced disease visible on radiograph.

Myalgia is reported by up to 85% of patients with SLE, but frank myositis occurs in only about 10%. Histologically and clinically, SLE myositis resembles polymyositis. Medications such as antimalarials and glucocorticoids can cause drug myopathies that must be ruled out in SLE patients with weakness. Fibromyalgia co-occurs in 30% of patients with SLE and is important to diagnose to avoid unnecessary use of immunosuppressive medications.

Kidney Involvement

Lupus nephritis occurs in up to 70% of patients with SLE; the presence of anti–double-stranded DNA antibodies is a marker for risk. All patients with SLE should be evaluated for possible nephritis with baseline serum creatinine, urine protein-creatinine ratio for proteinuria, and urinalysis with microscopic evaluation. Minor abnormalities (proteinuria <500 mg/24 h, minimal hematuria, no casts) should be monitored regularly (3-month intervals), whereas significant initial abnormalities (especially cellular casts) require immediate further evaluation. Patients with inadequately treated lupus nephritis may progress

to need dialysis or transplant. Signs and symptoms defining more severe lupus nephritis include hypertension, lower extremity edema, active urine sediment (proteinuria, hematuria, cellular casts), and elevated serum creatinine. Kidney biopsy is frequently warranted to define the histological subtype and the degree of disease activity and chronicity essential for planning appropriate therapy. Indications for kidney biopsy are as follows: increasing serum creatinine without explanation, proteinuria >1000 mg/24 h, proteinuria >500 mg/24 h with hematuria, and proteinuria >500 mg/24 h with cellular casts.

SLE patients with hypercoagulable states (for example, the antiphospholipid antibody syndrome, the nephrotic syndrome) may be at risk for renal artery or vein thrombosis.

See Glomerular Diseases in MKSAP 17 Nephrology for more information on the six classes and treatment of lupus nephritis. **H**

Neuropsychiatric Involvement

The American College of Rheumatology 1999 SLE classification criteria recognize 19 possible manifestations attributable to neuropsychiatric systemic lupus erythematosus (NPSLE) (**Table 18**). The most common manifestations are headache,

TABLE 18. Neuropsychiatric Manifestations of Systemic Lupus Erythematosus

Central Nervous System
Aseptic meningitis
Cerebrovascular disease
Demyelinating syndrome
Headache
Movement disorder (such as chorea)
Seizure disorder
Myelopathy
Acute confusional state
Anxiety disorder
Cognitive dysfunction
Mood disorder
Psychosis
Peripheral Nervous System
Acute inflammatory demyelinating polyradiculoneuropathy (such as Guillain-Barré syndrome)
Autonomic neuropathy
Mononeuropathy (single or multiplex)
Myasthenia gravis
Cranial neuropathy
Plexopathy
Polyneuropathy

Adapted with permission from John Wiley & Sons, from American College of Rheumatology nomenclature and case definitions for neuropsychiatric lupus syndromes. Arthritis Rheum. 1999;42(4):599-608. [PMID: 10211873] Copyright 1999 American College of Rheumatology.

cognitive dysfunction, and mood disorder. NPSLE prevalence is as high as 75%; prevalence of more acute presentations (for example, seizures and psychosis) is significantly lower. In addition to central manifestations, peripheral neuropathy occurs in up to 14% of SLE patients, with the majority due to the disease itself and the remainder due to non-SLE causes (medications, other diseases such as diabetes mellitus, spinal radiculopathies).

NPSLE pathophysiology may include vascular inflammation and/or occlusion, the effects of cytokines on neuronal function, or antibodies directed against various neuronal or glial components. The blood-brain barrier generally prevents passage of antibodies into the central nervous system (CNS) but with inflammation becomes permeable. Some of the antibodies/cytokines in NPSLE may also be produced within the CNS itself.

The general approach to suspected NPSLE is to first exclude an infection or medication effect. Evaluation of more severe manifestations such as seizures or meningitis requires CNS imaging, cerebrospinal fluid (CSF) analysis, and measurement of NPSLE-associated autoantibodies. Autoantibodies that may be found in the serum and/or CSF in patients with NPSLE include antineuronal, anti-NMDA receptor, antiribosomal P, and antiphospholipid antibodies/lupus anticoagulant (APLA/LAC). For patients with suspected peripheral neuropathies, electromyography (EMG) and nerve conduction studies (NCS) are useful in the diagnosis and potential cause of the neuropathy. EMG/NCS should be able to distinguish a spinal radiculopathy (non-SLE cause) from a mononeuritis (likely associated with SLE), for example.

Imaging of the patient with NPSLE should be influenced by the clinical manifestations and is often done to rule out other possibilities. Imaging may include CT to rule out CNS bleeding or stroke; MRI to identify infection, white matter lesions, or myelopathy in a patient with suspected transverse myelitis; and PET to evaluate functional abnormalities in patients with cognitive impairment. Neuropsychologic testing may help identify organic versus functional cognitive changes.

Cardiovascular Involvement

Up to 40% of patients with SLE experience pericarditis, which is often asymptomatic. Pericarditis may be associated with a neutrophilic pericardial effusion that can rarely lead to tamponade. Antinuclear antibodies (ANA), anti–double-stranded DNA antibodies, and so-called lupus erythematosus cells (neutrophils engulfing extruded cell nuclei) can be detected in the fluid but rarely alter diagnosis or management. Constrictive pericarditis may also occur. Pericardial disease can be demonstrated by CT or MRI.

Myocarditis occurs in 5% to 10% of patients with SLE, more commonly among black patients. Presentations can be dramatic, with acute onset of heart failure. Echocardiogram-measured ejection fractions of less than 20% are not uncommon. Rapid response to high-dose glucocorticoids supports a pathogenic role for SLE inflammation/autoimmunity. Cardiac MRI is increasingly used to detect myocardial inflammation.

Cardiac valves are abnormal on transesophageal echocardiogram in many patients with SLE, most characteristically those with APLA/LAC. Thickening of the mitral and aortic valve leaflets are the most common abnormalities, but vegetations, regurgitation, and stenosis also occur. Libman-Sacks endocarditis, the classic designation for noninfectious verrucous vegetations, favors the mitral valve. These verrucous masses can embolize, leading to downstream occlusion.

Patients with SLE have a 2- to 10-fold increased prevalence of ischemic heart disease, the most common cause of death among older patients with SLE. Severe SLE disease activity and prednisone doses of more than 20 mg/d are independent risk factors for early myocardial infarction. Traditional risk factors such as hypertension and total cholesterol levels also play a role and require clinical management.

Pulmonary Involvement

Pleuritis occurs in 45% to 60% of patients who have SLE, with or without pleural effusion. When present, effusions are exudative, and lupus erythematosus cells and ANA may be present.

Parenchymal lung involvement is relatively uncommon in SLE; lung infiltrates are more likely to be infectious than directly associated with SLE. Nonetheless, interstitial lung disease occurs in 3% to 8% of patients with SLE. Acute lupus pneumonitis is a potentially serious inflammatory airway disease characterized by fever, cough, shortness of breath, hypoxemia, and pleuritic chest pain. Chest radiograph may show unilateral or bilateral infiltrates. Mortality rates approach 50%, and aggressive respiratory support combined with immunosuppression is required. An even rarer manifestation is diffuse alveolar hemorrhage, which typically presents with shortness of breath, hypoxemia, diffuse alveolar infiltrates on chest radiograph, a dropping hematocrit, and a high DLCO on pulmonary function tests, all in the setting of active SLE. Bronchoscopy with bronchoalveolar lavage and biopsy is used to demonstrate hemorrhage and rule out infection. Chest MRI may detect blood as changes on T2-weighted images. Aggressive immunosuppressive therapy and respiratory support are required, but mortality rates are as high as 50% to 90%.

When evaluating a patient with SLE who has pulmonary infiltrates, it is usually prudent to treat empirically for a possible infectious cause. Antibiotics and immunosuppressive therapy are generally started simultaneously and modified in response to additional diagnostic data. Opportunistic infections should be considered in a patient who is immunosuppressed and/or not responding appropriately to therapy.

Shrinking lung syndrome is characterized by pleuritic chest pain and shortness of breath, with progressive decrease in lung volumes on chest radiograph and pulmonary function tests. Aggressive immunosuppression may reverse the process. The cause is uncertain, but pleuropulmonary disease or diaphragmatic dysfunction is believed to contribute.

Hematologic Involvement

All three bone marrow cell lines can be affected in SLE. Leukopenia occurs in 50% of patients, with lymphopenia predominating. Whereas hemolytic anemia with direct antiglobulin (Coombs) test positivity is seen in only 10%, up to 80% of patients with SLE have normocytic, normochromic anemia of chronic disease. Thrombocytopenia occurs in 30% to 50% and is generally mild. Severe thrombocytopenia (<50,000/μL [50 × 10^9/L]) occurs in 10% of SLE patients in isolation or in conjunction with hemolytic anemia (Evans syndrome); isolated idiopathic thrombocytopenic purpura may be a clue to underlying SLE. APLA/LAC is also associated with thrombocytopenia. In patients with quiescent SLE, mild cytopenias do not require intervention.

SLE cytopenias are driven by both immune and nonimmune mechanisms. Immune-mediated hematologic conditions seen in SLE include autoimmune hemolytic anemia, Evans syndrome, aplastic anemia, and pure red cell aplasia. Nonimmune causes include chronic SLE inflammation, infections, medications, myelodysplasia, and myelofibrosis. It may be difficult to distinguish disease activity from drug effect, and empiric withdrawal of a drug may be required. Indications for bone marrow biopsy include the following: no obvious explanation for cytopenia, elevated serum iron, elevated mean corpuscular volume unexplained by medication effect, serum monoclonal spike, and the antiphospholipid antibody syndrome.

APLA/LAC antibodies are detected in 40% of patients with SLE, but fewer than 40% of these patients are clinically affected. The APLA/LACs are autoantibodies that interact with endothelial cells, monocytes, platelets, and complement to cause a prothrombotic state. The common clinical manifestations include venous and arterial thrombosis, miscarriage (especially second trimester), livedo reticularis, cytopenias, and cardiac valve thickening/vegetations. LAC carries a higher risk of thrombosis than other APLAs; however, the highest risk is in patients who are triple positive for LAC, anti-β_2-glycoprotein I, and anticardiolipin antibodies, who have a 30% rate of thrombosis. Patients with SLE are at increased risk for thrombosis even in the absence of detectable APLA/LAC.

See Thrombotic Disorders in MKSAP 17 Hematology and Oncology for a discussion on the antiphospholipid antibody syndrome.

Gastrointestinal Involvement

Gastrointestinal disease occurs in 25% to 40% of patients with SLE and may be underrecognized. Esophageal dysmotility and/or reflux occurs in 5% of patients, especially those with Raynaud phenomenon and anti-U1-ribonucleoprotein antibodies. Sterile peritonitis is a potential cause of abdominal pain. Mesenteric vasculitis can occur, often accompanied by cutaneous vasculitis. Mesenteric thrombosis can occur in patients with the antiphospholipid antibody syndrome. Hepatic involvement occurs in 10% and is distinguished from primary autoimmune hepatitis by lower aminotransferase levels, lack of autoimmune hepatitis-associated autoantibodies (anti–smooth muscle, anti-liver/kidney microsomal), different histology on biopsy, and the presence of antiribosomal

P antibodies in SLE hepatitis. Very rarely, pancreatitis associated with SLE has been reported due to thrombosis, vasculitis, or medication complications.

Malignancy

In patients with SLE, there is a sevenfold increased risk of non-Hodgkin lymphoma, especially diffuse large B-cell lymphoma, compared with the general population. This increased risk may relate to chronic B-cell activation and/or use of medications (for example, azathioprine or cyclophosphamide) that promote hematologic malignancies. Hodgkin lymphomas and leukemias are also more common in SLE, presumably for similar reasons. Lung cancer rates are increased by 1.4 times the general population risk, and patients with SLE who develop lung cancer are invariably smokers.

Cervical cancer risk is increased and associated with both immunosuppressive (cyclophosphamide) use and increased prevalence of human papillomavirus in women with SLE. Women with SLE are less likely to undergo cervical screening than women in the general population, possibly related to care by specialists who are less likely to provide such screening. Certain solid organ tumors, notably breast, endometrial, prostate, and ovarian, may be less common in patients with SLE.

KEY POINTS

- The characteristic skin manifestation of systemic lupus erythematosus is acute cutaneous lupus erythematosus (also known as malar or butterfly rash), which is characterized by erythema and edema over the cheeks and bridge of the nose.

- Musculoskeletal involvement, including joint manifestations (most commonly inflammatory polyarthralgia) and myalgia, is common in patients with systemic lupus erythematosus.

- All patients with systemic lupus erythematosus should be evaluated for nephritis with baseline serum creatinine, urine protein-creatinine ratio, and urinalysis with microscopic evaluation.

- The most common neuropsychiatric manifestations of systemic lupus erythematosus are headache, cognitive dysfunction, and mood disorder.

- Pericarditis is the most common acute cardiac manifestation of systemic lupus erythematosus (SLE); ischemic heart disease is the most common cause of death for older patients with SLE.

Diagnosis

SLE should be considered in any patient who presents with unexplained multisystem disease. The most common early SLE manifestations include constitutional symptoms (fever, weight loss, or severe fatigue), arthralgia/arthritis, and skin disease. SLE should be included in the differential of a patient (especially a young woman) with any of the following manifestations: persistent rash, particularly if it is photosensitive; polyarticular arthritis; pleuritis; pericarditis; unexplained cytopenias, especially lymphopenia; a nephritic urine sediment; or thromboembolic disease. The American College of Rheumatology has defined 11 criteria, with the presence of any 4 serially or simultaneously sufficient to support the diagnosis of SLE, typically including a positive ANA (**Table 19**). Myalgia, arthralgia, and fatigue are insufficient reasons to test for ANA unless accompanied by objective SLE findings. Patients with these nonspecific symptoms should first be evaluated for more common conditions such as anemia, thyroid disease, and fibromyalgia. If unexplained findings such as cytopenias or organ involvement are found, SLE should then be added to the differential diagnosis.

Laboratory Studies

Initial laboratory studies for SLE include an ANA test to screen for nuclear-directed autoantibodies. The traditional indirect

immunofluorescence ANA is highly sensitive (95%) for SLE and may convey additional information based on the immunofluorescence pattern observed, but its specificity is limited because it can be positive in patients with other autoimmune diseases or in those without clinical autoimmune disease (usually at low titer). Therefore, ANA should always be interpreted in the context of pretest probability.

If ANA is positive, SLE-specific autoantibodies (anti–double-stranded DNA, anti-Smith, anti-U1-ribonucleoprotein, and anti-La/SSB), as well as tests for other autoimmune diseases under consideration, should be obtained to further characterize the disease (**Table 20**). Anti-Ro/SSA antibody testing may simultaneously occur because a small percentage of patients with SLE are negative for ANA but positive for anti-Ro/SSA antibodies. Conversely, a negative ANA plus a negative anti-Ro/SSA essentially rules out SLE. In many commercial

TABLE 19. American College of Rheumatology Criteria for the Diagnosis of Systemic Lupus Erythematosus

Criteria[a]	Definition
Malar rash	Fixed erythema, flat or raised, over the malar eminences
Discoid rash	Erythematous, circular, raised patches with keratotic scaling and follicular plugging; atrophic scarring may occur
Photosensitivity	Rash after exposure to ultraviolet light
Oral ulcers	Oral and nasopharyngeal ulcers (observed by physician)
Arthritis	Nonerosive arthritis of ≥2 peripheral joints, with tenderness, swelling, or effusion
Serositis	Pleuritis or pericarditis (documented by electrocardiogram, rub, or evidence of effusion)
Kidney disorder	Urinalysis: 3+ protein or urine protein >500 mg/24 h; cellular casts
Neurologic disorder	Seizures or psychosis (without other cause)
Hematologic disorder	Hemolytic anemia or leukopenia (<4000/μL [4.0×10^9/L]) or lymphopenia (<1500/μL [1.5×10^9/L]) or thrombocytopenia (<100,000/μL [100×10^9/L]) in the absence of offending drugs
Immunologic disorder	Anti–double-stranded DNA, anti-Smith, and/or antiphospholipid antibodies
ANA	An abnormal titer of ANA by immunofluorescence or an equivalent assay at any point in the absence of drugs known to induce ANA

ANA = antinuclear antibodies.

[a]Any combination of 4 or more of the 11 criteria, well documented at any time during a patient's history, makes it likely that the patient has systemic lupus erythematosus (specificity and sensitivity are 95% and 75%, respectively).

Adapted with permission from John Wiley & Sons, from Hochberg MC. Updating the American College of Rheumatology revised criteria for the classification of systemic lupus erythematosus. Arthritis Rheum. 1997;40(9):1725. [PMID: 9324032] Copyright 1997 American College of Rheumatology.

TABLE 20. Common Autoantibodies in Systemic Lupus Erythematosus

Autoantibody	Frequency in SLE	Comments
Antinuclear	95%	Useful as an initial screening test
Anti–double-stranded DNA	50%	Found in more severe disease, especially kidney disease; antibody levels commonly follow disease activity and are useful to monitor
Anti-Ro/SSA	40%	Associated with photosensitive rashes, discoid lupus, and neonatal SLE, including congenital heart block; also common in Sjögren syndrome
Anti-U1-ribonucleoprotein	35%	Associated with Raynaud phenomenon and esophageal dysmotility; also seen in MCTD
Anti-Smith	25%	Specific for SLE; often associated with more severe disease
Anti-La/SSB	15%	Common in Sjögren syndrome; less common in SLE and neonatal SLE
Antiribosomal P	15%	Associated with CNS lupus and lupus hepatitis

CNS = central nervous system; MCTD = mixed connective tissue disease; SLE = systemic lupus erythematosus.

laboratories, the sequential testing of autoantibodies has recently been automated. Although these new test sequences may simplify physician assessment, they often use a different method for assessing the initial ANA (ELISA rather than indirect immunofluorescence) that may have reduced sensitivity and specificity.

A complete blood count, chemistry panel, and urinalysis (including microscopy) should be ordered, along with an erythrocyte sedimentation rate (ESR) and potentially a C-reactive protein level (CRP). ESR is preferred over CRP initially because some patients with SLE do not generate CRP during SLE flares. However, monitoring CRP in patients with SLE and defining those who do or do not generate CRP during flares may be helpful in distinguishing flares from infection. Complements should also be assessed (most commonly, C3 and C4) because these levels are reduced during SLE activity, reflecting immune complex formation that provokes complement activation. These studies may help define the presence of organ involvement and the level of inflammation as well as provide a baseline for following disease activity.

Differential Diagnosis

The differential diagnosis of SLE includes other autoimmune multisystem diseases, many of which are similarly more common in women: ANCA-associated vasculitis, rheumatoid arthritis, adult-onset Still disease, dermatomyositis, Sjögren syndrome, and mixed connective tissue disease. Severe viral infection can also mimic SLE (fever, myalgia, rash, cytopenias).

Drug-Induced Lupus Erythematosus

Drug-induced lupus erythematosus (DILE) occurs when a medication triggers immune-mediated disease with manifestations mimicking SLE. Common symptoms include malaise, fever, arthritis, and rash; kidney and CNS disease are uncommon. ANA is often transiently positive, along with antihistone antibodies. Diagnosis is confirmed when symptoms resolve after discontinuing the offending agent. Patients with SLE are at no more risk of DILE than the general population.

High-risk medications for DILE include procainamide, methyldopa, quinidine, and hydralazine; all but hydralazine are now rarely used in current practice. Some drugs are lower risk (for example, minocycline), but because of frequent use, more cases develop. **Table 21** lists medications associated with DILE, the autoantibodies detected, and clinical manifestations. 🄷

Undifferentiated Connective Tissue Disease

Undifferentiated connective tissue disease (UCTD) refers to syndromes with objective abnormalities that do not meet sufficient criteria to be categorized as SLE or another specific connective tissue disease. Patients who have two or three criteria for SLE can be diagnosed as having UCTD or alternatively may be designated as having incomplete SLE.

KEY POINTS

- The most common early manifestations of systemic lupus erythematosus include constitutional symptoms, arthralgia/arthritis, and skin disease.

- Initial testing for systemic lupus erythematous (SLE) begins with antinuclear antibodies; if positive, SLE-specific autoantibodies (anti–double-stranded DNA, anti-Smith, anti-U1-ribonucleoprotein, and anti-La/SSB) should be obtained to further characterize the disease.

- In addition to antinuclear antibody and other autoantibody testing, laboratory studies for evaluating systemic lupus erythematosus include a complete blood count, chemistry panel, complement levels, erythrocyte sedimentation rate, and urinalysis.

(Continued)

TABLE 21.	Medications Commonly Associated with Drug-Induced Lupus Erythematosus	
Medication	**Antibodies Detected**	**Comments**
Procainamide	ANA; antihistone	75% ANA positive; 20% develop DILE; fever; arthritis; serositis
Hydralazine	ANA; antihistone	20% ANA positive; 5%-8% develop DILE; fever; arthritis; rare vasculitis and kidney disease
Minocycline	ANA; ANCA; anti-dsDNA rare	Arthritis; vasculitis; autoimmune hepatitis
Antithyroid drugs	ANA; ANCA; antihistone	Vasculitic rash; rare pulmonary and kidney disease
Statins	ANA; antihistone; anti-dsDNA	SLE, SCLE, dermatomyositis, and polymyositis all reported
Calcium channel blockers	ANA; anti-Ro/SSA; antihistone rare	SCLE
Thiazide diuretics	ANA; anti-Ro/SSA; antihistone rare	SCLE
ACE inhibitors	ANA; anti-Ro/SSA; antihistone rare	SCLE
TNF-α inhibitors	ANA in 23%-57%; chromatin and anti-dsDNA common; antihistone rare	DILE most common with infliximab, uncommon for etanercept; SLE, SCLE, DLE all reported

ANA = antinuclear antibodies; DILE = drug-induced lupus erythematosus; DLE = discoid lupus erythematosus; dsDNA = double-stranded DNA; SCLE = subacute cutaneous lupus erythematosus; SLE = systemic lupus erythematosus; TNF = tumor necrosis factor.

KEY POINTS *(continued)*

- Drug-induced lupus erythematosus occurs when a medication triggers immune-mediated disease with manifestations mimicking systemic lupus erythematosus; treatment includes discontinuing the offending agent.

- Undifferentiated connective tissue disease refers to syndromes with objective abnormalities that do not meet sufficient criteria to be categorized as systemic lupus erythematosus or another specific connective tissue disease.

Management

In virtually all cases, SLE management requires pharmacologic therapy (**Table 22**). Serial monitoring of disease-responsive laboratory studies (complete blood count, ESR, anti–double-stranded DNA antibodies, complements [C3 and C4], urinalysis, and urine protein-creatinine ratio) is mandatory to track disease activity, identify warning signs of disease flare, and monitor response to therapy. Frequency of monitoring depends upon current level of disease activity. Modification of therapy should generally be done with input from the patient's rheumatologist and/or nephrologist.

Hydroxychloroquine is an anchor drug for SLE and should be initiated in every patient with SLE who can tolerate the medication. This agent can prevent SLE flares, improve outcomes in high-risk pregnancies, reduce the risk of thrombosis and myocardial infarction, reduce disease-associated damage in general, and improve survival. It is particularly useful for arthritis and the skin manifestations. Hydroxychloroquine may be the only medication needed for mild disease.

For many acute manifestations of SLE, glucocorticoids are the initial treatment based on their efficacy and rapid onset of action. Glucocorticoid dose should be appropriate to the disease severity and the organs involved. For SLE-related arthritis, rash, pleuritis, pericarditis, or mild cytopenias, a dose of 20 to 40 mg/d of prednisone may be appropriate. Patients with more severe disease (for example, class II-IV nephritis, more severe cytopenias, or severe pleural or pericardial disease) may require high-dose glucocorticoids (40 to 60 mg/d of prednisone). The most severe manifestations (for example, rapidly progressive class III-IV nephritis, psychosis, seizures, diffuse alveolar hemorrhage, or myocarditis) should generally be treated in the hospital with high-dose intravenous glucocorticoids (1000 mg/d for 3 days) followed by 40 to 60 mg/d of oral prednisone. Given the many adverse effects associated with glucocorticoid use, glucocorticoids alone are generally not used for chronic therapy, and additional therapy is quickly added for disease control and glucocorticoid sparing. Prednisone is generally tapered as tolerated after the first month of therapy with the goal of reducing the dose to less than 10 mg/d by 3 months.

For severe SLE, the goal is to control autoimmunity and inflammation and induce disease remission with potent medications, then substitute with less potent and less toxic therapy to maintain the remission. For active lupus nephritis, mycophenolate mofetil is currently the preferred oral agent; dosage is 2000 to 3000 mg/d and may take 4 to 6 weeks to reach full efficacy. For the most severe disease (severe active nephritis, acute CNS lupus, pulmonary hemorrhage, myocarditis), intravenous cyclophosphamide in a dosage of 500 mg every 2 weeks for 6 doses or 750 mg/m² every month for 6 months is usually used to induce remission, followed by mycophenolate mofetil or possibly azathioprine as maintenance therapy. The biologic agent belimumab is approved for

TABLE 22. Medications Commonly Used to Treat Systemic Lupus Erythematosus

Medication	Common Uses in SLE	Important Side Effects
NSAIDs	Painful, non-organ-threatening manifestations such as arthritis	Hypertension; GI bleeding; AKI
Prednisone	Used for all manifestations in varying doses	Hypertension; glucose intolerance; weight gain; infection; osteonecrosis
Hydroxychloroquine	Used for mild to moderate disease; especially useful for skin involvement and to prevent disease flares	Rash; retinopathy; vacuolar myopathy
Mycophenolate mofetil	Moderate to severe disease; as effective as cyclophosphamide for remission induction for nephritis	Bone marrow suppression; elevation of liver enzymes; infection
Azathioprine	Moderate to severe disease	Bone marrow suppression; elevation of liver enzymes; hematologic malignancy
Cyclophosphamide	Severe organ or life-threatening disease	Bone marrow suppression; hemorrhagic cystitis; infection; malignancy
Belimumab	Add-on therapy for moderate to severe disease	Infusion reactions; infections

AKI = acute kidney injury; GI = gastrointestinal; SLE = systemic lupus erythematosus.

CONT.

patients with incomplete responses to conventional treatments. See Glomerular Diseases in MKSAP 17 Nephrology for details on the treatment of lupus nephritis.

NSAIDs can be useful for management of patients with arthritis, pleuritis, or pericarditis. These agents should be avoided in patients with kidney disease and/or uncontrolled hypertension. H

See Principles of Therapeutics for additional information on SLE medication toxicities, monitoring parameters, and more.

KEY POINTS

- Serial monitoring of disease-responsive laboratory studies (complete blood count, erythrocyte sedimentation rate, anti–double-stranded DNA antibodies, complements, urinalysis, and urine protein-creatinine ratio) is mandatory to track disease activity, identify warning signs of disease flare, and monitor response to therapy.

- Hydroxychloroquine should be initiated in every patient with systemic lupus erythematosus who can tolerate the medication.

- Glucocorticoids are usually the initial therapy for acute manifestations of systemic lupus erythematosus, with dosing based on disease severity.

- For severe systemic lupus erythematosus, the goal is to control autoimmunity and inflammation and induce disease remission with potent medications, then substitute with less potent and less toxic therapy to maintain the remission.

Pregnancy and Childbirth Issues

Women with SLE experience miscarriage, stillbirth, and premature delivery two to five times more often than women without the disease. SLE pregnancies are at an eightfold risk for intrauterine growth retardation. Active disease, especially nephritis, and the presence of anti-Ro/SSA and/or APL antibodies are risk factors for fetal morbidity and mortality. Conception should ideally be deferred until SLE disease is quiescent.

Proteinuria may increase during pregnancy in patients with SLE, rendering differentiation from preeclampsia/eclampsia a challenge. Increases in anti–double-stranded DNA antibody levels or the acute development of an active urine sediment implicates SLE as the cause. In contrast, serum urate rises in preeclampsia but not during lupus flares.

Fetuses of mothers who are positive for anti-Ro/SSA or anti-La/SSB antibodies are at risk for developing neonatal lupus erythematosus. Arthritis and rash are common manifestations; in 2% of these pregnancies, congenital heart block may occur and cause mortality or require permanent pacing. Risk of neonatal lupus erythematosus rises to 12% after a first child born with the condition. Recent studies suggest that maternal hydroxychloroquine use may reduce the risk of neonatal lupus erythematosus.

Medications that are safe for use during SLE pregnancies include hydroxychloroquine, prednisone, and azathioprine (if an immunosuppressive agent is absolutely needed). Cyclophosphamide-induced infertility is age- and dose-dependent and should be discussed with female patients of reproductive age before administering this medication. See Principles of Therapeutics for more information on medications and pregnancy.

KEY POINTS

- Women with systemic lupus erythematosus (SLE) experience miscarriage, stillbirth, and premature delivery two to five times more often than women without the disease; furthermore, SLE pregnancies are at an eightfold risk for intrauterine growth retardation.

- Fetuses of mothers who are positive for anti-Ro/SSA or anti-La/SSB antibodies are at risk for developing neonatal lupus erythematosus.

Prognosis

SLE prognosis has improved significantly from the 1960s (50% 5-year survival rate) to the present (>90% 5-year survival rate). Nonetheless, there continues to be a bimodal mortality for SLE, with early deaths related to SLE and infections and late mortality associated with cardiovascular disease. Factors adversely affecting survival include myocarditis, nephritis, low socioeconomic status, male gender, and age over 50 years at diagnosis.

A complete 5-year remission in SLE is uncommon, occurring in only 2% of patients. Current data suggest 20% to 40% of patients have an incomplete response to available therapies, indicating the need for better therapeutic approaches.

KEY POINT

- Factors adversely affecting survival of patients with systemic lupus erythematosus include myocarditis, nephritis, low socioeconomic status, male gender, and age over 50 years at diagnosis.

Sjögren Syndrome
Introduction

Sjögren syndrome is an immune-mediated disease of unknown cause manifesting as infiltrative inflammation that damages exocrine glands, including the major and minor salivary glands, lacrimal glands, and, less commonly, other exocrine glands such as the pancreas.

Pathophysiology

Biopsied glandular tissue from patients with Sjögren syndrome reveals inflammatory infiltrates composed of

CD4-positive T lymphocytes, accompanied by lesser populations of B and plasma cells. Immune system dysregulation, including B-cell hyperactivity and hypergammaglobulinemia, is commonly reported.

Epidemiology

The prevalence of Sjögren syndrome ranges from 0.19% to 1.39%, depending upon the classification criteria used. However, Sjögren syndrome may be underdiagnosed, such that its prevalence may be higher than reported. Incidence peaks around the fifth decade, and there is a female predominance (9:1 ratio).

Clinical Manifestations

The prominent clinical feature of Sjögren syndrome is sicca, or dryness, particularly of the eyes (keratoconjunctivitis sicca) and mouth (xerostomia). Keratoconjunctivitis sicca can result in corneal damage and visual impairment. Xerostomia can result in dental caries due to loss of antibacterial features of saliva. Dryness of mucosal surfaces (such as the vagina, skin, or bronchi) and exocrine gland hypertrophy are common findings. Sjögren syndrome can also cause extraglandular manifestations as a result of autoimmune/inflammatory mechanisms (**Table 23**).

Presumably because of preexisting lymphocyte activation, patients with Sjögren syndrome have an increased risk of lymphoma, with diffuse large B-cell and mucosa-associated lymphoid tissue (MALT) lymphomas being the most common

(See MKSAP 17 Hematology and Oncology). Sjögren syndrome lymphoma risk is 16- to 44-fold that of the general population. Hypocomplementemia and lymphopenia at the time of Sjögren diagnosis may predict lymphoma development. New and persistent adenopathy or other symptoms suggestive of lymphoma should prompt further evaluation with lymph node biopsy.

Diagnosis

Diagnosis of Sjögren syndrome is based primarily on typical sicca symptoms as well as glandular (enlarged lacrimal and/or parotid glands) and extraglandular manifestations. It is helpful to confirm eye and mouth dryness in an objective manner, for example, by documenting reduced tear production utilizing the Schirmer test (decreased wetting of tear test strips) or with special stains and slit-lamp examination. Rarely, gallium scanning or sialography may be warranted to characterize the exocrine gland involvement.

Laboratory findings include positive autoimmune serologies (rheumatoid factor, antinuclear, anti-Ro/SSA, and anti-La/SSB antibodies) and hypergammaglobulinemia. Anti-Ro/SSA and anti-La/SSB antibodies are characteristic for Sjögren syndrome but are also common in patients with systemic lupus erythematosus, mothers of infants with neonatal lupus, and, occasionally, healthy persons. Rheumatoid factor levels are typically higher than those seen in rheumatoid arthritis. In the presence of classic historical and physical findings, the presence of anti-Ro/SSA and anti-La/SSB antibodies may be sufficient to diagnose Sjögren syndrome. In unclear cases, a lip biopsy demonstrating minor salivary gland inflammation is considered the gold standard for diagnosis.

Other autoimmune diseases, including rheumatoid arthritis, systemic lupus erythematosus, and autoimmune thyroiditis, are commonly associated with Sjögren syndrome. This has traditionally been called secondary Sjögren syndrome, although recent classification criteria do not make this distinction. Conditions that mimic Sjögren syndrome include IgG4-related disease, graft versus host disease, amyloidosis, sarcoidosis, AIDS (diffuse infiltrative lymphocytosis syndrome), hepatitis C virus infection, and history of head and neck irradiation. Many of these conditions share with Sjögren syndrome a predilection for infiltration of exocrine glands, sicca symptoms, and/or positive antinuclear antibodies or rheumatoid factor, rendering diagnosis difficult.

Management

Management of Sjögren syndrome consists of symptomatic, local, and systemic approaches (**Table 24**). Sicca symptoms are treated with hydration and lubrication, although other local measures and medications may be helpful. Avoidance of medications that worsen sicca (for example, anticholinergic agents) is recommended. Immunosuppressive therapy does not alleviate sicca symptoms but may suppress extraglandular

TABLE 23. Extraglandular Clinical Manifestations of Sjögren Syndrome	
Site/Organ	**Manifestation/Frequency**
General	Fatigue (70%), fever (6%)
Skin	Rash, cutaneous vasculitis: 10%-16%
Joint	Arthralgia/arthritis: 36%
Lung	Interstitial pneumonitis: 5%-9%
Kidney	Interstitial nephritis, distal (type 1) renal tubular acidosis, glomerulonephritis: 5%-6%
Neurologic	Central nervous system (CNS): demyelinating disease, myelopathy, cranial nerve neuropathy
	Peripheral nervous system: small-fiber neuropathy, mononeuritis multiplex, peripheral neuropathy: 8%-27% (for CNS and peripheral)
Gastrointestinal	Autoimmune hepatitis, primary biliary cirrhosis: 3%-20%
Hematologic	Lymphoma, cytopenia: 2%
Other	Systemic vasculitis (7%), cryoglobulinemia (4%-12%), Raynaud phenomenon (16%), thyroid disease (10%-15%)

TABLE 24.	Management of Sjögren Syndrome
Symptom	**Therapy**
Ocular sicca	Artificial tears; glasses with side panels to reduce exposure; punctal plugs/occlusion; topical cyclosporine
Oral sicca	Artificial saliva; sugar-free lozenges to promote salivation; good dental hygiene; muscarinic cholinergic receptor stimulators (e.g., pilocarpine, cevimeline)
Vaginal/Skin sicca	Topical lubrication
Extraglandular	Mild symptoms (e.g., arthralgia or rash): NSAIDs; hydroxychloroquine; topical or low-dose glucocorticoids
	Moderate to severe symptoms (e.g., lung, kidney, or nervous system involvement; vasculitis): high-dose glucocorticoids; immunosuppressive therapy such as methotrexate, azathioprine, mycophenolate mofetil, cyclophosphamide, or rituximab

manifestations. Biologic agents have not been proven to treat Sjögren syndrome, although some reports suggest responsiveness to the anti–B-cell antibody rituximab.

Prognosis

Most patients with Sjögren syndrome do not progressively worsen over time, and their mortality rate is similar to the general population. Increased mortality is associated with lymphoproliferative malignancy and/or other associated autoimmune disease. Low complement levels, lymphocytopenia, and cryoglobulinemia at diagnosis are predictive of unfavorable outcome due to lymphoma, severe disease manifestations (such as vasculitis), and premature death.

KEY POINTS

- Sjögren syndrome manifests as infiltrative inflammation of exocrine glands, characterized by dry eyes and dry mouth.

- Patients with Sjögren syndrome have a 16- to 44-fold increased risk of lymphoma, most commonly from diffuse large B-cell and mucosa-associated lymphoid tissue lymphomas.

- In patients with classic historical and physical findings, the presence of anti-Ro/SSA and anti-La/SSB antibodies may be sufficient to diagnose Sjögren syndrome; in unclear cases, a lip biopsy demonstrating minor salivary gland inflammation is considered the gold standard for diagnosis.

- Autoimmune diseases, including rheumatoid arthritis, systemic lupus erythematosus, and autoimmune thyroiditis, are commonly associated with Sjögren syndrome.

Mixed Connective Tissue Disease

Introduction

Mixed connective tissue disease (MCTD) is an overlap syndrome that includes features of systemic lupus erythematosus (SLE), systemic sclerosis, and/or polymyositis in the presence of anti-U1-ribonucleoprotein (RNP) antibodies.

Epidemiology

MCTD is rare (1:1,000,000). Age at onset is between 30 and 50 years, with a 9:1 female predominance. Most patients have no known risk factors.

Clinical Manifestations and Diagnosis

More than 50% of patients with MCTD have hand edema and synovitis at disease onset. About one third develop myositis, and nearly half develop decreased esophageal motility and fibrosing alveolitis. Pulmonary arterial hypertension occurs in 20%, with fatigue often the initial symptom. Patients suspected of having MCTD should undergo high-resolution CT of the chest, echocardiography, and pulmonary function testing. Clinical findings may evolve, such that a patient who initially appears to have a single disease (for example, SLE) may accrue features to support an MCTD diagnosis.

Skin manifestations include sclerodactyly, scleroderma, calcinosis, telangiectasias, photosensitivity, malar rash, and Gottron rash. Pleuropericarditis occurs in up to 60% of patients, and sicca symptoms in up to 50%. Trigeminal neuralgia occurs in up to 25% of patients. Kidney involvement occurs in 25% of patients, typically as membranous nephropathy.

In addition to overlapping features of SLE, systemic sclerosis, and/or polymyositis, MCTD diagnosis requires the presence of anti-U1-RNP antibodies. Laboratory studies may additionally show leukopenia, thrombocytopenia, and an elevated erythrocyte sedimentation rate. Antinuclear antibodies may be present, with a very high titer (≥1:1200) in a speckled pattern. The presence of anti-Smith or anti–double-stranded DNA antibodies should suggest SLE rather than MCTD.

Management

MCTD management is determined by the manifestations of the individual patient. Glucocorticoids, azathioprine, and methotrexate can be used for arthritis and myositis. Symptoms associated with Raynaud phenomenon may benefit from calcium channel blockers; patients with esophageal dysmotility should receive proton pump inhibitors. Cyclophosphamide may be tried for interstitial lung disease and phosphodiesterase inhibitors and/or anti-endothelin therapies for pulmonary arterial hypertension.

Prognosis

The course of MCTD is variable; the likelihood of developing interstitial lung disease, pulmonary arterial hypertension, and/or cardiovascular disease increases with disease duration. MCTD mortality is increased compared with SLE, mainly as a consequence of pulmonary arterial hypertension. Renovascular disease as seen in systemic sclerosis may uncommonly contribute to morbidity and mortality.

KEY POINTS

- Mixed connective tissue disease is an overlap syndrome that includes features of systemic lupus erythematosus, systemic sclerosis, and/or polymyositis in the presence of anti-U1-ribonucleoprotein antibodies.
- Typical findings of mixed connective tissue disease include hand edema, synovitis, myositis, decreased esophageal motility, and fatigue.
- Treatment for mixed connective tissue disease is determined by the manifestations of the individual patient.

Crystal Arthropathies

Introduction

In crystal arthropathies, metabolic abnormalities promote the formation and deposition of crystals that stimulate inflammation. This chapter discusses gout, calcium pyrophosphate deposition, and basic calcium phosphate deposition.

Gout

Gout is characterized by intermittent painful inflammatory joint attacks, resulting from crystallization of excessive levels of uric acid (hyperuricemia).

Epidemiology

Gout is the most common inflammatory arthritis in the United States (prevalence, 4%). Serum urate levels rise after puberty in men and after menopause in women; premenopausal women are therefore protected from gout except in cases of underlying disease or strong genetic factors. Gout becomes increasingly common among older individuals owing to accumulation of additional hyperuricemia risk factors (for example, chronic kidney disease). Approximately 13% of patients over the age of 80 years are affected.

Gout is typically associated with multiple comorbidities (hypertension, obesity, diabetes mellitus, chronic kidney disease, vascular disease, dyslipidemia, and nephrolithiasis) that may complicate treatment, either by posing contraindications to specific therapies or because treating some comorbid conditions can worsen hyperuricemia (for example, using diuretics to treat hypertension).

Despite important advances in understanding and treating gout, it remains a disease that is often suboptimally managed.

Pathophysiology

Uric acid is the end product of purine metabolism in humans. Free purines arise from nucleic acid breakdown during cell turnover, from adenosine triphosphate metabolism, and through dietary intake. Xanthine oxidase is the terminal enzyme in human uric acid synthesis. In contrast to most mammals, humans lack the enzyme uricase, which processes urate to the more soluble allantoin (**Figure 20**).

At physiologic conditions (pH, 7.4), uric acid exists primarily as its ionized form, urate; therefore, hyperuricemia technically refers to elevated serum urate. The saturation concentration of urate is 6.8 mg/dL (0.40 mmol/L), with monosodium urate crystals unlikely to form at concentrations below this level; hyperuricemia is therefore defined based on this physiologic parameter. Urate is cleared by the kidneys via both glomerular filtration and active urate secretion in the proximal tubule; resorption by other proximal tubule transporters occurs concurrently.

The most common risk factor for hyperuricemia is underexcretion of urate by the kidneys due to impaired glomerular filtration and/or defects of urate handling in the renal proximal tubule (**Table 25**). Alternatively, about 10% of patients with gout have genetic aberrancies causing excessive uric acid production. Hyperuricemia in the adult population is common (up to 20%) but usually asymptomatic; measurement of serum urate is therefore not a useful screening tool for gout in the absence of appropriate clinical signs and symptoms.

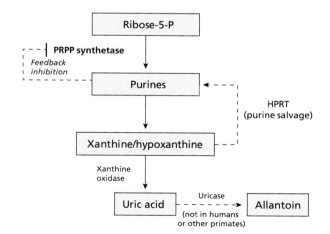

FIGURE 20. Purine biosynthesis and metabolism to uric acid. De novo purine synthesis can occur in human cells. Rarely, hereditary overactivity of phosphoribosylpyrophosphate (PRPP) synthetase results in excessive purine production. Purine salvage (to recover purines from the breakdown of nucleic acids for reuse) occurs through hypoxanthine-guanine phosphoribosyltransferase (HPRT); HPRT deficiency results in purine depletion and thus increased uric acid synthesis due to lack of negative feedback (as in Lesch-Nyhan syndrome). Humans lack the gene for uricase; in most other mammals, this enzyme converts uric acid to the more soluble allantoin and results in much lower urate levels.

TABLE 25.	Causes of Hyperuricemia
Primary renal uric acid underexcretion (hereditary, renal tubular basis)	
Chronic kidney disease of any cause (secondary uric acid underexcretion)	
Uric acid overproduction due to primary defect in purine metabolism: PRPP synthetase overactivity; HPRT deficiency	
Conditions of cell turnover leading to purine/urate generation: leukemia/lymphoma; psoriasis; hemolytic anemia; polycythemia vera	
Drug-induced hyperuricemia (agents reducing renal glomerular filtration and/or tubular urate excretion): thiazide and loop diuretics; cyclosporine; low-dose salicylates; ethambutol; pyrazinamide; lead ingestion/toxicity	
Diet-induced hyperuricemia (agents high in purines or inducing purine/urate biosynthesis): alcohol; shellfish; red meat; high-fructose corn syrup-sweetened beverages and foods	

HPRT = hypoxanthine-guanine phosphoribosyltransferase; PRPP = phosphoribosylpyrophosphate.

Nonetheless, hyperuricemia is the primary risk factor for gout, with increasing incidence of gout in patients with higher serum urate levels. The mechanisms leading to urate crystallization are incompletely elucidated but depend on temperature, pH, and other physicochemical factors.

Once crystals form, resident tissue macrophages phagocytose them to initiate an inflammatory cascade. Interleukin (IL)-1β production fuels the process and promotes synthesis of additional cytokines (for example, tumor necrosis factor α, IL-6). Additionally, complement activation on the crystal surface generates split products that stimulate and attract neutrophils. Collectively, these signals promote neutrophil infiltration, the hallmark of an established gout attack.

Clinical Manifestations

Gout can be considered as having three phases: acute gouty arthritis, intercritical gout, and chronic recurrent or tophaceous gout (also known as chronic tophaceous gouty arthropathy).

Acute Gouty Arthritis

The classic gout presentation is podagra, in which the metatarsophalangeal joint of the great toe becomes painful, red, and swollen over 12 to 24 hours. First gout attacks typically are monoarticular and begin at night. Approximately 90% of first attacks present in this manner. First attacks in women are less likely to fit this classic picture.

Recurrent attacks can occur in nearly any joint, with either monoarticular or polyarticular presentation. Attacks in bursae also occur. In poorly controlled disease, flares become more frequent and involve an increasing number of joints. Systemic inflammation is common, including fever (typically <38.9 °C [102.0 °F]), peripheral leukocytosis (up to 13,000/µL [13 × 10⁹/L]), and elevated inflammatory markers (C-reactive protein and erythrocyte sedimentation rate). Systemic

findings tend to correlate with the severity of the attack and normalize rapidly with treatment.

Soft tissues adjacent to the joints can be affected during acute flares, becoming red, painful, and edematous. Soft-tissue inflammation can mimic cellulitis, tenosynovitis, or dactylitis, rendering the diagnosis of gout challenging.

Although a chronically elevated serum urate level is a hallmark of gout, serum urate levels can occasionally be low during acute attacks, possibly because cytokines promote renal urate excretion. Thus, when there is reasonable clinical suspicion for gout, treatment is indicated even with a normal serum urate level. The serum urate level should be reassessed after the flare has resolved for a more accurate characterization.

Intercritical Gout

The period between gout attacks is referred to as the intercritical phase, during which the patient is typically asymptomatic. Early in the course of disease, attacks tend to be infrequent, but most patients experience a recurrent attack within 2 years of their first attack. In long-standing or poorly controlled gout, the time between attacks tends to diminish.

Chronic Recurrent and Tophaceous Gout

Chronic recurrent gout refers to a disease state in which poorly controlled gout results in frequent flares and/or chronic gouty arthropathy, in which synovitis persists between acute attacks. Chronic recurrent gout is usually the consequence of ineffective therapy, medication noncompliance, or undertreatment. Chronic recurrent gout poses a significant economic burden in terms of health care costs and lost time from work. Patients with this degree of gout severity should be referred to a rheumatologist for management.

Tophi (stone-like deposits of monosodium urate surrounded by a fibrous and inflammatory rind) may form in the joints and soft tissues (**Figure 21**). Tophi can form in any joint,

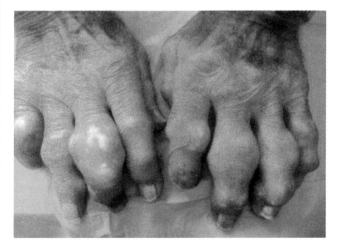

FIGURE 21. Numerous, bulky deposits of monosodium urate crystals form tophi, a sign of late-stage gout that has not been adequately treated with urate-lowering therapy.

leading to bone erosion, chronic joint damage, skin ulceration, infection, disability, and impaired quality of life.

Diagnosis

Gout should be suspected in the setting of acute monoarticular or polyarticular inflammation in an at-risk patient (see Epidemiology). Infectious arthritis must be actively excluded, given its high rate of morbidity and mortality. The differential diagnosis of acute gout is listed in **Table 26**. A high C-reactive protein and/or erythrocyte sedimentation rate support an inflammatory process but are nonspecific. A high serum urate level supports the potential for gout, but most patients with hyperuricemia do not have gout, and serum urate may be low during some acute attacks.

The gold standard for diagnosing gout is joint aspiration and synovial fluid analysis. Synovial fluid analysis permits definitive diagnosis and can rule out other, clinically indistinguishable conditions. Under polarized light, monosodium urate crystals are needle shaped and negatively birefringent (yellow when parallel, blue when perpendicular to the polarizing axis). Synovial fluid leukocyte count should also be measured; gout fluid is typically inflammatory (2000/μL to >100,000/μL [2.0-100 × 10^9/L], neutrophil predominance of ≥50%). Whereas extracellular crystals confirm a chronic gout diagnosis, crystals within neutrophils define active, gout-induced inflammation. Gram stain and cultures must be obtained to exclude infection. Acute gout and joint infection occasionally coexist.

Because joint aspiration is not always feasible or successful, diagnosis is occasionally made on clinical grounds alone.

However, a clinical diagnosis does not permit the definite exclusion of infection or other inflammatory arthritis. The American College of Rheumatology preliminary classification criteria for acute gout serve as a helpful, albeit imperfect, tool for diagnosing gout (**Table 27**). Importantly, infection of the first metatarsophalangeal joint is uncommon.

Radiography is of limited utility in early gout but may be warranted to exclude fracture or other non-gout etiologies. In severe or long-standing gout, radiographs can demonstrate classic gouty erosions described as punched-out lesions, often with overhanging edges where the bones have been eaten away by tophaceous deposits (**Figure 22**).

Management

Gout management centers on two fundamental principles: 1) control of inflammation to treat or prevent acute gout attacks and 2) reduction of serum urate to treat the underlying hyperuricemia that leads to inflammatory disease. Both are essential for proper gout management.

Treatment of Acute Gouty Arthritis

Acute gout flares should be treated with pharmacologic intervention, ideally within 24 hours of onset to maximize treatment efficacy. In patients with classic podagra or other mild to moderate presentations, monotherapy with colchicine (1.2 mg followed by 0.6 mg 1 hour later), full-dose NSAIDs (such as naproxen 500 mg twice daily), or glucocorticoids (for

TABLE 26. Differential Diagnosis of Acute Gouty Arthritis	
Condition	**Comments**
Infectious arthritis	Presentation may be identical to gout. Infectious arthritis is usually monoarticular but can be polyarticular. Gout and infectious arthritis can also coexist.
Acute calcium pyrophosphate crystal arthritis (also known as pseudogout)	Pseudogout is less likely to present in the great toe (podagra), but acute presentations may still be identical to gout. Synovial fluid analysis can distinguish these entities.
Basic calcium phosphate deposition	Because of their small size, basic calcium phosphate crystals are unlikely to be seen in synovial fluid on light microscopy except as aggregates stained with alizarin red.
Trauma	Trauma can lead to local pain and swelling, with or without a fracture, and can also trigger a gout attack.
Other forms of inflammatory arthritis (e.g., reactive arthritis, rheumatoid arthritis, psoriatic arthritis, acute rheumatic fever)	Clinical context, affected joints, and pattern of arthritis are all helpful in distinguishing these entities. Synovial fluid analysis is particularly important when there is diagnostic uncertainty.

TABLE 27. American College of Rheumatology Criteria for the Classification of Acute Arthritis of Primary Gout
Criteria
The presence of six of the following clinical, laboratory, and radiographic findings, even in the absence of crystal identification:
More than one attack of acute arthritis
Maximum inflammation developed within 1 day
Monoarthritis attack
Redness observed over joints
First metatarsophalangeal joint painful or swollen
Unilateral first metatarsophalangeal joint attack
Unilateral tarsal joint attack
Tophus (suspected)
Hyperuricemia
Asymmetric swelling within a joint visible on physical examination or radiography
Subcortical cysts without erosions visible on radiography
Monosodium urate monohydrate microcrystals in joint fluid during attack
Joint fluid culture negative for organisms during attack

Adapted with permission from John Wiley & Sons, from Wallace SL, Robinson H, Masi AT, et al. Preliminary criteria for the classification of the acute arthritis of primary gout. Arthritis Rheum. 1977;20(3):895-900. [PMID: 856219] Copyright 1977 American College of Rheumatology.

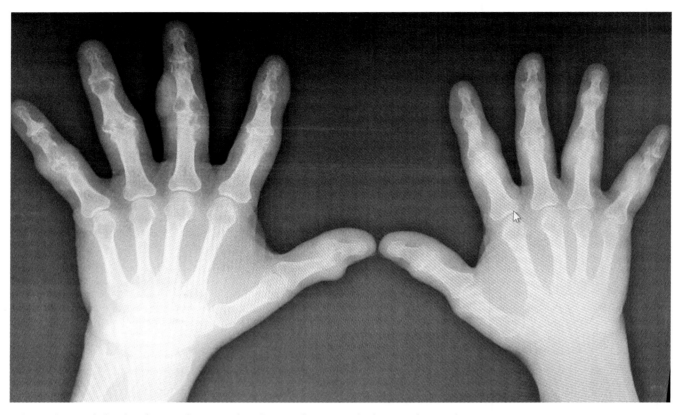

FIGURE 22. Punched-out bone lesions and erosions with overhanging edges associated with severe or long-standing gout.

Courtesy of Elaine Karis, MD.

H CONT. example, prednisone, 0.5 mg/kg) are all recommended. Selection should account for patient preferences, comorbidities, and concomitant medication use. Any NSAID, including selective cyclooxygenase-2 inhibitors, may be employed. Intra-articular glucocorticoid injection is an excellent option for monoarticular attacks, with fewer systemic toxicities than oral glucocorticoids, but requires expertise and prior synovial fluid assessment to rule out infection. Ice can reduce pain and swelling, particularly in flares involving one or two joints.

In refractory cases, switching to a different anti-inflammatory class may be attempted. For severe and/or polyarticular flares, combination therapy with two anti-inflammatory classes may be needed, but additive toxicities should be considered. Off-label use of the interleukin-1β inhibitors anakinra or canakinumab can be considered in severe cases when standard therapies are ineffective, contraindicated, or not tolerated. Patients already taking urate-lowering therapy should continue at the same dose throughout a flare because changes in serum urate can exacerbate attacks. **H**

Urate-Lowering Therapy and Prophylaxis

All patients with gout should be educated on lifestyle modifications to reduce serum urate, including weight loss if appropriate (see Table 25). Intake of high-purine (for example, meat and seafood) and high-fructose (for example, soft drinks and processed foods with added high-fructose corn syrup) foods as well as alcoholic beverages (especially beer) should be limited because all contribute to increased serum urate levels. Dairy intake may lower urate through uricosuric effects, and low-fat dairy products may thus offer benefit to patients with gout. Hydration and substitution of urate-lowering for urate-raising medications can further reduce baseline urate. For example, use of a calcium channel blocker or losartan instead of a diuretic for hypertension can promote decreased serum urate; notably, the former two agents should be used preferentially to treat hypertension in patients at risk for gout attacks.

The American College of Rheumatology (ACR) guidelines currently indicate that urate-lowering therapy should be initiated in patients with gout who have had two or more attacks within a 1-year period, one attack in the setting of chronic kidney disease of stage 2 or worse, one attack with the presence of tophi visible on examination or imaging, or one attack with a history of urolithiasis. Urate-lowering therapy should usually be initiated during the intercritical phase to avoid exacerbating active attacks. Treatment to a target serum urate level of less than 6.0 mg/dL (0.35 mmol/L) is mandatory; still lower targets may be needed to improve symptoms or signs of gout or to resolve tophi. First-line therapy for urate lowering is typically the xanthine oxidase inhibitor allopurinol. An appropriate alternative is the newer xanthine oxidase inhibitor, febuxostat, which is equally or more efficacious (and causes less hypersensitivity) but significantly more expensive.

The uricosuric agent probenecid blocks renal uric acid resorption and may be added to, or substituted for, a xanthine oxidase inhibitor if xanthine oxidase monotherapy is inadequate or not tolerated; however, probenecid may raise the risk of kidney stones and has limited efficacy in patients with impaired kidney function. In chronic refractory gout or when patients experience severe gout disease burden and standard urate-lowering therapy has been unsuccessful or not tolerated, the potent intravenous agent pegloticase is a treatment option. Pegloticase provides uricase activity, enzymatically converting urate to the more soluble compound allantoin. See Principles of Therapeutics for more information on urate-lowering therapy.

Gout flare prophylaxis should be initiated along with urate-lowering therapy because urate reduction can provoke attacks (owing to sloughing of microcrystals within the joint). Prophylaxis should continue in the presence of any active disease. In the absence of active disease, the ACR currently recommends that prophylaxis should be continued for the greater of the following: 6 months; 3 months after achieving the target serum urate level for a patient without tophi; or 6 months after achieving the target serum urate level where there has been resolution of tophi. First-line options for gout prophylaxis include colchicine, 0.6 mg (or 0.5 mg) once or twice daily, adjusting for kidney function and consideration of drug-drug interactions (see Principles of Therapeutics). Low-dose NSAIDs (such as naproxen, 250 mg twice daily) are an equally recommended alternative, but the gastrointestinal and cardiac toxicity of NSAIDs must be considered. Current guidelines endorse ≤10 mg of daily prednisone as an acceptable second-line prophylactic agent, with monitoring for the side effects of chronic glucocorticoid use.

KEY POINTS

- Gout is characterized by intermittent painful inflammatory joint attacks resulting from crystallization of excessive levels of uric acid (hyperuricemia).

- In patients with suspected gout, synovial fluid analysis is used to identify monosodium urate crystals, and Gram stain and cultures are ordered to exclude infection.

- Treatment of acute gouty arthritis involves control of inflammation using colchicine, NSAIDs, or glucocorticoids.

- Urate-lowering therapy should be initiated in patients with gout who have had two or more attacks within a 1-year period, one attack in the setting of chronic kidney disease of stage 2 or worse, one attack with the presence of tophi visible on examination or imaging, or one attack with a history of urolithiasis.

- Gout flare prophylaxis should be initiated along with urate-lowering therapy because urate reduction can transiently provoke attacks; first-line options include colchicine and NSAIDs.

Calcium Pyrophosphate Deposition

Calcium pyrophosphate (CPP) crystals are a common cause of calcification in connective tissues in and near joints. Calcium pyrophosphate deposition (CPPD) is associated with four distinct clinical presentations. There has been inconsistency in the literature and in practice surrounding the terminology for these entities. The European League Against Rheumatism (EULAR) recently published guidelines to clarify the terminology, although these have not been universally adopted. EULAR advocates for using "calcium pyrophosphate deposition" or "CPPD" as a broad term to refer to all instances of calcium pyrophosphate deposition and redefines the terminology for the various presentations of CPPD. Here we use the EULAR terminology but also mention the common terms used to describe the subtypes of CPPD.

The four clinical presentations are cartilage calcification (also known as chondrocalcinosis), acute CPP crystal arthritis (also known as pseudogout), chronic CPP crystal inflammatory arthritis, and osteoarthritis with CPPD.

Pathophysiology

The pathophysiology of CPPD is poorly characterized. CPPD in the joints may result from excessive body calcium or other metabolic derangements, overproduction of pyrophosphate by cartilage chondrocytes, or other local factors. Risk factors for CPPD include previous joint injury and familial predisposition. Particularly in a young person, a diagnosis of CPPD should prompt an evaluation for diseases associated with CPPD, including hyperparathyroidism, hemochromatosis, hypomagnesemia, and hypothyroidism.

The mechanism of chronic low-grade joint damage seen in some patients with cartilage calcification is not fully elucidated. In contrast, acute CPP crystal arthritis is known to induce inflammation via pathways similar to those induced by monosodium urate crystals in acute gout, triggering interleukin-1β production by macrophages and leading to additional inflammation and neutrophil recruitment.

Clinical Manifestations
Cartilage Calcification

Cartilage calcification (also known as chondrocalcinosis) is a radiographic finding that is usually the result of CPPD. Cartilage calcification is typically asymptomatic but may be associated with acute CPP crystal arthritis and/or pyrophosphate arthropathy. In the knee, cartilage calcification is seen as a linear density within and parallel to the surface of the cartilage (**Figure 23**); in the wrist, it is often seen in the triangular fibrocartilage distal to the ulna. Cartilage calcification can be an isolated finding or can occur in association with osteoarthritis. Prevalence increases with age, with a prevalence of approximately 50% in patients aged ≥85 years.

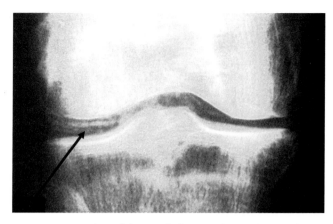

FIGURE 23. Cartilage calcification (also known as chondrocalcinosis) of the knee. This radiograph shows linearly arranged calcific deposits in the articular cartilage (*arrow*).

Acute Calcium Pyrophosphate Crystal Arthritis

Acute CPP crystal arthritis (also known as pseudogout) is characterized by painful inflammatory arthritis attacks reaching maximum intensity within 24 hours. The knee, wrist, and shoulder are typically affected; podagra is uncommon. Acute CPP crystal arthritis is generally indistinguishable from a gout flare; synovial fluid analysis is needed to make a definitive diagnosis (coexistence of the two diseases is possible). In contrast to monosodium urate crystals, CPP crystals are rhomboid shaped and positively birefringent. Cartilage calcification on radiograph suggests that an acute arthritis may be due to CPP crystals but is nondiagnostic. Acute CPP crystal arthritis occurs most commonly in patients over 65 years of age. ⧉

Pyrophosphate Arthropathy

Pyrophosphate arthropathy is a general term for joint damage attributed to CPPD and may present in two distinct patterns: chronic CPP crystal inflammatory arthritis and osteoarthritis with CPPD (both terms advocated by EULAR). In chronic CPP crystal inflammatory arthritis, there is ongoing inflammation with a pattern of joint involvement often resembling rheumatoid arthritis ("pseudo–rheumatoid arthritis"). In osteoarthritis with CPPD, patients exhibit accelerated osteoarthritis findings in joints not commonly involved with simple osteoarthritis (for example, wrist, metacarpophalangeal, or shoulder joints), with or without superimposed acute CPP crystal arthritis flares. It is presumed in these cases that the presence of crystals within the cartilage promotes a degenerative process not otherwise distinguishable from osteoarthritis.

Management

Management of CPPD centers on controlling symptoms and reducing inflammation (**Table 28**). In contrast to gout, no therapy is currently available to eliminate the pathogenic CPP crystals. Nonetheless, any underlying metabolic disorder that may contribute to CPPD should be addressed.

KEY POINTS

- Calcium pyrophosphate deposition can be associated with hyperparathyroidism, hemochromatosis, hypomagnesemia, and hypothyroidism.
- Acute calcium pyrophosphate crystal arthritis is generally indistinguishable from an acute gout flare; synovial fluid analysis is used to make a definitive diagnosis based on the characteristic rhomboid shape and positive birefringence of calcium pyrophosphate crystals.
- Management of calcium pyrophosphate deposition centers on control of symptoms and reduction of inflammation; any underlying metabolic disorder that may contribute should also be addressed.

Basic Calcium Phosphate Deposition

Basic calcium phosphate (BCP) crystals (including hydroxyapatite) are a common cause of cartilage calcification and may be radiographically indistinguishable from CPPD. Unlike CPP crystals, BCP crystals also commonly deposit in periarticular tendons, bursae, and other soft tissues. Patients are often

TABLE 28. Management of Calcium Pyrophosphate Deposition

Clinical Presentation	Treatment/Comments
Cartilage calcification (also known as chondrocalcinosis)	No specific treatment
Acute calcium pyrophosphate crystal arthritis (also known as pseudogout)	Local treatment: joint aspiration; intra-articular glucocorticoid injection; joint immobilization; ice packs
	Systemic treatment: NSAIDs; colchicine; glucocorticoids (oral or parenteral)
	Prophylaxis if recurrent attacks (three or more annual attacks): low-dose colchicine or daily NSAIDs (with gastrointestinal protection)
Chronic calcium pyrophosphate crystal inflammatory arthritis	Low-dose colchicine or daily NSAIDs (with gastrointestinal protection); low-dose glucocorticoids; methotrexate; hydroxychloroquine
Osteoarthritis with calcium pyrophosphate deposition (CPPD)	Same treatment as osteoarthritis without CPPD (e.g., physical therapy; pain control; local glucocorticoids)

asymptomatic, but BCP crystals can cause destructive arthropathy. Although not always visible on radiographs, BCP crystals have been identified as a common feature of degenerative joint disease in osteoarthritis (on histological examination). BCP crystals also can stimulate inflammation via pathways similar to monosodium urate and CPP crystals. BCP deposition can cause Milwaukee shoulder syndrome, a painful, swollen, and often destructive process of the glenohumeral joint and rotator cuff; this condition typically occurs in women over the age of 70 years.

Diagnosis of BCP deposition is made clinically or by joint aspiration. The synovial fluid is characteristically non-inflammatory (<2000/µL [2.0×10^9/L]). BCP crystals are not visible on polarized microscopy but may be visualized on electron microscopy or under light microscopy as nonbirefringent clumps that stain with alizarin red. Treatment for symptomatic BCP deposition includes NSAIDs, joint aspiration and tidal lavage, and intra-articular glucocorticoid injection.

KEY POINTS

- Basic calcium phosphate deposition can cause Milwaukee shoulder syndrome, which presents with a painful, swollen shoulder; is often associated with significant destruction of the glenohumeral joint and rotator cuff; and typically occurs in women over the age of 70 years.

- Diagnosis of basic calcium phosphate deposition is made clinically and/or by joint aspiration and staining with alizarin red.

- Management of symptomatic basic calcium phosphate deposition includes NSAIDs, joint aspiration and tidal lavage, and intra-articular glucocorticoid injection.

Infectious Arthritis

Introduction

Infectious arthritis is caused by bacteria, fungi, or viruses and should be considered in any patient with one or more inflamed joints. Significant morbidity and mortality can result from inadequate or delayed management.

Pathophysiology

Bacterial or fungal joint infections arise from hematogenous seeding (most cases), direct inoculation (for example, with surgery or, rarely, glucocorticoid injection), or contiguous spread from neighboring osteomyelitis, cellulitis, or septic bursitis. Some bacteria produce toxins or enzymes that directly damage tissues. Bacteria also trigger inflammatory responses characterized by neutrophilic infiltration into the joint space. If unresolved, these processes can rapidly progress to joint damage or destruction.

In some forms of viral-induced and other infectious arthritis, joint inflammation may develop as a consequence of immune complexes elicited by the pathogen, rather than direct infection.

Diagnosis

Infection should be considered in the differential diagnosis of any acutely or chronically inflamed joint. Joint infection should be suspected based on clinical history, presence of risk factors (**Table 29**), and initial laboratory studies. Although elevated inflammatory markers (leukocyte count, erythrocyte sedimentation rate [ESR], and C-reactive protein [CRP]) may suggest infectious arthritis, they cannot confirm the diagnosis or exclude other inflammatory causes.

Clinical Manifestations

The hallmarks of a joint infection are warmth, erythema, pain, and swelling. The typical bacterial infectious arthritis develops over days; onset is more indolent for fungal or mycobacterial infections. Joint infections are commonly limited to a single joint; the knee is the most common site, but the hip, wrist, and ankle are also commonly affected. In approximately 20% of cases, bacterial or fungal arthritis presents with polyarthritis

TABLE 29. Risk Factors for Infectious Arthritis
General Risk Factors
Age >80 years or very young children
Alcoholism
Cutaneous ulcers or other skin infections
Diabetes mellitus
End-stage kidney disease
History of intra-articular glucocorticoid injection
Injection drug use
Low socioeconomic status
Patients receiving immunosuppressive agents
Prosthetic joint or recent joint surgery
Sickle cell disease
Underlying malignancy
Risk Factors for Gonococcal Infection
Younger, sexually active patients
Risk Factors for Lyme Arthritis
Travel or residence in an endemic area
Documented tick bite or erythema chronicum migrans
Risk Factors for Mycobacterial or Fungal Infection
Patients with HIV infection or other immunosuppression
Patients receiving tumor necrosis factor α inhibitors
Travel or residence in an endemic area

CONT. and a worse prognosis. Fever and rigors may occur but are not universally present (60% of patients); absence of fever therefore does not exclude an infected joint.

Laboratory Studies and Imaging

When infectious arthritis is suspected, the synovial fluid must be aspirated and assessed for leukocyte count, Gram stain, culture (bacterial and, depending on index of suspicion, mycobacterial and fungal), and crystal analysis (to rule out alternative or concomitant etiologies). Joint aspiration should be performed before initiating antibiotics whenever possible to maximize the likelihood of positive cultures. In bacterial infection, the synovial fluid leukocyte count is markedly increased (usually >50,000/µL [50 × 10⁹/L] with neutrophil predominance). Because synovial fluid cultures have a sensitivity of approximately 80% and may be negative due to antibiotics, a fastidious organism, or other reasons, clinical assessment must ultimately guide treatment.

Cultures of blood and other possible sources of infection (such as urine or sputum) should be obtained if infectious arthritis is under consideration, ideally before starting antibiotics. Peripheral leukocyte count, ESR, and CRP should be measured.

Radiographs are nonspecific early in infectious arthritis but may reveal local swelling or joint destruction if the infection has been left untreated, whether in bacterial, mycobacterial, or fungal infections. MRI, CT, and ultrasonography are not routinely indicated but may help identify early erosions, concurrent osteomyelitis, or joint effusions that are difficult to assess on examination (for example, in the hip). Imaging may also help guide arthrocentesis.

Cultures of the genitourinary tract, rectum, and/or pharyngeal sites should be obtained when disseminated gonococcal infection is suspected. Diagnosis of Lyme disease and viral infections relies on serologic testing. ⊞

KEY POINTS

- Infectious arthritis is caused by bacteria, fungi, or viruses and should be considered in any patient with one or more inflamed joints.
- The hallmarks of a joint infection are warmth, erythema, pain, and swelling.
- Diagnosis of infectious arthritis is confirmed by joint aspiration and aided by clinical history, physical examination, and laboratory studies.
- In bacterial infection, the synovial fluid leukocyte count is markedly increased (usually >50,000/µL [50 × 10⁹/L] with neutrophil predominance).

Causes

Common causes of infectious arthritis are discussed in the following sections. For more information on the specific infections/diseases, refer to MKSAP 17 Infectious Disease.

Infection with Gram-Positive Organisms

Gram-positive organisms are the most common causes of infectious arthritis in adults. *Staphylococcus aureus* is the most common infecting organism, regardless of age or risk factors. *S. aureus* damages joints directly via toxic effects and indirectly via inflammatory responses. Symptoms develop rapidly and escalate within hours to days. The emergence of methicillin-resistant *S. aureus* poses treatment challenges. *Streptococcus pneumoniae* is another common pathogen. Polymicrobial infections occur uncommonly but may indicate a worse prognosis.

Infection with Gram-Negative Organisms

Nongonococcal Gram-Negative Organisms

Nongonococcal gram-negative bacterial arthritis is more common in patients who are immunosuppressed, are elderly, or have a history of injection drug use, recent trauma, or gastrointestinal infection. *Escherichia coli* and *Pseudomonas aeruginosa* are the most common gram-negative organisms to infect the joints. Injection drug users are at particular risk for *Pseudomonas*. Patients with sickle cell anemia are predisposed to *Salmonella* infection. *Haemophilus influenzae*, previously a common cause of infectious arthritis, has declined due to *H. influenzae* vaccine. Gram-negative bacterial joint infections cause rapid onset of symptoms and potential joint destruction if not promptly and appropriately treated.

Disseminated Gonococcal Infection

Disseminated gonococcal infection occurs in up to 3% of patients with *Neisseria gonorrhoeae* and can cause two distinct clinical presentations. Risk is highest in young, sexually active adults.

Patients with disseminated gonococcal infection and bacteremia present with vesiculopustular or hemorrhagic macular skin lesions (**Figure 24**), fever, chills, and polyarthralgia. Knees,

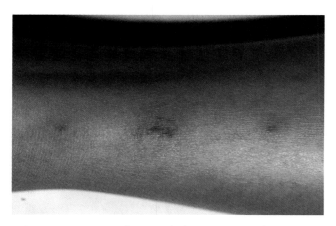

FIGURE 24. Disseminated gonococcal infection presents as a febrile arthritis-dermatitis syndrome with migratory polyarthralgia evolving into frank arthritis with or without tenosynovitis that involves one or more joints. Skin lesions are found in approximately 75% of cases, classically presenting as a small number of necrotic vesicopustules on an erythematous base.

elbows, and distal joints are typical sites of involvement. Tenosynovitis of the dorsa of the hands and/or feet is a characteristic feature. Synovial fluid leukocyte counts are lower than in other bacterial infections (<25,000/μL [25 × 10⁹/L]). Blood cultures or cultures of the genitourinary tract (for example, cervical or urethral specimens), rectum, or pharynx are often positive, but synovial fluid cultures are usually negative. Special media are required to culture *N. gonorrhoeae*.

Gonococcal infection can also present as a purulent arthritis without the rash or other features of bacteremia. In this case, one or two joints are typically involved, most commonly the knee followed by the wrist, ankle, and elbow. Synovial fluid cultures are more often positive for *N. gonorrhoeae* in this setting.

Lyme Arthritis

Lyme disease is caused by infection with *Borrelia* species. There are three phases of Lyme disease: early localized, early disseminated, and late. Although arthralgia is common in early Lyme disease, Lyme arthritis generally refers to frank inflammation of the joints as a manifestation of late Lyme disease. Late Lyme arthritis frequently causes impressively large effusions, most often a knee monoarthritis with prominent stiffness but relatively little pain. Asymmetric oligoarticular presentations also occur. Lyme arthritis can occur as a transient event, follow an intermittent pattern, or develop into a chronic arthritis. Diagnosis is made by serologic testing (enzyme-linked immunosorbent assay followed, if positive, by Western blot) indicating an immune response to *Borrelia burgdorferi*. Joint aspiration demonstrates a moderately inflammatory synovial fluid (leukocyte count typically 20,000-25,000/μL [20-25 × 10⁹/L], neutrophil predominant). Synovial fluid cultures are negative, but *B. burgdorferi* DNA can be detected by polymerase chain reaction. Permanent joint damage is less common than in gram-positive or gram-negative pyogenic infections.

Mycobacterial Infections

Several mycobacterial species can affect the musculoskeletal system, the most important being *Mycobacterium tuberculosis*.

Mycobacterium tuberculosis

Mycobacterium tuberculosis infection exhibits extrapulmonary symptoms in nearly 20% of patients, with bone or joint involvement occurring in approximately 2% overall. Patients at particular risk include persons who have lived in or visited an endemic area, patients with untreated HIV infection, and patients with immunosuppression for any other reason, including biologic therapy for autoimmune diseases. Musculoskeletal *M. tuberculosis* can develop early after infection or after an extended latency, with reactivation often triggered by immunocompromise. Patients with musculoskeletal *M. tuberculosis* infection typically manifest a chronic, indolent course, often without constitutional symptoms. Musculoskeletal *M. tuberculosis* infection most commonly presents as spondylitis (Pott disease) or vertebral osteomyelitis. Tuberculous osteomyelitis of almost any other bone is also possible.

Arthritis caused by *M. tuberculosis* is usually monoarticular, often involving the hip or knee. Joint destruction is possible but occurs slowly. Synovial fluid analysis usually suggests a nonspecific inflammatory process; imaging may be normal or show erosions that cannot be readily distinguished from other infections. Acid-fast smears of synovial fluid are positive only in a minority of cases; synovial fluid culture or synovial biopsy with granuloma identification are more likely to be diagnostic. Tuberculin skin tests are not uniformly positive, especially in immunosuppressed individuals; therefore, a negative test does not definitively exclude infection. Although signs of pulmonary tuberculosis or tuberculosis of other sites should be sought, many patients present with isolated musculoskeletal disease.

Mycobacterium marinum

Mycobacterium marinum is a freshwater and saltwater organism that enters the skin through breaks or abrasions. Common scenarios include anglers and aquarium hobbyists with bare hand exposure to water. *M. marinum* infections typically begin as red or violaceous plaques, nodules, or abscesses in the skin, and may spread locally to involve the hand joints. Therapy requires multidrug regimens such as rifampin and ethambutol.

Fungal Infections

Fungal infections are a rare cause of infectious arthritis but are important to consider, particularly in immunocompromised patients and/or endemic areas. Fungal arthritis is most likely to be caused by *Coccidioides* (endemic in the southwestern United States), *Sporothrix* (found in farm and garden soil), *Cryptococcus*, *Blastomyces* (endemic in the central United States), and *Candida*. Infections are typically monoarticular, follow an indolent course, and derive most often from hematogenous spread. Direct inoculation of the joint due to trauma or extension from a nearby site of infection is also possible. Both arthritis and osteomyelitis can occur. Diagnosis is often challenging. Synovial fluid analysis typically reveals inflammatory fluid with negative bacterial cultures. Appropriate fungal cultures or synovial biopsy may yield a diagnosis.

Viral Infections

Various viral infections can lead to musculoskeletal symptoms. Symptoms may occur via direct invasion, immune complex deposition, or less well-defined mechanisms.

Hepatitis

Hepatitis B virus (HBV) and hepatitis C virus (HCV) infections frequently cause musculoskeletal symptoms. Acute HBV infection causes symmetric polyarthritis (especially in the hands and knees) during the prodromal stage of disease, often accompanied by rash; joint pain lasts days or weeks and then resolves. In chronic HBV, arthritis may persist, possibly due to immune complex formation. Chronic HCV causes a wide array of musculoskeletal symptoms ranging from arthralgia to arthritis (oligoarticular or polyarticular presentations). Both HBV and especially HCV infection may provoke cryoglobulinemia, resulting in arthritis, glomerulonephritis, and other signs of vasculitis such as palpable purpura. Diagnosis of HBV and HCV is by serologic and polymerase chain reaction testing.

Parvovirus B19

Parvovirus B19, which causes the childhood condition known as fifth disease (also known as erythema infectiosum), is a DNA virus with a tropism for erythrocyte precursors. Adults usually contract the virus from children; individuals at risk include school workers and parents. Infection may be asymptomatic or produce a flu-like illness. As the host mounts a response, a classic "slapped cheek" rash and arthritis may occur. In adults, the rash may be absent or atypical. The arthritis begins acutely, with symmetric swelling and stiffness of the small joints of the hands and feet, as well as wrists and knees, often mimicking rheumatoid arthritis. Parvovirus B19 arthritis typically lasts for several weeks, but occasionally many months, before resolving. The presence of circulating anti-parvovirus IgM antibodies provides evidence of active disease; IgG antibodies indicate prior infection and are found in many healthy persons. Management is supportive, using anti-inflammatories (such as NSAIDs) and analgesics.

Rubella

Rubella (German measles) has become uncommon in countries with vaccine programs; nonvaccinated populations remain at risk. Infection can cause rash, fever, and lymphadenopathy. A polyarthritis of sudden onset may occur, affecting medium and small joints (hands, wrists, knees), usually resolving within 2 weeks. Synovial fluid is inflammatory. Diagnosis is made by documenting IgM anti-rubella antibodies or by isolating the virus from synovial fluid or the nasopharynx. Arthritis can also occur in response to the rubella vaccine.

Chikungunya

Chikungunya virus is an alphavirus endemic to Asia and Africa, where it is transmitted by mosquito vectors; however, cases are increasingly seen in the United States secondary to travel to endemic countries. Chikungunya virus causes fever, rash, and myalgia, along with thrombocytopenia and/or leukopenia. Chikungunya arthritis is self-limited, but severe polyarthritis/tenosynovitis can persist for as long as 6 months. Diagnosis is by clinical context, travel history, and identification of IgM anti-Chikungunya antibodies and/or viral isolation by polymerase chain reaction. Treatment is supportive.

Prosthetic Joint Infections

Prosthetic joint infection is a rare but serious complication of joint replacement. Infection rates are highest in knee replacements (up to 2%) and lower in hip and shoulder replacements. Coagulase-negative staphylococci (for example, *Staphylococcus epidermidis*) are common infecting organisms. Risk factors include superficial surgical site infection, malignancy, revision arthroplasty, inflammatory arthritis, immunosuppression, obesity, and chronic illness. Infections are most likely to occur within the first 2 years after surgery. Infections may be of early (<3 months after surgery), delayed (3-12 months), or late (>12 months after surgery) onset. Early and delayed onset infections are acquired during prosthesis implantation, whereas late-onset infections arise de novo from hematogenous seeding of the joint. Prosthetic joint infection is promoted by the development of a biofilm (coalescence of bacteria) on the artificial joint surface; biofilms are resistant to treatment both because of lack of perfusion and because biofilm bacteria develop antimicrobial resistance as a consequence of their limited exposure to treatment agents.

Early-onset infections present with joint swelling, erythema, wound drainage, and/or fever. Delayed-onset infections present insidiously with prolonged joint pain, often without fever. Late-onset infections may present as acute pain and swelling, often after hematogenous seeding from a vascular catheter or a site of infection distant from the affected joint.

Prompt orthopedic consultation should be sought for patients with suspected prosthetic joint infection because treatment nearly always requires surgical intervention (in addition to antibiotics). ESR and CRP are typically elevated. Plain radiographs are mandatory and may show erosion or loosening around the implantation site. Aspiration of the affected joint can confirm the diagnosis but may be deferred if surgical intervention is imminent. Synovial fluid cultures and blood cultures should always be obtained prior to antibiotic initiation in a stable patient. Surgical options include debridement, primary replacement of the affected hardware, or complete removal of the artificial joint and replacement after the infection is fully resolved.

Infections in Previously Damaged Joints

Joints that have been previously damaged by trauma, inflammatory arthritis, degenerative arthritis, surgical procedures, or other causes are inherently more susceptible to infection. In patients with a history of joint damage or radiographic evidence of prior damage, acute pain and swelling in a joint should raise suspicion for the possibility of an infected joint.

KEY POINTS

- Gram-positive organisms are the most common causes of infectious arthritis in adults, with *Staphylococcus aureus* being the most common infecting organism.
- Patients with disseminated gonococcal infection present with one of two syndromes: arthritis, tenosynovitis, and dermatitis or a purulent monoarthritis or oligoarthritis.
- Nongonococcal gram-negative bacterial arthritis is more common in patients who are immunosuppressed, are elderly, or have a history of injection drug use, recent trauma, or gastrointestinal infection.

(Continued)

KEY POINTS *(continued)*

- Musculoskeletal *Mycobacterium tuberculosis* typically presents as a chronic, indolent process, often without constitutional symptoms and most commonly as spondylitis, vertebral osteomyelitis, or hip or knee arthritis.
- Prompt orthopedic consultation should be sought for patients with suspected prosthetic joint infection because treatment typically requires surgical intervention.

Management
Pharmacologic Therapy

Pharmacologic therapy is the cornerstone of treatment for infectious arthritis. Bacterial or fungal joint infections require antimicrobial or antifungal agents (**Table 30**). Particularly for bacterially infected joints, antibiotic therapy should be initiated rapidly to prevent joint damage and other adverse outcomes. Whenever possible, synovial fluid culture

TABLE 30. Infectious Arthritis Treatment Based on the Suspected Pathogen

Likely or Identified Pathogen	First-Line Therapy	Second-Line Therapy	Comments
Gram-Positive Cocci			
If MRSA is a concern (risk factors or known MRSA carrier)	Vancomycin or linezolid	Clindamycin, daptomycin	—
MSSA	Oxacillin/nafcillin or cefazolin	—	Narrow treatment to MSSA coverage based on sensitivity data.
Gram-Negative Bacilli			
Enteric gram-negative bacilli	3rd generation cephalosporin (e.g., ceftriaxone or cefotaxime)	Fluoroquinolones	—
Pseudomonas aeruginosa	Ceftazidime with an aminoglycoside (e.g., gentamicin)	Carbapenems, cefepime, piperacillin-tazobactam, fluoroquinolones	—
Gram-Negative Cocci			
Neisseria gonorrhoeae	IV ceftriaxone × 7-14 days	Fluoroquinolones (only if culture sensitivities support this)	If suspected gonococcal arthritis, treat for co-infection with chlamydia empirically (azithromycin or doxycycline); in the absence of specific culture sensitivity data, "stepping down" to oral therapy of any type is no longer recommended due to increasing resistance of *N. gonorrhoeae* to commonly used oral agents.
Gram Stain Unavailable or Inconclusive			
Likely pathogen depends on patient risk factors: consider MRSA, and gram-negative organism if immunocompromised, at risk for gonococcal infection, or with joint trauma	E.g., vancomycin, or vancomycin + 3rd generation cephalosporin	—	Appropriate to start with broad antibiotic coverage and narrow coverage if culture data become available.
Borrelia burgdorferi (Lyme arthritis)	Oral doxycycline or amoxicillin × 28 days	—	If concurrent neurologic findings, IV ceftriaxone × 28 days.
Mycobacterium tuberculosis	3- to 4-drug treatment (e.g. isoniazid, pyrazinamide, rifampin, ethambutol, streptomycin)	—	Duration may vary from 6 months or longer depending on drug regimen (shorter treatment if rifampin is used).
Fungal infections	Amphotericin B, azoles (fluconazole, itraconazole, voriconazole, posaconazole), depending on suspected organism or culture data	—	Prolonged treatment courses of several months may be needed; maintenance therapy may be required in high-risk patients.

IV = intravenous; MRSA = methicillin-resistant *Staphylococcus aureus*; MSSA = methicillin-sensitive *Staphylococcus aureus*.

results should guide treatment. However, if the patient is unstable or culture data are unavailable, empiric therapy should be initiated. Duration of treatment for bacterial arthritis is variable. Commonly, 2 weeks of intravenous therapy is followed by 2 weeks of oral therapy. However, patient response, organism sensitivities, and severity of infection (number of joints involved, associated bacteremia) may alter the treatment course.

Management of arthritis due to viral infections is usually supportive, awaiting resolution of the underlying infection. Arthritis due to HCV (with or without cryoglobulinemia) may improve with antiviral treatment.

Surgical Therapy

Drainage of purulent fluid from a bacterially infected native joint is a critical component of successful treatment. Infected native joints that can be drained fully with aspiration can be managed with either serial (usually daily) arthrocentesis or surgical drainage. For joints that are less easily accessed (such as the hip) or when needle drainage proves inadequate, arthroscopic or open surgical drainage is required. Surgical management of prosthetic joint infections is discussed in Prosthetic Joint Infections. **H**

KEY POINTS

- For bacterially infected joints, antibiotics should be initiated promptly to prevent joint damage.
- Synovial fluid culture results should guide treatment of bacterial or fungal infections; however, if the patient is unstable or culture data are unavailable, empiric therapy should be initiated.
- Management of viral arthritis is generally supportive, awaiting resolution of the underlying infection.
- Drainage of purulent fluid from a bacterially infected native joint is a critical component of successful treatment.

Idiopathic Inflammatory Myopathies

Introduction

The idiopathic inflammatory myopathies (IIMs) are characterized by autoimmunity and inflammatory involvement of muscle fibers (frequently termed *myositis*), resulting in muscle weakness. The three IIMs are polymyositis (PM), dermatomyositis (DM), and inclusion body myositis (IBM).

Pathophysiology

Although all three IIMs cause muscle weakness, they have different underlying immunologic mechanisms. PM is a CD8-positive T-cell–mediated immune disease with direct myocyte injury. DM is considered an immune complex disease with vascular inflammation in muscle and subsequent muscle damage. IBM is most likely a myodegenerative disorder with vacuolar inclusions and a related T-cell response.

Epidemiology

The IIMs are rare (prevalence, 5-22/100,000). Overall female-to-male ratio is 2:1. DM has a bimodal distribution of onset, with the highest incidence in the second and fourth decades. PM incidence peaks in the fourth decade. IBM typically affects men older than 50 years of age.

KEY POINT

- The idiopathic inflammatory myopathies include polymyositis, dermatomyositis, and inclusion body myositis and are associated with inflammatory involvement of muscle fibers and resultant weakness.

Clinical Manifestations

The IIMs affect various sites and organs. PM and DM may also be associated with systemic symptoms (fever, fatigue, weight loss), Raynaud phenomenon, and arthritis. About 30% of patients with DM and PM may present with an acute onset of significant constitutional symptoms and a constellation of features called the antisynthetase syndrome. This syndrome is defined by the presence of autoantibodies to aminoacyl-transfer (t)RNA synthetase enzymes (such as anti-Jo-1) plus two of the following clinical features: inflammatory myositis, interstitial lung disease, Raynaud phenomenon, nonerosive inflammatory arthritis, and mechanic's hands.

IBM is rarely associated with extramuscular manifestations.

Muscular Involvement

Symmetric painless proximal weakness of the arms and legs is the classic feature of DM and PM. Onset is acute or subacute, with disease progressing over weeks. The deltoids, arm/hip flexors, and neck flexors are characteristically involved. Patients report difficulty combing hair, rising from a chair, and climbing stairs (classic triad of hair, chair, stair), and difficulty with routine activities such as cooking, cleaning, and shopping. Muscle atrophy is absent initially but may occur in long-standing disease.

In contrast to DM and PM, muscle weakness in IBM characteristically affects both distal and proximal muscles. Although typically symmetric, IBM muscle involvement may be asymmetric in up to 15% of patients. Onset is insidious and slowly progressive, often over years.

Cutaneous Involvement

DM is associated with multiple cutaneous manifestations. Gottron sign/papules are symmetric erythematous/violaceous macules, patches, or papules located on the extensor surfaces of the metacarpophalangeal joints (**Figure 25**).

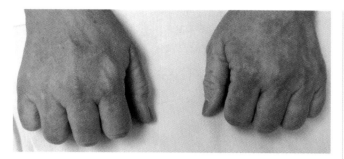

FIGURE 25. Gottron papules. Erythematous papular and patchy eruption with overlying scaling on the extensor surface of metacarpophalangeal joints in a patient with dermatomyositis.

Common rashes include heliotrope rash (edematous lilac discoloration of periorbital tissue) (**Figure 26**) as well as photodistributed rashes such as the shawl sign (upper back) (**Figure 27**) and V sign (neck/upper chest) (**Figure 28**). Poikiloderma (mottled pigmentation, epidermal atrophy, and telangiectasia) can occur in both sun-exposed and unexposed

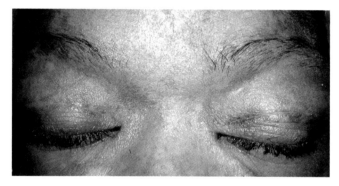

FIGURE 26. Heliotrope rash. Violaceous erythematous papular eruption with hyperkeratosis on the upper eyelids in a patient with dermatomyositis.

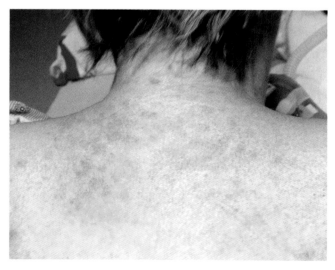

FIGURE 27. Shawl sign. Poikilodermatous (demonstrating a variety of different shades) erythematous patchy rash on the upper back in a patient with dermatomyositis.

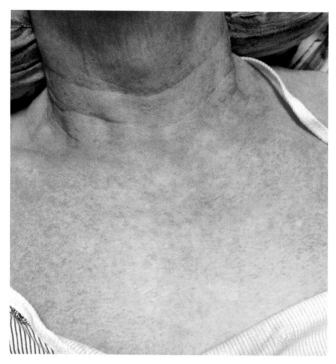

FIGURE 28. V sign. Violaceous erythema and redness present on the neck and upper chest in a patient with dermatomyositis.

areas. Gottron sign/papules and heliotrope rash are considered pathognomonic for DM. Nail changes such as cuticular hypertrophy or nailfold capillary abnormalities can occur. Amyopathic DM refers to classic cutaneous findings occurring in the absence of muscle involvement. Mechanic's hands, characterized by hyperkeratotic fissuring of the palmar and lateral surfaces of the fingers, is seen in both DM and PM (**Figure 29**). See MKSAP 17 Dermatology for more information on the cutaneous manifestations of DM.

The skin is generally uninvolved in PM and IBM.

Cardiopulmonary Involvement

Interstitial lung disease (ILD) is common in DM and PM. ILD is symptomatic in 10% to 25% of patients with DM and PM and

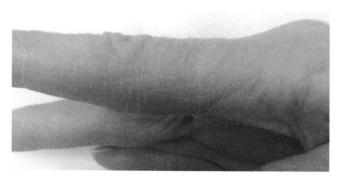

FIGURE 29. Mechanic's hands. Hyperkeratotic, fissured skin on the palmar and lateral aspects of fingers, seen in patients with polymyositis and dermatomyositis.

can be recognized in up to 65% of patients screened with high-resolution CT. ILD may precede muscle symptoms, may be asymptomatic, and is associated with poor prognosis. ILD occurrence is often associated with antisynthetase antibodies, including anti–Jo-1, and may cause rapidly progressive respiratory failure and death. Routine screening for ILD with imaging such as chest radiography or CT is appropriate in asymptomatic patients in the presence of antisynthetase antibodies. ILD is not commonly seen in IBM.

All of the IIMs can cause chest wall and diaphragm muscle weakness, resulting in shortness of breath and, occasionally, respiratory failure. Pharyngeal muscle involvement can lead to aspiration pneumonia, which can worsen ILD.

Symptomatic cardiac disease is uncommon, but minor electrocardiogram changes (arrhythmias and conduction abnormalities), presumably due to subclinical myocarditis, are commonly observed.

Gastrointestinal Involvement

Weakness of the striated muscle of the upper esophagus and/or oropharynx is common in IIM and can lead to dysphagia, aspiration, regurgitation, and associated pneumonitis. Esophageal disease is more common among older patients and those with IBM. Gastrointestinal hypomotility may occur and promote malabsorption. **H**

KEY POINTS

- Symmetric painless proximal muscle weakness of the arms and legs is the classic feature of dermatomyositis and polymyositis; onset is acute or subacute.

- The muscle weakness associated with inclusion body myositis affects both distal and proximal muscle groups; onset is insidious and slowly progressive.

- Dermatomyositis is associated with Gottron papules/sign, heliotrope rash, photodistributed rashes, and nailfold changes; skin is generally spared in polymyositis and inclusion body myositis.

- Interstitial lung disease in patients with dermatomyositis or polymyositis may be asymptomatic, may precede muscle symptoms, is often associated with antisynthetase antibodies, including anti–Jo-1, and is associated with poor prognosis.

Association with Malignancy

Increased malignancy rates are seen in both DM and PM. Relative risk for malignancy is 2.4 to 7.7 for DM and 1.7 to 2.1 for PM, compared with the general population. Malignancy risk is highest during the first year after DM/PM diagnosis and declines thereafter but remains elevated even after 5 years. Cutaneous necrosis, vasculitis, and older age at diagnosis may be risk factors.

Cancers associated with DM and PM are similar to those seen in the general population, including adenocarcinomas of the bladder, cervix, lung, ovaries, pancreas, and stomach. Ovarian cancer risk may be especially increased. Age-appropriate screening is recommended for all patients with PM or DM, with consideration of additional testing for ovarian cancer using imaging such as transvaginal pelvic ultrasonography. Routine additional testing is not cost effective, but chest and abdominal CT and/or PET scanning should be considered if there is strong suspicion or additional risk factors are present.

Any relationship between malignancy and IBM remains poorly defined.

KEY POINT

- Age-appropriate cancer screening is recommended for patients with dermatomyositis or polymyositis, with consideration of additional testing for ovarian cancer; additional CT or PET scanning to look for underlying malignancy is not cost effective unless the patient has additional risk factors. **HVC**

Diagnosis

IIM is a clinical diagnosis supported by tissue and laboratory studies. The unifying feature is muscle weakness; the pattern of muscle and extramuscular involvement suggests the specific type. Once IIM is suspected, muscle enzyme and autoantibody studies, as well as electromyography and/or imaging studies, are performed. Muscle biopsy should be performed in most patients. **Table 31** lists common and differentiating features of the IIMs.

Muscle-Related Enzymes

Muscle enzyme elevations occur in more than 90% of patients with DM and PM, especially during active disease. Creatine kinase and aldolase are the most important, but others (for example, lactate dehydrogenase and aspartate aminotransferase) also may be elevated. In DM and PM, muscle enzyme elevation is dramatic (usually 10- to 50-fold the upper limit of normal) but may or may not correlate with degree of weakness. Normal muscle enzymes may be present in 5% to 10% of patients with DM or PM, particularly in chronic disease with loss of muscle mass. Amyopathic DM refers to DM with cutaneous involvement and normal muscle enzyme levels in the absence of muscle manifestations.

Patients with IBM typically have mildly elevated levels of muscle enzymes, in the range of one to threefold the upper limit of normal.

Autoantibodies

A number of characteristic autoantibodies are seen in DM and PM. Antinuclear antibodies (ANA) are detected in approximately 80% of patients with DM and PM.

Myositis-specific autoantibodies (MSA) are found in approximately 30% of patients with PM and/or DM and include antibodies to aminoacyl-transfer (t)RNA synthetases

TABLE 31. Features of the Idiopathic Inflammatory Myopathies

	Dermatomyositis	Polymyositis	Inclusion Body Myositis
Epidemiology			
Sex	Childhood: female = male; Adult: female > male	Female > male	Male > female
Age of onset	All	<50 years	>50 years
Familial association	No	No	Yes
Clinical Presentation			
Onset of symptoms	Acute or subacute	Acute or subacute	Insidious
Weakness	Proximal	Proximal	Proximal and distal
Course	Rapid	Rapid	Slowly progressive
Skin rash	Yes	No	No
Diagnostic Findings			
Muscle enzymes	>10 times normal	>10 times normal	<10 times normal
Electromyography	Myopathic	Myopathic	Myoneuropathic
Muscle biopsy	Microinfarctions; myofibril grouping	Myofibril necrosis	Rimmed vacuoles; inclusions
Treatment			
Response	Good	Good	Poor

(antisynthetase antibodies, including anti–Jo-1), antibodies to signal recognition particle (SRP), and antibodies to Mi-2, a nuclear helicase.

Myositis-associated autoantibodies (MAA), commonly anti-PM-Scl, anti-Ku, anti-Ro/SSA, anti-La/SSB, and anti-U1-ribonucleoprotein (RNP) antibodies, are found in approximately 30% of patients with PM and/or DM.

In clinical practice, ANA testing is usually done initially during diagnostic work-up. Positive ANA supports the diagnosis of IIM, although negative tests do not exclude it. MSA testing is usually performed during initial diagnostic evaluation or once diagnosis is established because MSA may be associated with particular clinical syndromes, patterns of organ involvement, certain histopathologic findings, and prognosis. MAA testing is usually ordered if previous testing has been inconclusive. Positive anti-U1-RNP antibodies suggest an overlap syndrome with mixed connective tissue disease.

To date, no autoantibodies characteristic of IBM have been identified.

Imaging Studies

Imaging studies are sensitive but nonspecific for the IIMs and cannot definitively differentiate among inflammatory, metabolic, traumatic, and other myopathies. Muscle imaging can identify affected sites for biopsy, aid in clinical diagnosis, and help follow the response to treatment and course of disease. MRI is usually the preferred modality and can show active inflammation of muscle and follow its course; edema, active myositis, fibrosis, and calcification in advanced disease can also be detected. Because of limited specificity, the pattern of muscle involvement on MRI is usually reported as either consistent or likely inconsistent with IIM.

Electromyography

Electromyography (EMG) is obtained in most patients with IIM due to almost universal availability and high sensitivity. EMG can identify characteristic abnormalities and exclude neuropathic disease. The characteristic triad of EMG findings includes short duration small, low-amplitude polyphasic potentials; fibrillation potentials at rest; and bizarre, high frequency, repetitive discharges. As with MRI, these findings are not adequately specific for definitive diagnosis alone because they may also be seen in infectious, toxic, or metabolic myopathies.

Muscle Biopsy

Biopsy of an affected muscle is the gold standard for diagnosis and should be obtained initially in most patients to distinguish between DM, PM, and IBM as well as nonimmune, noninflammatory myopathic disorders. Muscle biopsy is also sometimes needed during the course of disease to evaluate treatment response or rule out a new or alternative cause of weakness.

DM is typically associated with a mixed B and CD4-positive T-cell perivascular infiltrate, vasculitis with microinfarction and grouping of muscle fibers, and perifascicular muscle atrophy. PM infiltrates primarily consist of CD8-positive T cells, involving all layers of muscle fibers with invasion and myophagocytosis. The primary target seems to be the vascular endothelium in DM and the myofibrils themselves in PM. IBM demonstrates a mild T-cell predominant inflammatory infiltrate (similar to PM), along with the presence of rimmed vacuoles and eosinophilic and basophilic inclusions within muscle fibers. Filamentous tubules seen on electron microscopy are highly specific for IBM.

KEY POINTS

- Dermatomyositis and polymyositis are associated with elevation of muscle enzymes such as creatine kinase and aldolase as well as autoantibodies such as antinuclear antibodies, myositis-specific autoantibodies, and myositis-associated autoantibodies.

- In the idiopathic inflammatory myopathies, muscle imaging can identify sites for biopsy, aid in clinical diagnosis, and help assess the response to treatment.

- Biopsy of an affected muscle is the gold standard for diagnosis to distinguish between dermatomyositis, polymyositis, and inclusion body myositis as well as nonimmune, noninflammatory myopathic disorders.

Differential Diagnosis

The differential diagnosis for myopathy is broad (**Table 32**) and includes hereditary diseases, infection, and endocrine and drug-induced myopathies. Colchicine and hydroxychloroquine, both used frequently in rheumatologic disease, may cause myopathy. Glucocorticoids, used in treating IIMs, can themselves cause muscle weakness that may require withdrawal of therapy. Statins are a frequent cause of myalgia and/or asymptomatic creatine kinase elevations; many cases are mild, and not all will require discontinuation. Rarely, statin use can result in an autoimmune myopathy associated with antibodies to the enzyme HMG-CoA reductase. See MKSAP 17 Neurology for more information on myopathy.

KEY POINT

- The differential diagnosis of the idiopathic inflammatory myopathies includes other myopathies that present with muscle weakness, toxic myopathies, and disorders that present with weakness but without muscle involvement.

Management

IIM management requires a comprehensive approach combining aggressive pharmacotherapy, physical therapy to maintain muscle strength, and supportive interventions. Glucocorticoids, initiated at high doses and tapered once serum muscle enzymes normalize, are the mainstay treatment for PM and DM. Clinical symptoms may take months to improve.

TABLE 32. Differential Diagnosis of Myopathy

Myopathy[a]	Common Examples	Comments
Idiopathic inflammatory myopathies	Dermatomyositis (DM); polymyositis (PM); inclusion body myositis (IBM)	DM and PM: acute/subacute, symmetric proximal weakness, pathognomic rash in DM; IBM: insidious, proximal and distal weakness
Connective tissue disease	Systemic lupus erythematosus; mixed connective tissue disease; systemic sclerosis	Prominent extramuscular features typical of underlying disorder
Endocrine disease	Hypothyroidism; Addison disease; vitamin D deficiency	Subtle extramuscular features; routine testing to evaluate
Infection-induced myopathies	Bacterial: Lyme disease; pyomyositis Viral: influenza; HIV; hepatitis B; hepatitis C Parasitic: toxoplasmosis; trichinosis	Detailed history and physical usually gives clue; difficult to diagnose
Drug- or toxin-induced myopathies	Glucocorticoids; ethanol; statins; colchicine; hydroxychloroquine	Lack of typical symptoms; muscle biopsy is useful
Metabolic myopathies	Acid maltase deficiency; McArdle disease	Typical history; associated with exercise/exertion; ischemic forearm testing
Mitochondrial myopathies	Kearns-Sayre syndrome; Leigh syndrome	Difficult to diagnose; muscle biopsy needed to evaluate
Muscular dystrophies	Duchenne dystrophy; Becker dystrophy	Suggestive history; onset typically in young adulthood
Neurologic and neuromuscular disorders	Amyotrophic lateral sclerosis; myasthenia gravis; Guillain-Barré syndrome; cerebrovascular accident; multiple sclerosis	Suggestive history; some are weakness mimickers (lack of direct involvement of muscle)

[a]Asymptomatic elevation in serum muscle enzymes, especially creatine kinase, is fairly common, may occur without any underlying disease, and is more frequent in black persons. Although usually benign, it must be distinguished from an actual myopathic disorder if weakness and other suggestive features are present.

Immunosuppressive therapy with methotrexate or azathioprine is used for glucocorticoid-resistant disease or glucocorticoid sparing; it is also used in poor prognosis groups and patients with extramuscular disease such as ILD. Other immunosuppressive agents (such as mycophenolate mofetil and leflunomide) have also been used. Intravenous immune globulin (IVIG) therapy is recommended as an alternative treatment for DM.

IBM is generally resistant to pharmacotherapy, although glucocorticoids, methotrexate, and/or IVIG are often tried.

KEY POINTS

- Management of the idiopathic inflammatory myopathies combines pharmacotherapy, physical therapy to maintain muscle strength, and supportive interventions.
- Glucocorticoids are the mainstay therapy for dermatomyositis and polymyositis, with high doses used until serum muscle enzymes normalize.
- In dermatomyositis and polymyositis, immunosuppressive therapy is used for glucocorticoid-resistant disease and for glucocorticoid sparing; it is also used in poor prognosis groups or in patients with severe extramuscular disease such as interstitial lung disease.
- Inclusion body myositis is generally resistant to treatment, although glucocorticoids, methotrexate, and/or intravenous immune globulin are often tried.

Prognosis

DM and PM are responsive to early aggressive treatment, with symptomatic and histologic improvement in most cases and a 5-year survival rate of 95%. Older age, underlying malignancy, pulmonary fibrosis, and esophageal dysmotility are associated with poorer prognosis; the most common causes of death are malignancies, infections (particularly aspiration pneumonia), profound muscle weakness, cardiovascular disease, and respiratory failure.

Patients with IBM tend to experience a long slow decline of muscle function regardless of therapy, with a large impact on daily activities but little impact on overall survival.

KEY POINT

- The most common causes of death in patients with polymyositis and dermatomyositis are malignancies, infections, profound muscle weakness, cardiovascular disease, and respiratory failure.

Systemic Vasculitis
Introduction

Vasculitis refers to inflammation of arteries, veins, or capillaries. Involved vessels may be large, intermediate, or small. Vasculitis can be idiopathic, or secondary to an antigen trigger or other

autoimmune condition (**Table 33**). Vasculitis can mimic, or be mimicked by, other systemic conditions (**Table 34**). Discussion here is limited to diseases in which vasculitis is the primary disorder.

Large-Vessel Vasculitis

Giant cell arteritis (GCA) and Takayasu arteritis (TA) constitute the large-vessel vasculitides. Although not a vasculitis,

TABLE 33. Causes of Secondary Vasculitis
Medications
Antimicrobial agents
Vaccines
Antithyroid agents
Anticonvulsant agents
Antiarrhythmic agents
Diuretics
Other cardiovascular drugs
Anticoagulants
Antineoplastic agents
Hematopoietic growth factors
NSAIDs
Leukotriene inhibitors
Psychotropic drugs
Sympathomimetic agents
Allopurinol
Tumor necrosis factor modulatory agents
Interferon alfa
Infections
Hepatitis A, B, and C virus
HIV
Bacterial endocarditis
Parvovirus B19
Neoplasms
Hairy cell leukemia (associated with polyarteritis nodosa)
Other hematologic and solid malignancies
Autoimmune Diseases
Systemic lupus erythematosus
Rheumatoid arthritis
Sjögren syndrome
Inflammatory myopathies
Systemic sclerosis
Relapsing polychondritis
Inflammatory bowel disease
Primary biliary cirrhosis

TABLE 34. Differential Diagnosis of Vasculitis	
Disease	Comments
Infection (sepsis, endocarditis, hepatitis)	Heart murmur, rash, and/or musculoskeletal symptoms can occur in bacterial endocarditis or viral hepatitis.
Drug toxicity/poisoning	Cocaine, amphetamines, ephedra alkaloids, and phenylpropanolamine may produce vasospasm, resulting in symptoms of ischemia.
Coagulopathy	Occlusive diseases (disseminated intravascular coagulation, the antiphospholipid antibody syndrome, thrombotic thrombocytopenic purpura) can produce ischemic symptoms.
Malignancy	Paraneoplastic vasculitis is rare. Any organ system may be affected, but the skin and nervous system are the most common. Vasculitic symptoms may precede, occur simultaneously with, or follow diagnosis of cancer. Lymphoma occasionally may involve the blood vessels and mimic vasculitis. Consider malignancy in patients with incomplete or no response to therapy for idiopathic vasculitis.
Atrial myxoma	Classic triad of symptoms: embolism, intracardiac obstruction leading to pulmonary congestion or heart failure, and constitutional symptoms (fatigue, weight loss, fever). Skin lesions can be identical to those seen in leukocytoclastic vasculitis. Atrial myxomas are rare but are the most common primary intracardiac tumor. Myxomas also can occur in other cardiac chambers.
Multiple cholesterol emboli	Typically seen in patients with severe atherosclerosis. Embolization may occur after abdominal trauma, aortic surgery, or angiography. May also occur after heparin, warfarin, or thrombolytic therapy. Patients may have livedo reticularis, petechiae and purpuric lesions, and localized skin necrosis.

polymyalgia rheumatica (PMR) is discussed here because of its close association with GCA.

Giant Cell Arteritis

Epidemiology and Pathophysiology

GCA is the most common primary vasculitis (10 cases/100,000). GCA is most common among white persons, especially northern Europeans. Women are affected more often than men (2:1 ratio). Median age of onset is 70 years; GCA in patients under age 50 is rare.

GCA characteristically affects the second- to fifth-order branches of the aorta. Affected arteries include the external carotids, temporal arteries (hence the alternative designation *temporal arteritis*), and ciliary and ophthalmic arteries. Subclavian and brachial arteries can be affected. Uncommonly, intracranial arteritis may occur.

In GCA, dendritic cells in the vessel adventitia become activated and recruit T cells and monocytes into the vessel wall. Within the media, macrophages coalesce into multinucleated giant cells and secrete metalloproteinases, disrupting the internal elastic lamina. Simultaneously, intimal proliferation can reduce blood flow and induce partial or complete ischemia of the affected tissue bed.

Clinical Manifestations and Diagnosis

Patients with GCA classically report scalp pain, headache, or tenderness over the temporal artery, which is usually unilateral. Systemic inflammation results in malaise, weight loss, and low-grade fever. Patients may experience pain in the muscles of mastication during chewing (jaw claudication). The most feared outcome is blindness, caused by ophthalmic and/or posterior ciliary artery occlusion. Blindness can be sudden or preceded by transient visual loss (amaurosis fugax). Diplopia is common. In some patients, brachial artery involvement causes decreased pulses and hand or forearm ischemia. Aortic aneurysm is a potential complication as is aortic dissection, which may occur with or without preceding aneurysm formation. Of patients with GCA, 30% to 50% concurrently have PMR (see Polymyalgia Rheumatica).

GCA should be considered in any individual ≥50 years of age with temporal or other atypical headache, jaw claudication, or visual changes, with or without PMR. Nearly all patients with GCA have a markedly elevated erythrocyte sedimentation rate (ESR), which is typically elevated to greater than 50 mm/h. On examination, the temporal artery may be erythematous, swollen, and tender. Definitive diagnosis should be pursued whenever possible via biopsy of a temporal artery segment. However, the presence of skip lesions and the need for expert examination of the biopsied specimen may sometimes lead to false-negative results. In such cases, biopsy of the contralateral artery may be warranted. Angiography of the arms is indicated in patients with peripheral vascular insufficiency.

Management

Treatment of suspected GCA should never be deferred pending biopsy because 1) treatment is rapidly effective and prevents blindness, and 2) biopsy specimens remain interpretable for at least 2 weeks after treatment initiation. In virtually all instances, patients with GCA should receive oral prednisone (60 mg/d [or 1 mg/kg/d]). In patients with visual loss, intravenous (IV) pulse glucocorticoids (typically methylprednisolone, 1000 mg/d for 3 days) may be tried, although restoration of vision should not be anticipated. Prednisone should generally be administered for approximately 1 month (or until resolution of signs and symptoms), with subsequent dose reduction at a rate of about 10% every few weeks. The ESR usually responds rapidly and can then serve as a marker of disease activity.

Patients should be monitored for relapse, in which case prednisone should be transiently increased; treatment duration may range from 6 to 18 months. Data from observational studies support that the coadministration of low-dose aspirin (80 mg/d) further reduces the risk of blindness and deserves consideration.

When prednisone is contraindicated or in cases where GCA has failed to respond to glucocorticoid therapy, methotrexate, the anti–interleukin-6 agent tocilizumab, and cyclophosphamide have been used, although evidence of their effectiveness is limited.

The long-term outcomes of adequately treated GCA are good, with recurrences uncommon.

Polymyalgia Rheumatica
Epidemiology and Pathophysiology
PMR is not a vasculitis but is discussed here because of its relationship with GCA; most experts consider that GCA and PMR exist on a spectrum of a single unifying disease. Of patients with GCA, 30% to 50% have concurrent PMR; conversely, 10% to 15% of patients with PMR, but no clinical GCA, show occult GCA on blind temporal artery biopsy. PMR epidemiology is similar to GCA, but PMR is 2 to 3 times more common.

Clinical Manifestations and Diagnosis
Patients with PMR experience symmetric pain and stiffness in the shoulder, neck, and hip regions, without actual joint arthritis. Common symptoms include the inability to comb hair or rise from a chair unassisted. In some cases, mild synovitis occurs in the wrists and hands. Strength and muscle enzymes (creatine kinase, aldolase) are generally normal.

PMR is a clinical diagnosis based on the characteristic symptoms in a patient older than 50 years. Patients with PMR demonstrate systemic inflammation (for example, elevated ESR), along with low-grade fever, malaise, and fatigue. In the absence of GCA signs and symptoms, temporal artery biopsies are not routinely performed.

Management
In contrast to GCA, PMR responds well to low-dose prednisone (10-20 mg/d). Most patients respond with dramatic improvement in their symptoms within 3 days, and failure to do so suggests an alternative diagnosis. Patients with PMR frequently experience partial relapses during prednisone tapering, requiring transient up-titration. PMR treatment is therefore commonly of long duration; some patients need several years to completely discontinue prednisone, whereas others remain on prednisone indefinitely.

Takayasu Arteritis
Epidemiology and Pathophysiology
In Takayasu arteritis (TA), the affected arteries are primarily the aorta (ascending, descending thoracic, and abdominal aorta) and its major branches. In contrast to GCA, TA is rare (2 cases/million patient-years) and mainly affects young women (9:1 ratio) with a typical age at onset between 15 and 25 years.

Histologically, the pathophysiologic processes of TA and GCA are similar, with infiltration of T cells, macrophages, and giant cells in the vessel wall.

Clinical Manifestations and Diagnosis
Clinical manifestations of TA result from inflammation and/or the consequences of large artery disease. Fever, fatigue, malaise, and weight loss, along with arthralgia and myalgia, often precede the onset of specific signs and symptoms. Patients may have diminished or absent pulses in the brachial, femoral, axillary, carotid, ulnar, and radial distributions, often accompanied by bruits. Blood pressure measurements may differ on the left and right sides. Aortic coarctation may cause decreased kidney perfusion, compensatory renin/angiotensin release, and hypertension. Wall weakness may lead to aneurysms of the aorta and other vessels; aortic root aneurysm can result in aortic valve incompetence. Central nervous system involvement is uncommon but can lead to syncope, stroke, and ocular findings.

TA should be suspected in patients younger than 40 years with unexplained systemic inflammation and/or signs and symptoms of large-vessel impairment. Angiogram demonstrates focal arterial narrowing and/or aneurysms (**Figure 30**). Laboratory testing is nonspecific but typically reveals an elevated ESR.

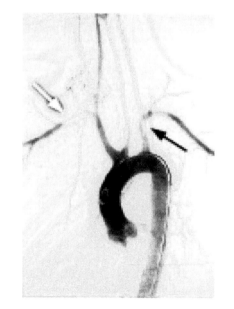

FIGURE 30. Takayasu arteritis. This angiogram of the aorta demonstrates high-grade stenosis of the proximal right subclavian artery (*white arrow*) as well as the left subclavian artery just below the origin of the left vertebral artery (*black arrow*). Incidentally noted is anatomic variation with a common origin of the right brachiocephalic artery and the left common carotid artery.

Management

CONT.

Untreated TA conveys significant morbidity and mortality; early recognition and management are therefore critical. Standard TA treatment is high-dose prednisone (1 mg/kg/d), followed by taper. Patients with structural damage to affected vessels may require angioplasty to improve blood flow, or, in severe cases, arterial bypass or reconstruction. **H**

KEY POINTS

- Giant cell arteritis should be considered in any individual older than age 50 years with temporal or other atypical headache, jaw claudication, or visual changes.
- Although temporal artery biopsy is indicated to make a definitive diagnosis of giant cell arteritis, initiation of prednisone should not be delayed; treatment can prevent blindness, and biopsy specimens remain interpretable for at least 2 weeks after treatment initiation.
- Patients with polymyalgia rheumatica experience symmetric pain and stiffness in the shoulders, neck, and hips, along with low-grade fever, malaise, and fatigue; standard treatment is low-dose prednisone.
- Takayasu arteritis should be suspected in patients younger than age 40 years with unexplained systemic inflammation and/or signs and symptoms of large-vessel impairment; standard treatment is high-dose prednisone.

Medium-Vessel Vasculitis

Polyarteritis Nodosa

Epidemiology and Pathophysiology

Polyarteritis nodosa (PAN) is rare (5-10 patients/million); men and women are affected equally. In approximately 30% of cases, PAN is associated with hepatitis B virus infection; hepatitis B vaccination reduces PAN incidence. The remainder of cases are idiopathic. PAN characteristically affects medium and small arteries; arterial inflammation results in vessel narrowing and, characteristically, aneurysms and microaneurysms. The classic features of PAN result from ischemia and/or aneurysm rupture. Organs typically affected include the kidneys, gastrointestinal tract (especially the mesenteric artery and small intestine), peripheral nervous system, and skin. Involvement of the testicles, ovaries, and breasts can occur. Coronary arteries can also be affected.

Clinical Manifestations and Diagnosis

Patients with PAN usually present with nonspecific inflammatory symptoms (fatigue, malaise, fever, myalgia, arthralgia). Renal artery vasculitis can cause decreased kidney blood flow, resulting in decreased glomerular filtration, renin/angiotensin overproduction, and hypertension. Glomerulonephritis does not occur. Abdominal symptoms include chronic or intermittent ischemic pain, especially after eating (abdominal angina);

bowel infarction may ensue. Neurologic involvement commonly takes the form of mononeuritis multiplex. Skin findings include livido reticularis, purpura, and painful subcutaneous nodules.

Elevated inflammatory markers are typically present, and hepatitis B antigenemia is detectable in infected patients. Vascular imaging studies are most useful for diagnosis. Mesenteric and/or renal artery imaging with either angiography or CT angiography reveals medium-sized artery aneurysms and stenoses.

Management

PAN carries significant potential for poor outcome, including kidney disease and mortality. Treatment is aggressive, including high-dose prednisone and cyclophosphamide. Other disease-modifying antirheumatic drugs (methotrexate, azathioprine, mycophenolate mofetil) may be considered for milder disease or as maintenance therapy. Patients with hepatitis B should receive plasma exchange and antiviral therapy whenever feasible. **H**

Primary Angiitis of the Central Nervous System

Epidemiology and Pathophysiology

Primary angiitis of the central nervous system (PACNS) is exceedingly rare (2.4 cases/million person-years). Median age of onset is 50 years, with men affected twice as often as women. Progression may be insidious. Vascular involvement is limited to intracerebral vessels; a necrotizing granulomatous vasculitis is typical.

Clinical Manifestations and Diagnosis

The most common features of PACNS are recurrent headaches and progressive encephalopathy. Strokes, transient ischemic attacks, visual field defects, and seizures also occur. Systemic vasculitis is absent, and systemic inflammatory markers are not elevated. Diagnosis requires a high index of suspicion and aggressive evaluation, including lumbar puncture, MRI, cerebral angiography, and brain biopsy. Cerebrospinal fluid analysis reveals lymphocytosis and elevated protein. MRI reveals multiple diffuse and focal abnormalities but is nonspecific. Intracranial angiography typically reveals areas of ectasia and stenosis, but other entities (atherosclerosis, vasospasm) may produce similar pictures. The definitive test is a brain biopsy revealing granulomatous vasculitis. Brain biopsy also permits identification and/or elimination of other important diagnoses, including infection and malignancy. Because vascular involvement in PACNS is patchy, a normal biopsy may sometimes represent a false negative. Nonetheless, brain biopsy is nearly always necessary.

Management

PACNS can lead inexorably to cognitive decline, dementia, and death. Management is aggressive and includes high-dose glucocorticoids and daily oral cyclophosphamide. **H**

Kawasaki Disease
Epidemiology and Pathophysiology
Kawasaki disease (KD) is a medium-vessel vasculitis of infants and children, most commonly boys of Asian origin. A seasonal predominance (late winter-spring) suggests an as-yet unidentified infectious trigger.

Clinical Manifestations and Diagnosis
Symptoms of KD include high spiking fevers, conjunctivitis, and mucositis of the lips and oral cavity, including a strawberry-like tongue. A polymorphous truncal rash is accompanied by palmar and plantar erythema, induration, and desquamation. Cervical lymphadenopathy is common. Most concerning is vasculitic involvement of the coronary arteries, resulting in coronary artery aneurysms and/or thrombosis, and potentially myocardial infarction and mortality. Other cardiac manifestations include myocarditis and pericarditis.

Management
Standard KD treatment consists of intravenous immune globulin (2 g/kg) plus aspirin (30-100 mg/kg/d). This regimen reduces inflammation and the risk of coronary aneurysms. Patients who develop medium-large coronary artery aneurysms during the acute phase of the illness are at increased risk of coronary artery stenosis and require close follow-up with periodic testing that may include electrocardiography, echocardiography, and ischemic stress testing.

KEY POINTS

- In approximately 30% of cases, polyarteritis nodosa (PAN) is associated with hepatitis B virus infection; hepatitis B vaccination reduces PAN incidence.

- Treatment of polyarteritis nodosa includes high-dose prednisone and cyclophosphamide.

- Primary angiitis of the central nervous system presents with recurrent headaches and progressive encephalopathy.

- Kawasaki disease occurs in infants and young children; symptoms include high spiking fevers, conjunctivitis, rash, and mucositis of the lips and oral cavity.

Small-Vessel Vasculitis

Small-vessel vasculitis affects post-capillary venules, arterioles, and capillaries. Because these vessels are ubiquitous, small-vessel vasculitides present with a wide range of manifestations. Two major categories of small-vessel vasculitis are discussed here: ANCA-associated vasculitis and immune complex–mediated vasculitis.

ANCA-Associated Vasculitis

ANCA-associated vasculitis constitutes three diseases: granulomatosis with polyangiitis (formerly known as Wegener granulomatosis), microscopic polyangiitis, and eosinophilic granulomatosis with polyangiitis (formerly known as Churg-Strauss syndrome). In addition, rapidly progressive glomerulonephritis may sometimes present as an ANCA-associated process (see MKSAP 17 Nephrology, Glomerular Diseases). ANCAs were first recognized when sera from patients with vasculitis were noted to bind to fixed neutrophils in vitro in two distinct patterns—either perinuclear (p-ANCA) or diffusely throughout the cytoplasm (c-ANCA). These patterns were found to reflect distinct antibody types, with p-ANCA mainly directed toward the neutrophil enzyme myeloperoxidase (MPO), and c-ANCA toward the neutrophil proteinase 3 (PR3). These antibodies are now specifically identified using enzyme-linked immunosorbent assays.

Specific ANCA-associated diseases are classically associated with one or the other, but not both, ANCA types. Although the clinical pictures of c-ANCA and p-ANCA vasculitides differ, investigators have proposed a common process through which all ANCA may promote vasculitis (**Figure 31**). Based on the proposed model, the extent of ANCA deposition need not be large to cause disease. Thus, on immunofluorescence of histopathologic specimens, little antibody staining is seen, leading

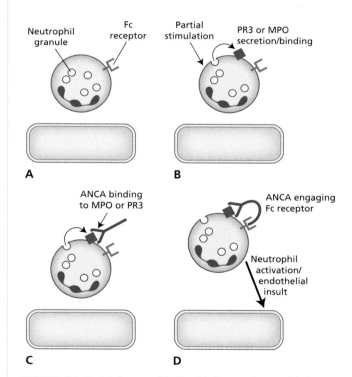

FIGURE 31. Model of presumed ANCA activity in promoting vasculitis. A, Quiescent neutrophil and adjacent endothelial cell. B, Low-level activation of the neutrophil ("priming") results in early partial neutrophil degranulation (release of granule contents to the extracellular environment), allowing de novo exposure of MPO and/or PR3, which result in humoral immunity and the formation of anti-MPO or anti-PR3 autoantibodies. C, Adherence of secreted MPO/PR3 on the neutrophil surface permits ANCA binding to the neutrophil. D, ANCA bound to neutrophil surface engages the neutrophil Fc receptor, fully stimulating the neutrophil and leading to release of enzymes such as metalloproteinases, as well as toxic oxygen radicals, that damage the endothelium. MPO = myeloperoxidase; PR3 = proteinase 3.

to the designation of ANCA vasculitides as *pauci-immune*. In all ANCA vasculitides, fever, malaise, weight loss, myalgia, and arthralgia are common. H

Granulomatosis with Polyangiitis
Epidemiology and Pathophysiology
Granulomatosis with polyangiitis (GPA) is the most common ANCA-associated vasculitis (8-10 cases/million). GPA typically affects middle-aged to older patients (mean age, approximately 55 years). White persons, typically northern Europeans, are more commonly affected. Of note, 80% to 90% of patients with GPA demonstrate a c-ANCA pattern and anti-PR3 antibody positivity.

Clinical Manifestations and Diagnosis
Classic GPA affects the upper respiratory tract (including sinuses and ears), lungs, and kidneys. Nasal and/or sinus pain and stuffiness, rhinitis, and/or epistaxis are common. Nasal inflammation can cause cartilage damage and collapse (saddle nose deformity). Hearing loss may occur, usually due to eustachian tube damage. Inflammation can damage the trachea, causing airway narrowing and obstruction. Ocular inflammation may lead to blindness. In the lungs, nodules and infiltrates occur (**Figure 32**); capillaritis may result in alveolar hemorrhage and hemoptysis. In the kidneys, rapidly progressive crescentic glomerulonephritis may ensue. Other organ systems commonly involved include the skin (painful cutaneous nodules, palpable purpura, urticarial and ulcerative lesions) and peripheral nerves.

Diagnosing GPA requires the appropriate clinical and serological picture. In the setting of a classic GPA picture,

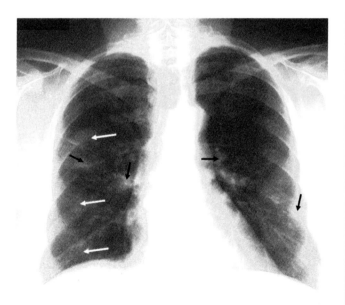

FIGURE 32. A frontal chest radiograph showing both patchy alveolar infiltrates (*white arrows*) and nodules (*black arrows*) in a patient with granulomatosis with polyangiitis (formerly known as Wegener granulomatosis).

positivity for c-ANCA/anti-PR3 is considered by many rheumatologists to be adequate to initiate treatment. However, because all effective treatments have toxicity, most experts recommend that a tissue diagnosis is essential in all but the most clear-cut cases. Tissues available for biopsy include skin, lung, sinuses, sural nerve, and kidneys. Lung biopsy is invasive but most reliably provides the characteristic histopathologic findings, including both vasculitis and necrotizing granulomas (characteristic of GPA but not the other ANCA diseases). Kidney biopsy is high yield when kidney involvement is apparent, but because granulomas are absent, the biopsy will not distinguish GPA from the other ANCA conditions. Skin biopsies are less often nondiagnostic but are readily obtained.

Management
For severe or generalized disease, treatment of GPA consists of high-dose glucocorticoids plus cyclophosphamide for approximately 6 months, followed by maintenance therapy with methotrexate, azathioprine, or mycophenolate mofetil. Glucocorticoids alone are insufficient to control GPA. Recent studies suggest that the anti-B-cell antibody rituximab is as efficacious as cyclophosphamide, possibly with less toxicity. For limited disease (no kidney disease and only mild lower airway disease), methotrexate and glucocorticoids alone may be sufficient; such patients should be carefully monitored for treatment failure necessitating the more aggressive regimen. Using these approaches, GPA mortality has declined from 90% to around 10%. H

Microscopic Polyangiitis
Epidemiology and Pathophysiology
Microscopic polyangiitis (MPA) shares features with GPA but differs with regard to organ involvement and autoimmunity. MPA occurs about half as frequently as GPA. Men are affected more commonly than women (2:1 ratio). Patients tend to develop MPA in their fourth to fifth decades, but earlier and later cases occur. Patients with MPA classically express p-ANCA and anti-MPO antibodies.

Clinical Manifestations and Diagnosis
The typical organ involvement in MPA is vasculitis of the kidneys and lungs. Kidney involvement is nearly ubiquitous; as in GPA, the lesions are those of necrotizing glomerulonephritis. Crescent formation is common, and immune deposits are sparse or absent. Lung involvement occurs in more than half of cases, consisting of non-granulomatous alveolar infiltrates that may be fleeting or persistent and are histologically reflected as pulmonary capillaritis with neutrophilic infiltrates. Most ominous is diffuse alveolar hemorrhage, which can be fatal if not adequately managed. Upper airways remain uninvolved. Skin rashes (especially palpable purpura) are common.

Diagnosis requires the appropriate conjunction of symptoms and serologies. Most patients are positive for p-ANCA and

CONT.

anti-MPO antibodies. Biopsy of an affected organ reveals capillaritis, glomerulonephritis, and/or leukocytoclastic vasculitis in the absence of granulomas.

Management
Like GPA, MPA treatment requires high-dose glucocorticoids plus cyclophosphamide for 6 months, followed by maintenance therapy with methotrexate, azathioprine, or mycophenolate mofetil. As in GPA, rituximab for MPA has recently shown promise. **H**

Eosinophilic Granulomatosis with Polyangiitis
Epidemiology and Pathophysiology
Eosinophilic granulomatosis with polyangiitis (EGPA) is the rarest ANCA-associated vasculitis. Strong association of EGPA with asthma and eosinophilia suggests an atopic trigger.

Clinical Manifestations and Diagnosis
Patients with EGPA report a preceding history of atopy, including allergic rhinitis, nasal polyps, or asthma. The symptomatology of EGPA depends upon localization of the vasculitis. Lung disease is common, manifested as infiltrates and capillaritis. Peripheral nerve disease is more common in EGPA than in other ANCA vasculitides, presenting as mono- or polyneuropathy or mononeuritis multiplex. Kidney disease is somewhat less common than in other ANCA diseases. Hypereosinophilia, in both the peripheral blood and involved tissues, is characteristic; a diagnosis of EGPA should be revisited in the absence of eosinophils. Tissue biopsy shows necrotizing vasculitis with eosinophilic infiltrates. Eosinophilic granulomas may be seen in the tissues as well as the vessels. IgE levels are frequently elevated. EGPA patients who are ANCA-positive typically display the p-ANCA/anti-MPO pattern. Because up to 40% of patients are ANCA-negative, a negative ANCA test should not eliminate EGPA as a diagnosis.

Management
One unique aspect of EGPA may be the sensitivity of eosinophils to glucocorticoids. In patients with mild or limited disease, glucocorticoid treatment alone may therefore be sufficient. In more severe disease, glucocorticoids plus cyclophosphamide is preferred, followed by maintenance therapy with a less toxic immunosuppressive agent. As in all ANCA diseases, the potential for permanent tissue damage mandates an early and aggressive approach if full return to function is to be anticipated. **H**

KEY POINTS

- Granulomatosis with polyangiitis (formerly known as Wegener granulomatosis) typically affects the upper respiratory tract, lungs, and kidneys and is associated with c-ANCA and antiproteinase 3 (PR3) antibody positivity. *(Continued)*

KEY POINTS *(continued)*

- Microscopic polyangiitis typically involves the kidneys and lungs, and patients classically express p-ANCA and antimyeloperoxidase (MPO) antibodies.

- Treatment of both granulomatosis with polyangiitis and microscopic polyangiitis consists of high-dose glucocorticoids plus cyclophosphamide for approximately 6 months, followed by maintenance therapy.

- Eosinophilic granulomatosis with polyangiitis is associated with atopy, hypereosinophilia, lung disease, and peripheral nerve disease; glucocorticoids may be sufficient for mild/limited disease, and more severe disease may be treated with glucocorticoids plus cyclophosphamide, followed by maintenance therapy.

Immune Complex-Mediated Vasculitis
Several vasculitides arise from the formation of immune complexes. If not cleared, such complexes deposit in small vessels, activate complement, and recruit neutrophils. Any organ may be affected, but skin and joint involvement is common. Dermal capillaritis characteristically allows erythrocyte extravasation (palpable purpura), worse in dependent areas. Influxed neutrophils undergo cell death and breakup (clasis) as well as release of pyknotic nuclei (nuclear dust), a process designated as leukocytoclastic vasculitis (**Figure 33**).

Cryoglobulinemic Vasculitis
Epidemiology and Pathophysiology
In cryoglobulinemic vasculitis, antibodies have the special characteristic of precipitating in vitro at temperatures below normal body temperature (37.0 °C [98.6 °F]). The immune complex formation that typically occurs in vivo in these diseases may not relate to this cryoglobulinemic property because body core temperature is sufficient to prevent cold-induced precipitation. However, severe cold exposure of the fingertips, ear helices, and tip of the nose may result in cold-related precipitation, vascular ischemia, and infarction.

Three types of cryoglobulins are recognized (**Table 35**). Type I is a monoclonal antibody, often resulting from hematologic malignancy. Type I cryoglobulins rarely form immune complexes in vivo but may cause hyperviscosity. Type II cryoglobulins consist of a polyclonal IgG antibody together with a monoclonal IgM with rheumatoid factor activity (that is, binds to other immunoglobulins, contributing to immune complex formation). Type II cryoglobulins precipitate ex vivo in the cold but also form immune complexes in vivo to generate vascular inflammation. Ninety percent of patients with type II cryoglobulinemia have chronic hepatitis C virus infection, which furnishes the antigen(s) for immune complex formation; the remaining 10% are idiopathic and designated as

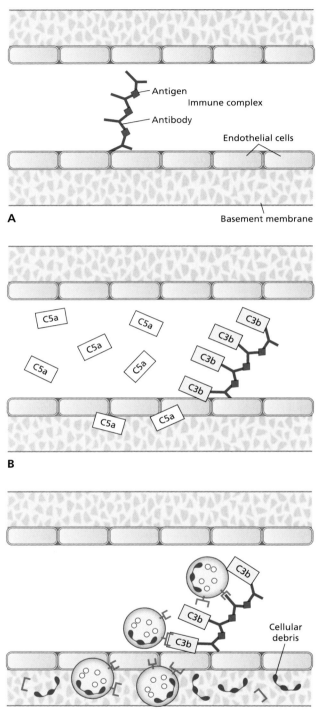

TABLE 35. Types of Cryoglobulins

Type	Composition	Common Underlying Conditions
I	Monoclonal IgM	Hematologic malignancy (e.g., Waldenstrom macroglobulinemia, multiple myeloma)
II	Polyclonal IgG + monoclonal IgM rheumatoid factor	Chronic hepatitis C infection; HIV infection; idiopathic (essential mixed)
III	Polyclonal IgG + polyclonal IgM rheumatoid factor	Autoimmune disease (e.g., systemic lupus erythematosus, rheumatoid arthritis)

essential mixed cryoglobulinemia. Type III cryoglobulins are also mixed but consist of polyclonal IgG together with polyclonal IgM rheumatoid factor. Type III cryoglobulins typically occur secondary to other autoimmune diseases and resolve with appropriate disease treatment.

Clinical Manifestations and Diagnosis

As in all immune complex vasculitides, palpable purpura is the characteristic rash in type II cryoglobulinemia. Other organs characteristically involved include peripheral nerves and the kidneys (glomerulonephritis). Less commonly, gastrointestinal, central nervous system, and other organ involvement occurs.

Diagnosis depends upon recognition of palpable purpura in the setting of other relevant organ involvement. Positivity for hepatitis C suggests but does not prove a diagnosis of type II cryoglobulinemia. Characteristically, patients with cryoglobulinemic vasculitis manifest evidence of complement activation, with C4 disproportionately low relative to C3. Inflammatory markers are typically elevated. Absence of rheumatoid factor argues against type II or type III cryoglobulinemia. Cryoglobulins can be assessed directly in serum from blood that has been allowed to clot at 37.0 °C (98.6 °F). In patients with cryoglobulinemia, such serum, when incubated at 4.0 °C (39.2 °F), forms cryoprecipitates, the extent of which can be expressed as a volume-percent (cryocrit).

Management

Definitive cryoglobulinemia treatment requires clearance of the driving antigen. For patients with hepatitis C–related type II cryoglobulinemia, this means resolving the hepatitis C infection with antiviral therapy. However, if the vasculitic organ involvement is severe, reduction of cryoglobulins themselves is imperative. Classic treatment involves glucocorticoids, cyclophosphamide, and plasmapheresis. More recently, anti–B-cell therapy with rituximab has demonstrated efficacy at reducing cryoglobulinemia and may provide a less toxic alternative. **H**

FIGURE 33. The process of classic immune complex–mediated small-vessel vasculitis. A, In the setting of antigen/antibody balance, immune complexes form that may become trapped in small vessels. B, The formation of immune complexes lead to complement activation by the classical pathway, particularly including the generation of C3b (an opsonin) and C5a (a chemoattractant). C, The presence of C5a attracts neutrophils, which engage C3b and antibody Fc tails to undergo further activation. Neutrophils also invade the vascular wall. Some neutrophils undergo cell death and breakdown (leukocytoclasis), resulting in the presence of cellular fragments within the vessel wall.

Henoch-Schönlein Purpura

Epidemiology and Pathophysiology

Henoch-Schönlein purpura (HSP) is the most common childhood vasculitis (incidence, 20/100,000) and tends to appear after upper respiratory infections. HSP is rarer among adults. The HSP antigen is unknown, but the immune complex antibodies are unique in belonging to the IgA subfamily.

Clinical Manifestations and Diagnosis

The characteristic symptoms of HSP are abdominal pain and palpable purpura. Purpuric lesions commonly occur on palms and soles. Gastrointestinal ischemia may be severe enough to cause intestinal bleeding. Arthritis is common, and other organ systems may be involved; patients with HSP may present with glomerulonephritis.

The diagnosis is based on the clinical picture in both children and adults. Laboratory studies are nonspecific but confirm systemic inflammation. Diagnosis is established by biopsy of the affected organ. Skin biopsy will show leukocytoclastic vasculitis and, on immunofluorescence, IgA and C3 complement deposition. Kidney biopsy will show IgA nephropathy. Serum IgA levels may be elevated.

Management

Pediatric HSP is typically self-limiting, and treatment usually requires only supportive care. When more severe organ involvement occurs, glucocorticoids may be considered but have limited benefit on the purpura and nephritis. Adults tend to experience a more severe course, are more likely to relapse, and are typically treated with glucocorticoids.

Hypersensitivity Vasculitis

Epidemiology and Pathophysiology

Hypersensitivity vasculitis represents a hypersensitivity response to a known or unknown antigen, such as a drug or infection. As in the other small-vessel vasculitides, hypersensitivity vasculitis typically results from immune complex formation and deposition. Complement is activated, and neutrophils accumulate in capillaries, arterioles, and postcapillary venules, often resulting in the classic pathologic appearance of a leukocytoclastic vasculitis. In contrast to HSP, IgA is usually not involved.

Clinical Manifestations and Diagnosis

As in all immune complex vasculitides, the characteristic rash of hypersensitivity vasculitis is palpable purpura (**Figure 34**). Other rashes, including vesicles, pustules, maculopapular lesions, and urticaria, may occur. Other organ systems are usually spared.

Management

Definitive hypersensitivity vasculitis management consists of removing the offending antigen, after which the rash should resolve within weeks. When the rash is severe, or if removal of

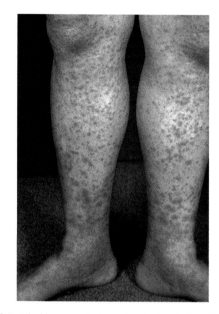

FIGURE 34. Palpable purpura is shown, the classic rash of small-vessel, immune complex–mediated vasculitides. The lesions are nonblanching and represent extravasations of blood from damaged vessels. Purpuric lesions are typically more prominent on the lower extremities, a consequence of the superimposed effect of gravity on oncotic pressure.

the antigen is not readily accomplished, most clinicians consider prednisone to resolve the inflammatory component. Other agents that may help improve hypersensitivity vasculitis include colchicine, dapsone, and NSAIDs.

KEY POINTS

- Ninety percent of patients with type II cryoglobulinemia have chronic hepatitis C virus infection.

- Palpable purpura is the characteristic rash in type II cryoglobulinemia; other organs characteristically involved include peripheral nerves and the kidneys.

- Henoch-Schönlein purpura occurs mainly in children, and characteristic symptoms are abdominal pain and palpable purpura; this disease is typically self-limiting.

- Hypersensitivity vasculitis presents as palpable purpura and represents a hypersensitivity response to an antigen that typically resolves when the offending agent is removed.

Systemic Sclerosis

Introduction

Systemic sclerosis (SSc) is an autoimmune disease characterized by fibrosis, with resultant thickening and hardening of the skin (scleroderma). Internal organ involvement is common and causes significant morbidity and mortality.

Pathophysiology

Deposition of increased amounts of structurally normal collagen is the classic finding of SSc and the cause of most clinical manifestations. This fibrosing phenotype is accompanied by autoimmunity as well as small artery endothelial damage and dysfunction. Fibroblast activation and collagen deposition lead to tissue fibrosis in skin and other organs due to the complex interactions between the immune system, interstitium, and vasculature. The impact of each of these factors is variable and leads to heterogeneity in the clinical features.

The triggering and initial proliferating events of SSc remain undefined. No consistent environmental trigger has been identified. A role for heredity is supported by genetic loci associated with the disease, but these are shared with other autoimmune diseases and provide limited insight into the generation of the SSc phenotype.

Epidemiology

Annual incidence of SSc is 1 to 2/100,000 persons, and prevalence is 19 to 75/100,000. Peak age of onset occurs between 30 and 50 years, with a female predominance (3:1 ratio). SSc is more common (and perhaps more severe) in black persons.

Classification

SSc is the most characteristic of the scleroderma spectrum disorders, a group of diseases sharing the feature of skin hardening. The scleroderma spectrum disorders include SSc, localized scleroderma (in which fibrosis is histopathologically identical to SSc but limited to a single patch of the skin), and scleroderma-like conditions (which include other disorders associated with thickened, sclerotic skin). SSc is further characterized as two distinct subsets based on skin involvement: diffuse cutaneous systemic sclerosis (DcSSc) and limited cutaneous systemic sclerosis (LcSSc).

Table 36 describes the common manifestations and features of the scleroderma spectrum disorders.

KEY POINTS

- Diffuse cutaneous systemic sclerosis is characterized by extensive distal and proximal skin thickening (chest, abdomen, and arms proximal to wrists) and is commonly accompanied by internal organ fibrosis.
- Limited cutaneous systemic sclerosis is characterized by distal (face, neck, and hands), but not proximal, skin thickening; it is usually unaccompanied by internal organ fibrosis but is more likely to be associated with pulmonary arterial hypertension.

Diagnosis

SSc should be suspected in the presence of symmetric skin induration on the hands, arms, face, and/or torso. Isolated skin induration without any other features occurs in less than 10% of patients with SSc. Sclerodactyly (skin fibrosis of the fingers or toes) and characteristic extracutaneous features are often present and support the diagnosis. Skin induration plus one or more of the following extracutaneous features strongly suggests the diagnosis of SSc: Raynaud phenomenon, digital infarction, and/or pitting; heartburn, dysphagia, or diarrhea; hypertension and/or kidney disease; dyspnea on exertion, interstitial lung disease, or pulmonary arterial hypertension; or mucocutaneous telangiectasias. Skin thickening confined to a single area suggests localized scleroderma in its various forms; internal organ involvement is extremely rare in these limited conditions (see Table 36).

In patients with skin thickening and clinical features suggestive of SSc, autoantibody testing is done to further support the diagnosis. Antinuclear antibodies are often present (70% prevalence). Anticentromere antibodies are associated with LcSSc (15%-40% prevalence) and the CREST (calcinosis, Raynaud phenomenon, esophageal dysmotility, sclerodactyly, and telangiectasia) syndrome, whereas anti–Scl-70 antibodies are associated with DcSSc (15%-40% prevalence). Patients who have DcSSc without anti–Scl-70 antibodies may instead have antibodies to an alternative antigen, RNA polymerase III. Still other autoantibodies have been identified whose sensitivity for SSc is low (20%) but whose specificity is high (>95%) (**Table 37**).

A skin biopsy is usually not needed to confirm the diagnosis because the findings are classic and characteristic.

KEY POINT

- In patients with skin thickening and clinical features suggestive of systemic sclerosis, autoantibody testing (antinuclear, anti–Scl-70, anticentromere, and anti–RNA polymerase III) is done to further support the diagnosis.

Clinical Manifestations and Management

Treatments addressing the underlying mechanisms of SSc have yet to be developed. Instead, therapeutic options currently focus on managing individual organ manifestations.

Cutaneous Involvement

Skin thickening occurs in most patients with SSc. Skin involvement varies in both the extent of body surface involved and the severity of induration. In LcSSc, scleroderma is restricted to the hands and, to a lesser extent, the face and neck. Scleroderma involving the chest, abdomen, forearms, upper arms, and shoulders indicates DcSSc.

In early SSc, swelling, edema, and erythema of the hands and forearms may precede skin induration. Pruritus may be a significant symptom. Sclerodactyly may develop (**Figure 35**, on page 80), and vascular involvement (see Vascular Involvement)

TABLE 36. Common Manifestations/Features of the Scleroderma Spectrum Disorders

Disorder	Manifestation/Feature	Comments
Systemic Sclerosis		
Diffuse cutaneous systemic sclerosis (DcSSc)	Distal and proximal skin thickening (chest, abdomen, arms proximal to wrists); commonly has visceral organ involvement	Skin involvement is extensive and is commonly accompanied by internal organ fibrosis and ILD
Limited cutaneous systemic sclerosis (LcSSc)	Distal (face, neck, hands), but not proximal, skin thickening; typically not accompanied by internal organ fibrosis	More likely to develop PAH and Raynaud phenomenon early in disease and display features of the CREST syndrome
Systemic sclerosis sine scleroderma	Fibrosing organ involvement without skin thickening	Difficult to diagnose; prognosis may be similar to LcSSc
Localized Scleroderma		
Morphea	Plaques generally on the trunk	Systemic manifestations or Raynaud phenomenon is extremely rare
Linear scleroderma	Streaks/lines of thickened skin	Same as above
Scleroderma-like Conditions[a]		
Eosinophilic fasciitis	Orange peel induration (peau d'orange) of proximal extremities with sparing of hands and face; peripheral eosinophilia; skin retraction over the superficial veins may be more apparent with elevation of an affected limb	Full-thickness skin biopsy demonstrates lymphocytes, plasma cells, and eosinophils infiltrating the deep fascia; glucocorticoids are the mainstay of treatment
Nephrogenic systemic fibrosis	Secondary to gadolinium in patients with kidney disease; brawny, wood-like induration of extremities, sparing the digits	Skeletal muscle fibrosis with contractures and/or cardiac muscle involvement can occur, with cardiomyopathy and increased mortality; changes in use and formulation of gadolinium have reduced incidence
Scleredema	Indurated plaques/patches on back, shoulder girdle, and neck	Typically seen in long-standing diabetes mellitus
Scleromyxedema	Waxy, yellow-red papules over thickened skin of face, upper trunk, neck, and arms; deposition of mucin with large numbers of stellate fibroblasts in the dermis	Associated with paraproteinemia (IgGλ) and may therefore occur in the setting of multiple myeloma or AL amyloidosis; more frequent in men
Chronic graft versus host disease	Lichen planus–like skin lesions or localized or generalized skin thickening	Occurs most commonly after hematopoietic stem cell transplantation; may occasionally be seen after blood transfusion in an immunocompromised host
Drug and toxin exposure	Can produce scleroderma-like tissue changes	Examples: bleomycin, docetaxel, pentazocine, L-tryptophan, organic solvents

CREST = calcinosis cutis, Raynaud phenomenon, esophageal dysmotility, sclerodactyly, and telangiectasia; ILD = interstitial lung disease; PAH = pulmonary arterial hypertension.

[a]Sclerderma-like skin changes may also occur as a manifestation of systemic endocrine, kidney, or infiltrative disorders.

TABLE 37. Autoantibodies and Their Associations in Systemic Sclerosis

Autoantibody	Clinical Associations	Comments
Antinuclear	DcSSc; LcSSc	Overall prevalence in SSc: 70%; not associated with specific manifestations
Anticentromere (kinetochore proteins)	LcSSc ± PAH	Overall prevalence in SSc about 30%; highly associated (>90%) with CREST variant of LcSSc
Anti–Scl-70 (DNA topoisomerase-1)	DcSSc; ILD	Overall prevalence in SSc: about 30%; highly associated with DcSSc
Anti-RNA polymerase III	DcSSc; kidney disease	Useful in DcSSc with negative Scl-70
Anti-U3-RNP (fibrillarin)	DcSSc; PAH; myositis	Associated with poor outcome; more common in black men
Anti-PM-Scl	Myositis	Associated with overlap syndrome and polymyositis
Anti-Ku	Myositis	Rare occurrence
Anti-Th/To	LcSSc; PAH	Rare occurrence

CREST= calcinosis, Raynaud phenomenon, esophageal dysmotility, sclerodactyly, and telangiectasias; DcSSc = diffuse cutaneous systemic sclerosis; ILD = interstitial lung disease; LcSSc = limited cutaneous systemic sclerosis; PAH = pulmonary arterial hypertension; RNP = ribonucleoprotein; SSc= systemic sclerosis.

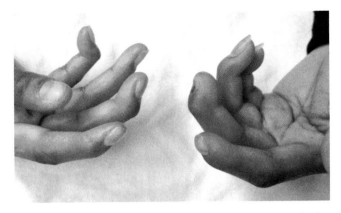

FIGURE 35. Sclerodactyly in a patient with systemic sclerosis. Indurated/tight skin of the fingers with resorption at the tips, leading to loss of pulp.

can result in digital ulcers and pitting of the fingertips (**Figure 36**). Some patients develop telangiectasias and calcinosis cutis. Scleroderma of the face may lead to the reduction of skin wrinkles and limitation of the oral aperture. Late in the disease, induration improves and skin may become soft and thin, making the diagnosis difficult.

SSc pruritus is managed symptomatically with antihistamines and skin emollients. Limited data suggest that the early inflammatory phases of skin disease may respond to systemic glucocorticoids, weekly methotrexate, or other immunosuppressive therapies, and a therapeutic trial can be considered. However, glucocorticoids may potentiate the risk of renal crisis (see Kidney Involvement) and should be administered cautiously. The indurated, thickened phase of skin involvement

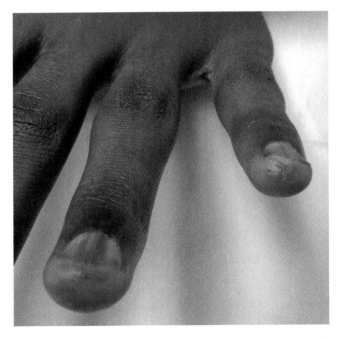

FIGURE 36. Digital pitting in a patient with systemic sclerosis. Digital pits and hyperkeratosis at the tips of the fourth and fifth fingers.

responds poorly to therapy; no treatment has been shown to be consistently effective.

Musculoskeletal Involvement

In addition to hand swelling, patients with early SSc (especially DcSSc) often develop arthralgia, myalgia, and fatigue. Inflammatory arthritis with palpable tenderness and joint swelling is atypical; joint erosions should suggest an overlap with rheumatoid arthritis. Later in the disease, fibrosis of the periarticular structures leads to joint pain, immobility, and contractures, especially in the fingers and extremities. Fibrosis around tendons is sometimes associated with palpable and/or audible deep tendon friction rubs, which occur more commonly in DcSSc and may connote aggressive disease and internal organ involvement. Fibrosis also occurs around nerves, causing cranial and peripheral entrapment neuropathies and occasionally producing autonomic neuropathy. Fibrosis within muscle can lead to myopathy; myositis has also been reported.

Low-dose systemic glucocorticoids, methotrexate, and leflunomide may help treat inflammatory arthritis and myositis but have limited efficacy for other SSc musculoskeletal manifestations. Surgical release of entrapped nerves can relieve compressive symptoms. Surgical tendon release and/or reconstruction may occasionally be an option.

Vascular Involvement

Raynaud phenomenon (sequential white, blue, and red color changes in the digits precipitated by cold or stress) occurs in almost all patients with SSc. Raynaud phenomenon is initially transient and reversible; later, structural changes develop within small blood vessels, resulting in permanently impaired flow that produces acrocyanosis, digital pitting, and/or ulcerations. In contrast, primary Raynaud disease is commonly seen in young women, has a benign and usually self-limiting course, and does not cause vascular damage and digital ulcerations. It can be followed periodically in the absence of digital pits or nailfold capillary abnormalities.

In patients with LcSSc, Raynaud phenomenon may precede other disease manifestations by years or decades. In contrast, Raynaud phenomenon among DcSSc patients usually coincides with the appearance of skin and/or musculoskeletal manifestations. Office-based examination of the nailfold capillaries of patients with SSc using a dermatoscope or ophthalmoscope reveals both capillary destruction and dilated capillary loops, which can distinguish SSc from primary Raynaud as well as nonvascular causes of tissue fibrosis (**Figure 37**).

Avoidance of cold exposure, keeping core temperature warm to increase shunting of blood flow peripherally, and avoiding smoking reduce the risk of Raynaud episodes. Calcium channel blockers, antiplatelet agents, and topical nitrates are first-line pharmacotherapy and can reduce the number and severity of episodes. Refractory patients may be treated with phosphodiesterase-5 inhibitors (sildenafil or tadalafil). Endothelin-1 blockers can also be effective and may prevent

FIGURE 37. A 40× magnification of the nailfold using wide-field microscopy revealing a capillary pattern characterized by dilatation in some areas and avascularity in others during the "active phase" of diffuse cutaneous systemic sclerosis.

recurrences of digital ulcerations. Regional sympathetic blockade or digital sympathectomy may be tried to reverse vasospasm and save an at-risk digit; localized injection of botulinum toxin A has also shown promise. Surgical debridement and amputations may be needed for severe ischemia and gangrene that does not respond to salvage therapy.

Gastrointestinal Involvement

More than 70% of patients with SSc have clinical gastrointestinal involvement. Upper involvement is common, with fibrosis causing pharyngeal dysfunction, esophageal hypomotility, and lower esophageal sphincter incompetence. Consequences include dysphagia, chronic gastroesophageal reflux, esophagitis, stricture, Barrett esophagus, and pulmonary microaspiration. Vascular abnormalities in the stomach cause angiodysplasias of the gastric antral mucosal lining (so-called watermelon stomach), resulting in recurrent bleeding and chronic anemia. Involvement of the intestines causes dysmotility, malabsorption, and blind loop formation. Patients may present with bloating, weight loss, alternating constipation and diarrhea, and pseudo-obstruction. Wide-mouthed diverticula may be seen on imaging studies of the colon but are rarely of clinical significance. Primary biliary cirrhosis may occur, especially in patients with LcSSc. Anal involvement can cause fecal incontinence.

H$_2$ blockers and proton pump inhibitors are effective therapies for esophagitis and gastritis. Dysmotility is managed with promotility agents such as metoclopramide; in refractory cases, octreotide can be tried. Malabsorption due to bacterial overgrowth is evaluated through glucose hydrogen breath testing and may be managed with rotating courses of antibiotics. Patients may also need nutritional support as well as enzyme and vitamin supplementation. Pseudo-obstruction is managed conservatively with bowel rest and proximal decompression as needed. Gastritis and vascular ectasia are evaluated with upper endoscopy; ectasias can be ablated with laser/photocoagulation.

Kidney Involvement

Kidney involvement is common in patients with SSc. Up to 50% of patients have mild proteinuria, elevation in the plasma creatinine concentration, and/or hypertension, but most do not progress to chronic kidney disease. Kidney involvement is more common and more severe in DcSSc. The most striking and life-threatening manifestation of kidney disease is scleroderma renal crisis (SRC). SRC occurs in 10% to 15% of patients, is more frequent in DcSSc, and tends to occur early in the disease course; if untreated, it carries a mortality rate approaching 90%. In SRC, involvement of afferent arterioles leads to glomerular ischemia and hyperreninemia. The typical presentation is acute kidney injury and severe hypertension, mild proteinuria, urinalysis with few cells or casts, microangiopathic hemolytic anemia, and thrombocytopenia. Some patients develop pulmonary edema and hypertensive encephalopathy. Occasionally, patients remain normotensive despite kidney dysfunction.

ACE inhibitors significantly improve kidney survival and decrease mortality among patients with SRC. The mechanism of action of ACE inhibitors is believed to be mitigation of the effect of interstitial fibrosis and vascular dysfunction in the glomerular arterial bed. Treatment with an ACE inhibitor should be initiated promptly in SSc patients with even mild hypertension or otherwise unexplained elevations in serum creatinine levels. The ACE inhibitor should be up-titrated until good control of blood pressure is achieved and continued even in the setting of kidney disease. Prophylactic use of ACE inhibitors in normotensive patients is controversial, with some studies suggesting worse overall outcomes. Angiotensin receptor blockers (ARBs) are an alternative for patients who cannot take ACE inhibitors, although ARBs are less effective for managing SRC.

Pulmonary Involvement

Pulmonary involvement is frequent (>70%) in patients with SSc and can be symptomatic and disabling. The two principal clinical manifestations are interstitial lung disease and pulmonary vascular disease. Other pulmonary manifestations include pleuritis, recurrent aspiration, organizing pneumonia, and hemorrhage from endobronchial telangiectasias. Patients with SSc also have an increased risk for developing lung cancer.

Interstitial Lung Disease

Interstitial lung disease (ILD) usually develops subacutely with progressive fibrosis. Patients with DcSSc and anti–Scl-70 antibodies are at higher risk for developing ILD. The most common symptom of ILD is slowly progressive dyspnea, at first on exertion, but later at rest. Other symptoms include nonproductive cough, decreased exercise tolerance, and chest pain. Auscultation reveals "Velcro"-like inspiratory crackles, most prominent at the lung bases. Some patients develop acute inflammatory response/alveolitis or early pulmonary fibrosis in the absence of respiratory symptoms or physical findings. Pulmonary function testing reveals decreased lung volumes and decreased D$_{LCO}$. High-resolution noncontrast chest CT reveals ground glass and reticular linear opacities in patients with alveolitis or fibrosis, and honeycombing in the later stages. Lung biopsy is rarely needed but may be useful in patients with atypical presentations or concern about other diseases such as infection or cancer.

Patients with SSc who have evidence of alveolitis and/or rapidly progressive lung disease may be treated with immunosuppressive agents. Oral or intravenous cyclophosphamide provides modest benefit in the first year, but these benefits are lost by 24 months of follow-up. Azathioprine may have a role as maintenance therapy following a 6-month course of cyclophosphamide. High-dose glucocorticoids are frequently used in SSc patients with ILD, but there is no clear evidence of their benefit, and their use may convey an increased risk of SRC.

Pulmonary Arterial Hypertension

Pulmonary vascular disease occurs in up to 40% of patients with SSc. Vascular disease leading to pulmonary arterial hypertension (PAH) may occur secondary to ILD (typically in DcSSC) or as an isolated process (typically in LcSSc). Patients are usually asymptomatic in early disease but later develop dyspnea on exertion and diminished exercise tolerance. Severe disease can lead to right-sided heart failure. Pulmonary artery thrombosis can also occur and is frequently fatal.

Pulmonary function tests and echocardiography are useful in the diagnosis and evaluation for PAH. Baseline and annual monitoring of PAH is recommended in all patients with SSc without advanced ILD. Pulmonary function tests demonstrate a reduced D_{LCO}, and echocardiogram can estimate pulmonary artery systolic pressure in the presence of tricuspid regurgitation. Right heart catheterization (RHC) should be performed prior to initiation of treatment. RHC can accurately document the pressure, follow the readings, assess responsiveness to vasodilators, and guide choice of treatment.

All patients with PAH should be considered for oxygen supplementation. Anticoagulation should be considered after bleeding risk assessment. Vasodilating agents, including phosphodiesterase-5 inhibitors (sildenafil or vardenafil) and prostacyclin analogues (iloprost, epoprostenol, or treprostinil), have demonstrated efficacy in relieving symptoms of PAH associated with SSc. Endothelin receptor antagonists (bosentan and ambrisentan) have also shown efficacy in improving symptoms and delaying progression of PAH in SSc. Select patients may benefit from a vasodilator in combination with an endothelin receptor antagonist. Patients with PAH must be closely monitored using 6-minute walk tests and serial RHC studies.

Cardiac Involvement

Cardiac involvement in SSc may be due to cardiac fibrosis or coronary artery disease or secondarily due to systemic or pulmonary hypertension. Intrinsic cardiac fibrosis is uncommon and usually asymptomatic. Symptomatic cardiac involvement in SSc is rare (10%-20% prevalence) but has a poor prognosis, with 5-year mortality rates of 75%. Pericarditis and pericardial effusion occur but are rarely symptomatic. Coronary artery vasospasm and structural disease lead to contraction band necrosis (pathologic finding of ischemia followed by reperfusion due to vasospasm) and patchy myocardial fibrosis, promoting cardiomyopathy and heart failure. Conduction disturbances and arrhythmias are common and probably relate to fibrosis of the conduction system. Many deaths among patients with SSc are sudden and possibly a result of ventricular arrhythmia.

There is no specific treatment for cardiac fibrosis. Management of the complications and consequences of SSc cardiac disease should be carried out in collaboration with an experienced cardiologist.

KEY POINTS

- In early systemic sclerosis, swelling, edema, and erythema of the hands and forearms may precede skin induration, and pruritus, sclerodactyly, and digital ulcers and pitting may develop.

- Upper gastrointestinal involvement is common in systemic sclerosis, with fibrosis causing pharyngeal dysfunction, esophageal hypomotility, and lower esophageal sphincter incompetence.

- Nailfold capillarioscopy can distinguish secondary Raynaud phenomenon associated with systemic sclerosis from primary Raynaud phenomenon.

- ACE inhibitors significantly improve kidney survival and decrease mortality among patients with scleroderma renal crisis.

- Baseline and annual monitoring of pulmonary arterial hypertension is recommended for all patients with systemic sclerosis without advanced interstitial lung disease.

Pregnancy and Systemic Sclerosis

Pregnancy in patients with SSc carries an increased risk of spontaneous miscarriage and abortion as well as increased rates of premature birth and low-birth-weight full-term infants. Pregnant patients with SSc may develop decompensated pulmonary arterial hypertension or scleroderma renal crisis, each carrying a high complication and/or mortality rate. It may be difficult to distinguish SSc kidney dysfunction from preeclampsia or eclampsia. Many medications useful in SSc are contraindicated in pregnancy. Management by an experienced physician is therefore imperative. See Principles of Therapeutics for more information on medications and pregnancy.

KEY POINT

- Pregnancy in patients with systemic sclerosis carries an increased risk of spontaneous miscarriage and abortion as well as increased rates of premature births and low-birth-weight full-term infants.

Other Rheumatologic Diseases

Behçet Syndrome

Behçet syndrome is a form of vasculitis that affects small to large arterial vessels and can affect veins as well. All patients with this syndrome have recurrent painful oral ulcerations; patients may also demonstrate additional distinctive features, including hypopyon (**Figure 38**) and pathergy (**Figure 39**). Behçet syndrome is more common among individuals living in or with ancestry from East Asia to Turkey; prevalence is 6.6/100,000 in the United States, but 300/100,000 in Turkey. A genetic role in Behçet pathogenesis is underlined by the increased prevalence of HLA-B51 among affected individuals. Diagnostic criteria are listed in **Table 38**.

Other major manifestations include pulmonary artery, aorta, and/or femoral artery inflammation (3%-12% of patients). Aneurysms and stenosis can occur. A rare variant of Behçet is Hughes-Stovin syndrome, characterized by pulmonary artery aneurysms and systemic thrombophlebitis. Central nervous system involvement occurs in 3% to 25% and can include headaches, stroke, pyramidal signs, behavioral changes, or, rarely, dural sinus thrombosis. Gastrointestinal involvement may be hard to distinguish from inflammatory

TABLE 38. The International Study Group Diagnostic Criteria for Behçet Syndrome
Recurrent painful oral ulceration (≥3 times in a 12-month period) is a mandatory feature for diagnosis. Ulcers can occur anywhere in the mouth or on the tongue and often resolve spontaneously within a few weeks.
At least two of the following are also required for diagnosis:
Recurrent painful genital ulceration: These ulcers are found on the scrotum in men or the labia in women and may lead to scarring.
Eye involvement: Panuveitis, isolated anterior uveitis or posterior uveitis, or retinal vasculitis can occur and be vision threatening. Hypopyon is a distinctive feature of the anterior uveitis of Behçet, in which a fluid collection of leukocytes is visible in the anterior chamber.
Skin involvement: Erythema nodosum, pseudofolliculitis, or acneiform lesions can occur. Acneiform lesion on trunk or thighs should raise a concern for Behçet and may demonstrate small-vessel vasculitis on biopsy.
Pathergy test: In some patients with Behçet, transient subcutaneous insertion of a sterile, large-bore needle under the skin results in the development of a pustule at the site 24-48 hours later. Positive pathergy tests occur more commonly in endemic areas and are rare in the United States.

bowel disease, but ulceration typically involves the ileum rather than the rectal or perianal regions and does not lead to fistula formation.

Treatment is commensurate with disease severity. Low-dose prednisone or colchicine is used for oral/genital ulcers, and high-dose prednisone and immunomodulating agents such as azathioprine are used for more severe disease. Tumor necrosis factor (TNF)-α inhibitors, interferon alfa, and anti-interleukin (IL)-1β therapy have been used in recalcitrant or severe cases.

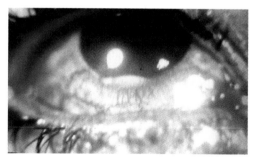

FIGURE 38. The eye of this patient with Behçet syndrome shows hypopyon, a layered collection of pus in the anterior chamber, representing a form of anterior uveitis. In addition to Behçet, hypopyon may indicate the presence of other autoimmune diseases, sight-threatening infectious keratitis, or endophthalmitis.

> **KEY POINT**
> - Behçet syndrome is characterized by recurrent painful oral ulcers plus at least two of the following: recurrent genital ulcers, eye involvement, skin involvement, and pathergy.

Relapsing Polychondritis

Relapsing polychondritis (RP) is an inflammatory disease affecting cartilaginous tissues and is thought to be driven by an autoimmune response to type II collagen. **Table 39** presents the McAdams criteria for RP. Auricular involvement affects the helix but spares the earlobes (**Figure 40**). Nasal chondritis can result in collapse of the nasal bridge (saddle nose deformity), which can also be seen in trauma, granulomatosis with polyangiitis (formerly known as Wegener granulomatosis), cocaine use, congenital syphilis, and leprosy. Airway stenosis from tracheal ring involvement and aortitis/large-vessel vasculitis may occur and be life-threatening. In 30% of patients, RP coexists with other inflammatory/autoimmune diseases.

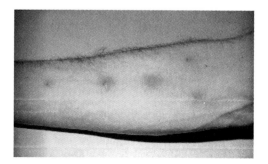

FIGURE 39. Pathergy, a pustule-like lesion or papule that appears 48 hours after a sterile skin prick by a 20- to 21-gauge needle in Behçet syndrome.

TABLE 39. McAdams Criteria for Diagnosis of Relapsing Polychondritis

Criteria[a]	Approximate Frequency
Recurrent bilateral auricular chondritis	90%
Nonerosive inflammatory polyarthritis	65%
Nasal chondritis	60%
Ocular inflammation (conjunctivitis, keratitis, scleritis/episcleritis, uveitis)	55%
Respiratory tract chondritis involving larynx or trachea	50%
Cochlear and/or vestibular dysfunction (neurosensory hearing loss, tinnitus, and/or vertigo)	10%

[a]Relapsing polychondritis is diagnosed when three of the six criteria are present.

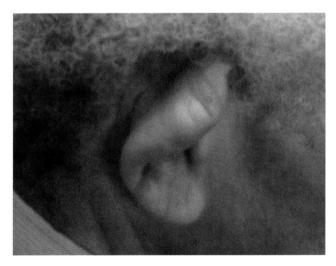

FIGURE 40. Floppy ears in a patient with relapsing polychondritis. Chronic inflammation of the upper section of the ear eventually results in loss of cartilage and structural collapse. The ear lobe, which does not contain cartilage, is unaffected.

Patients who develop RP in their 60s or 70s should be evaluated for myelodysplastic syndrome.

RP is diagnosed by its typical clinical manifestations. Laboratory tests are nonspecific; acute phase reactants are elevated in 80%, and mild anemia is present in 44%. Anti–type II collagen antibodies are present in 33% but are not considered diagnostic. Patients with RP should undergo imaging (CT or MRI) to evaluate the large airways for inflammation/stenosis. Cartilage biopsy is usually unnecessary.

Auricular chondritis typically responds to low-dose prednisone. For more severe manifestations (for example, laryngotracheal chondritis or aortitis), high-dose prednisone is initiated. For persistent disease and/or glucocorticoid sparing, dapsone, methotrexate, azathioprine, cyclosporine, and cyclophosphamide have all been used. Biologic agents such as tocilizumab (an IL-6 receptor antagonist) are currently being assessed.

KEY POINT

- Relapsing polychondritis is characterized by chondritis of the ears, nose, and/or respiratory tract; nonerosive inflammatory polyarthritis; ocular inflammation; and cochlear and/or vestibular dysfunction.

Adult-Onset Still Disease

Adult-onset Still disease (AOSD) is a multisystem inflammatory disease characterized by high spiking fevers, a salmon-colored rash, arthritis, and high neutrophil counts (**Table 40**). The cause is uncertain, but cytokines (for example, IL-1β, IL-6, TNF-α, and IL-18) are significantly elevated, reflecting macrophage hyperactivation.

Atypical manifestations that may influence prognosis include myocarditis, disseminated intravascular coagulation, fulminant hepatitis, and the hemophagocytic syndrome, a life-threatening process characterized by fever, splenomegaly, cytopenias, elevated ferritin, and evidence of hemophagocytosis on bone marrow biopsy.

AOSD diagnosis is clinically based and requires exclusion of infection, malignancy, or other rheumatologic diseases. Erythrocyte sedimentation rate and C-reactive protein can be markedly elevated. Serum ferritin is elevated in 78% of patients, often to extremely high levels, and

TABLE 40. Yamaguchi Criteria for the Diagnosis of Adult-Onset Still Disease

Major Criteria[a]	Approximate Frequency
Daily spiking fever to 39.0 °C (102.2 °F)	99%
Arthralgia/arthritis >2 weeks	85%
Nonpruritic salmon-colored macular/maculopapular rash on trunk or extremities	85%
Leukocyte count >10,000/µL (10 × 10⁹/L), >80% neutrophils	90%

Minor Criteria	Approximate Frequency
Sore throat	66%
Lymphadenopathy and/or splenomegaly	65%/50%
Elevated AST, ALT, or LDH	70%
Negative ANA and RF	N/A

ALT = alanine aminotransferase; ANA = antinuclear antibodies; AST = aspartate aminotransferase; LDH = lactate dehydrogenase; RF = rheumatoid factor.

[a]Diagnosis requires five criteria with at least two major criteria.

Adapted with permission from Yamaguchi M, Ohta A, Tsunematsu T, et al. Preliminary criteria for classification of adult Still's disease. J Rheumatol. 1992 Mar;19(3):424-30. [PMID: 1578458] implies macrophage activation. Lymph node biopsy shows a reactive process on histology.

Therapy for AOSD includes high-dose NSAIDs and/or prednisone, with methotrexate as a standard second-line agent. Recently, treatment approaches employing anti-IL-1β (for example, anakinra) or anti-IL-6 (for example, tocilizumab) therapies have shown significant promise.

KEY POINTS

- Characteristics of adult-onset Still disease include daily spiking fever, arthritis, a salmon-colored rash, and extremely elevated serum ferritin.

- Diagnosis of adult-onset Still disease is clinically based and requires exclusion of infection, malignancy, or other rheumatologic diseases.

Autoinflammatory Diseases

The autoinflammatory diseases (also known as periodic fever syndromes) are rare monogenic diseases characterized by autoactivation of the innate immune system, including myeloid leukocyte activation and overproduction of inflammatory cytokines. Patients experience regular episodes of systemic inflammation in the absence of infection or autoimmunity. Autoinflammatory diseases may be inherited or acquired through mutation. It is anticipated that more syndromes will be described in the coming years.

The classic autoinflammatory disease is familial Mediterranean fever (FMF), associated with mutation of the $MEFV_1$ gene that codes for pyrin, a regulator of IL-1β production. More than 40 different mutations in $MEFV_1$ have been identified that result in FMF. Attacks last 1 to 3 days and are characterized by polyserositis, arthritis, erysipeloid rash around the ankles, and elevation of acute phase reactants. AA amyloidosis is a potential long-term consequence of FMF and other autoinflammatory diseases due to the production and deposition of serum amyloid A. FMF management includes chronic daily treatment with colchicine. Increasingly, management of autoinflammatory diseases is being directed at specific cytokines that are implicated as pathogenic.

Table 41 lists the features of currently recognized autoinflammatory diseases.

TABLE 41. Autoinflammatory Diseases

	FMF	TRAPS	HIDS	FCAS	MWS	NOMID
Inheritance	Autosomal recessive	Autosomal dominant	Autosomal recessive	Autosomal dominant	Autosomal dominant	Autosomal dominant
Age at Onset	65% <10 years of age; 90% <20 years of age	50% <10 years of age; up to 5th decade	Usually <5 years of age	<1 year of age	Childhood	Neonatal period
Ethnicity	Mediterranean	All	Northern European	European	European	All
Clinical Manifestations						
Attack Duration	12-72 h	Days to weeks	3-7 days	12-24 h	1-2 days	Progressive
Abdominal	Pain; serositis	Pain; serositis	Pain; vomiting	Nausea	Pain	-
Pleuritis	Common	Common	Rare	-	Rare	Rare
Arthritis	Monoarthritis of lower extremities	Large joints	Symmetric polyarthritis of large joints	Arthralgia	Arthralgia; oligoarthritis	Epiphyseal overgrowth; contractures
Rash	Erysipeloid on lower legs	Migratory with underlying myalgia	Diffuse maculopapular	Cold-induced; urticaria-like	Urticaria-like	Urticaria-like
Other Manifestations	High risk for amyloidosis	Conjunctivitis; periorbital edema	Cutaneous vasculitis; lymphadenopathy; elevated IgD	Conjunctivitis; headache; amyloidosis	Sensorineural deafness; conjunctivitis; amyloidosis	Sensorineural deafness; aseptic meningitis; mental retardation
Treatment	Colchicine	Glucocorticoids; TNF-α inhibitors	NSAIDs; glucocorticoids	IL-1β inhibition	IL-1β inhibition	IL-1β inhibition

FCAS = familial cold autoinflammatory syndrome; FMF = familial Mediterranean fever; HIDS = hyperimmunoglobulinemia D with periodic fever syndrome; IL = interleukin; MWS = Muckle-Wells syndrome; NOMID = neonatal-onset multisystem inflammatory disease; TNF = tumor necrosis factor; TRAPS = tumor necrosis factor receptor-associated periodic syndrome.

KEY POINT

- Autoinflammatory diseases are characterized by episodes of systemic inflammation in the absence of infection or autoimmunity; these rare diseases may be inherited or acquired through mutation.

Sarcoidosis

Sarcoidosis is a multisystem disease characterized by noncaseating granulomas that form in tissues. Sarcoidosis most commonly affects the lungs and is therefore discussed in detail in MKSAP 17 Pulmonary and Critical Care Medicine. Although less common, the rheumatologic manifestations of sarcoidosis are important and discussed here.

Sarcoidosis can manifest as Löfgren syndrome, which is seen in younger adults and is characterized by acute arthritis, bilateral hilar lymphadenopathy, and erythema nodosum. When all three occur together, there is a 95% specificity for the diagnosis, and further diagnostic tests are unnecessary. The "arthritis" of Löfgren syndrome is actually a nondestructive periarthritis of the soft tissue, entheses, and tenosynovium. Symmetric ankle involvement is classic, but knees, wrists, and elbows can also be involved. Löfgren is more common among Europeans and is self-limited, with 90% of patients remitting within 12 months. Treatment is symptomatic and includes NSAIDs, colchicine, or low-dose glucocorticoids.

A more chronic form of true arthritis affects 1% to 4% of patients and occurs in more severe sarcoidosis. The arthritis is usually polyarticular, involving the shoulders, hands, wrists, knees, and ankles. An entire digit may be affected, leading to dactylitis. Black persons and those with sarcoid skin involvement are more likely to have chronic arthritis.

Granulomatous bone involvement occurs in 3% to 13% of patients, often those with more severe disease. The hands, feet, skull, ribs, sternum, nasal bones, pelvis, tibia, and femur may be affected. The radiographic pattern is lytic (focal areas of cyst formation), permeative (bone has a lacey appearance), or destructive.

Myopathy is a rare manifestation of systemic sarcoidosis. Acute myopathy can mimic polymyositis with proximal muscle weakness and muscle enzyme elevation. Chronic sarcoid myopathy affects older women, involves the proximal muscles, may have normal muscle enzymes, and occurs in the context of known disease. A nodular localized myopathy of sarcoidosis has also been described.

Granulomatous infiltration of the parotid glands may mimic Sjögren syndrome and produce sicca symptoms. The triad of sarcoid parotitis, uveitis, and fever is called uveoparotid fever or Heerfordt syndrome.

Sarcoid musculoskeletal involvement can be diagnosed via biopsy, and the extent and response to therapy can be gauged via gallium or PET scanning if needed. Treatment

involves glucocorticoids or other immunosuppressants such as methotrexate, azathioprine, or mycophenolate mofetil as dictated by the disease burden. TNF-α inhibitors may be useful in more severe disease or where glucocorticoid use is problematic.

KEY POINTS

- Sarcoidosis can manifest as Löfgren syndrome, which is characterized by acute arthritis, bilateral hilar lymphadenopathy, and erythema nodosum; when all three occur together, there is a 95% specificity for the diagnosis, and further diagnostic tests are unnecessary. **HVC**

- A chronic form of polyarticular arthritis can be found in severe sarcoidosis, which may affect the shoulders, hands, wrists, knees, and ankles; an entire digit may also be involved, leading to dactylitis.

True Connective Tissue Diseases

Ehlers-Danlos Syndrome

Ehlers-Danlos syndrome (EDS) defines a group of inherited genetic disorders of collagen-related (COL) genes or the procollagen lysyl hydroxylase (PLOD) gene, leading to defect(s) in the production, structure, or function of collagen. Most EDS variants are inherited as autosomal dominant mutations. EDS subcategories include the benign hypermobility type, the more severe kyphoscoliotic type, and the life-threatening vascular type in which large- to medium-sized vessels and organs such as the uterus or bowel can rupture.

EDS clinical characteristics include joint hypermobility, hyperextensible skin, atrophic scars, and velvety skin. Hypermobile joints may lead to joint dislocations or early osteoarthritis. Mitral, aortic, or tricuspid valve regurgitation may be present. Diagnosis is based on family history and clinical examination. Genetic consultation may be useful if the diagnosis is uncertain. Treatment is supportive. Patients with hypermobility should avoid activities that could lead to joint damage. Periodic echocardiography should assess cardiac status/aortic root size; invasive vascular procedures should be avoided for those with the vascular type of EDS.

EDS disorders require extensive counseling pertaining to issues of pregnancy both in terms of maternal complications of pregnancy and delivery as well as potential inherited disease in the child. Patients with vascular EDS should be evaluated promptly for any unexplained pain and should wear a medical alert identification bracelet.

Marfan Syndrome

Marfan syndrome (MFS) is an autosomal dominant condition characterized by a mutation in the gene for fibrillin 1 (FBN1). Fibrillin 1 is an important structural protein in tissues that contain elastic fibers, such as arteries, ligaments, and the structure that stabilizes the lens of the eye. Manifestations may relate to an overexpression of the cytokine transforming growth factor (TGF)-β. Clinical features include the following:

- Tall stature with short upper body to lower body ratio
- Arachnodactyly (long fingers; thumb and index finger overlap around the wrist)
- Anterior thoracic deformity: pectus excavatum or pectus carinatum
- Spinal curvature: scoliosis or kyphosis
- Hyperextensibility of skin
- Pes planus with a long narrow foot
- Myopia with dislocation of the lens (usually superiorly)
- Aortopathy of the ascending aorta: aortic regurgitation/dissection/aneurysm
- Mitral valve prolapse
- Pneumothorax from apical lung bullae
- Other: high arched palate, hernias, atrophic scarring over pectoral, deltoid, or lumbar areas

MFS diagnosis is made clinically, with genetic consultation if necessary. Testing for *FBN1* mutations is available. The 2012 revised Ghent criteria emphasize aortic root dilatation and lens dislocation for diagnosis but also include systemic features and *FBN1* mutations. Current guidelines recommend that echocardiography should be performed at the time of diagnosis to determine aortic root and ascending aortic diameters and 6 months later to determine their rate of enlargement. Annual imaging is recommended if stability of the aortic diameter is documented. If the maximal aortic diameter is 4.5 cm or greater, more frequent imaging should be considered.

For most patients with MFS, surgical repair of the dilated aortic root/ascending aorta is usually performed at a threshold of an external diameter of 5.0 cm. For women contemplating pregnancy, it is reasonable to prophylactically replace the aortic root and ascending aorta if the diameter is greater than 4.0 cm. β-Blockers are recommended to slow the aortopathy. Counseling regarding joint protection to prevent osteoarthritis is useful.

Osteogenesis Imperfecta

Osteogenesis imperfecta (OI) comprises four genetic syndromes characterized by autosomal dominant or recessive mutations in *COL* genes, leading to abnormalities in the structure of type I collagen. OI is associated with bone fractures, short stature, body deformity, hearing loss, and dental deformity. A characteristic feature of OI is blue sclerae (reflecting visibility of the underlying choroid) but is not specific to OI. Patients with pseudoxanthoma elasticum, ochronosis/alkaptonuria, Ehlers-Danlos syndrome, or Marfan syndrome may also have blue sclerae.

OI diagnosis is based on clinical findings and family history. Bisphosphonates may reduce fractures and improve skeletal growth, and orthopedic surgeons are often involved due to the fractures experienced by these patients.

KEY POINTS

- Clinical characteristics of Ehlers-Danlos syndrome include joint hypermobility, hyperextensible skin, atrophic scars, and velvety skin; diagnosis is based on family history and clinical examination.
- Marfan syndrome is associated with tall stature, arachnodactyly, anterior thoracic deformity, spinal curvature, and skin and ocular involvement; aortopathy and mitral valve prolapse are also common.
- Osteogenesis imperfecta is associated with bone fractures, short stature, body deformity, hearing loss, and dental deformity; blue sclerae is characteristic but nonspecific.

IgG4-Related Disease

IgG4-related disease is a recently recognized syndrome characterized by abundant IgG4-producing plasma cells seen on tissue biopsy; it unites an unlikely group of diseases under one banner (**Table 42**). Most of these conditions are characterized by infiltration of the affected tissue and the clinical consequences that infiltration entails. Almost any organ can be involved; lymph nodes are frequently affected. Most patients are men (60%-80%) older than age 50 years.

Diagnosis is made by tissue biopsy and the demonstration of a characteristic histology, which includes the following:

- Dense lymphoplasmacytic infiltrate
- CD4-positive T cells and plasma cells in germinal centers
- IgG4-staining plasma cells constituting more than 50% of the total plasma cells
- Storiform (spokes on a wheel–appearing) fibrosis
- Obliterative phlebitis
- Rare neutrophils and no granulomas

TABLE 42. Conditions Associated with IgG4-Related Disease

Condition	Organ Involved
Hypertrophic pachymeningitis	Dura mater
Lymphocytic hypophysitis	Pituitary gland
Idiopathic orbital inflammatory disease	Periocular mass
Mikulicz disease	Parotid glands
Dacryoadenitis	Lacrimal glands
Küttner tumor	Submandibular glands
Riedel thyroiditis	Thyroid
Inflammatory aortitis/vasculitis	Aorta/arteries
Autoimmune pancreatitis	Pancreas
Ormond disease (retroperitoneal fibrosis)	Periaortic mass
Tubulointerstitial nephropathy	Kidneys
Sclerosing cholangitis	Biliary tract

Because serum IgG4 levels are elevated in only 70% of patients, a normal level does not rule out the disease. PET scan may identify involvement that is not clinically apparent and can document response to therapy. Initial treatment is prednisone, 0.5-0.6 mg/kg/d for 2 to 4 weeks, followed by a slow taper over months. Azathioprine, mycophenolate mofetil, and methotrexate have been used as glucocorticoid-sparing agents. Recently, rituximab has shown significant benefit in patients with IgG4-related disease and appears to selectively affect IgG4 production; it may replace prednisone as the treatment of choice in severe or refractory disease. Treatment response may be limited by the amount of fibrosis present prior to therapy initiation.

See MKSAP 17 Gastroenterology and Hepatology for information on IgG4-related pancreatitis.

KEY POINTS

- The conditions comprising IgG4-related disease are characterized by abundant IgG4-producing plasma cells seen on tissue biopsy, enlargement of the affected tissue, and the clinical consequences that enlargement entails.
- Serum IgG4 levels are elevated in only 70% of patients with IgG4-related disease; therefore, a normal level does not rule out the disease.

Bibliography

Approach to the Patient with Rheumatologic Disease

Anderson J, Caplan L, Yazdany J, et al. Rheumatoid arthritis disease activity measures: American College of Rheumatology recommendations for use in clinical practice. Arthritis Care Res (Hoboken). 2012 May;64(5):640-7. [PMID: 22473918]

Brown A. How to interpret plain radiographs in clinical practice. Best Pract Res Clin Rheumatol. 2013 Apr;27(2):249-69. [PMID: 23731934]

Castro C, Gourley M. Diagnostic testing and interpretation of tests for autoimmunity. J Allergy Clin Immunol. 2010 Feb;125(2 Suppl 2):S238-47. [PMID: 20061009]

Colglazier C, Sutej P. Laboratory testing in the rheumatic diseases: a practical review. South Med J. 2005 Feb;98(2):185-91. [PMID: 15759949]

Joshua F. Ultrasound applications for the practicing rheumatologist. Best Pract Res Clin Rheumatol. 2012 Dec;26(6):853-67. [PMID: 23273796]

Qaseem A, Alguire P, Dallas P, et al. Appropriate use of screening and diagnostic tests to foster high-value, cost-conscious care. Ann Intern Med. 2012 Jan 17;156(2):147-9. [PMID: 22250146]

Yazdany J, Schmajuk G, Robbins M, et al; American College of Rheumatology Core Membership Group. Choosing Wisely: The American College of Rheumatology's top 5 list of things physicians and patients should question. Arthritis Care Res (Hoboken). 2013 Mar;65(3):329-39. [PMID: 23436818]

Principles of Therapeutics

Barnes PM, Bloom B. Complementary and alternative medicine use among adults and children: United States, 2007. Natl Health Stat Report. 2008 Dec 10;(12):1-23. [PMID: 19361005]

Cameron M, Gagnier JJ, Chrubasik S. Herbal therapy for treating rheumatoid arthritis. Cochrane Database of Syst Rev. 2011 Feb 16;(2):CD002948. [PMID: 21328257]

Chan ES, Cronstein BN. Methotrexate—how does it really work? Nat Rev Rheumatol. 2010 Mar;6(3):175-8. [PMID: 20197777]

Coxib and traditional NSAID Trialists' (CNT) Collaboration, Bhala N, Emberson J, et al. Vascular and upper gastrointestinal effects of non-steroidal anti-inflammatory drugs: meta-analyses of individual participant data from randomized trials. Lancet. 2013 Aug 31;382(9894):769-79. [PMID: 23726390]

Crittenden DB, Pillinger MH. New therapies for gout. Annu Rev Med. 2013;64:325-337. [PMID: 23327525]

Dixon WG, Watson KD, Lunt M, et al. Influence of anti-tumor necrosis factor therapy on cancer incidence in patients with rheumatoid arthritis who have had a prior malignancy: results from the British Society for Rheumatology Biologics Register. Arthritis Care Res (Hoboken). 2010 Jun;62(6):755-63. [PMID: 20535785]

Fleischmann R, Kremer J, Cush J, et al. Placebo-controlled trial of tofacitinib monotherapy in rheumatoid arthritis. N Engl J Med. 2012 Aug 9;367(6):495-507. [PMID: 22873530]

Furie R, Petri M, Zamani O, et al. A phase III, randomized, placebo-controlled study of belimumab, a monoclonal antibody that inhibits B lymphocyte stimulator, in patients with systemic lupus erythematosus. Arthritis Rheum. 2011 Dec;63(12):3918-30. [PMID: 22127708]

Genovese MC, McKay JD, Nasonov EL, et al. Interleukin-6 receptor inhibition with tocilizumab reduces disease activity in rheumatoid arthritis with inadequate response to disease-modifying antirheumatic drugs: the tocilizumab in combination with traditional disease-modifying antirheumatic drug therapy study. Arthritis Rheum. 2008 Oct;58(10):2968-80. [PMID: 18821691]

Hennekens CH, Dalen JE. Aspirin in the treatment and prevention of cardiovascular disease: past and current perspectives and future directions. Am J Med. 2013 May;126(5):373-8. [PMID: 23499330]

Jones RB, Tervaert JW, Hauser T, et al. Rituximab versus cyclophosphamide in ANCA-associated renal vasculitis. N Engl J Med. 2010 Jul 15;363(3):211-20. [PMID: 20647198]

Kamanamool N, McEvoy M, Attia J, Ingsathit A, Ngamjanyaporn P, Thakkinstian A. Efficacy and adverse events of mycophenolate mofetil versus cyclophosphamide for induction therapy of lupus nephritis: systemic review and meta-analysis. Medicine. 2010 Jul;89(4):227-35. [PMID: 20616662]

Khanna D, Fitzgerald JD, Khanna PP, et al; American College of Rheumatology. 2012 American College of Rheumatology guidelines for management of gout. Part 1: systematic nonpharmacologic and pharmacologic therapeutic approaches to hyperuricemia. Arthritis Care Res (Hoboken). 2012 Oct;64(10):1431-46. [PMID: 23024028]

Mariette X, Matucci-Cerinic M, Pavelka K, et al. Malignancies associated with tumour necrosis factor inhibitors in registries and prospective observational studies: a systematic review and meta-analysis. Ann Rheum Dis. 2011 Nov;70(11):1895. [PMID: 21885875]

Singh JA, Furst DE, Bharat A, et al. 2012 Update of the 2008 American College of Rheumatology recommendations for the use of disease-modifying antirheumatic drugs and biologic agents in the treatment of rheumatoid arthritis. Arthritis Care Res (Hoboken). 2012 May;64(5):625-39. [PMID: 22473917]

Van Assen S, Agmon-Levin N, Elkayam O, et al. EULAR recommendations for vaccination in adult patients with autoimmune inflammatory rheumatic diseases. Ann Rheum Dis. 2011 Mar;70(3):414-22. [PMID: 21131643]

Rheumatoid Arthritis

Huzinga TW, Pincus T. In the clinic. Rheumatoid arthritis. Ann Intern Med. 2010 Jul 6;153(1):ITC1-1-ITC1-15; quiz ITC1-16. [PMID: 20621898]

Jacobs JW. Optimal use of non-biologic therapy in the treatment of rheumatoid arthritis. Rheumatology (Oxford). 2012 Jun;51(Suppl 4):iv3-8. [PMID: 22513146]

Pavelka K, Kavanaugh AF, Rubbert-Roth A, Ferraccioli G. Optimizing outcomes in rheumatoid arthritis patients with inadequate responses to disease-modifying anti-rheumatic drugs. Rheumatology (Oxford). 2012 Jul;51(Suppl 5):v12-21. [PMID: 22718922]

Pisetsky DS, Ward MM. Advances in the treatment of inflammatory arthritis. Best Pract Res Clin Rheumatol. 2012 Apr;26(2):251-61. [PMID: 22794097]

Radner H, Neogi T, Smolen JS, Aletaha D. Performance of the 2010 ACR/EULAR classification criteria for rheumatoid arthritis: a systematic literature review. Ann Rheum Dis. 2013 Jan;73(1):114-23. [PMID: 23592710]

Sen D, Brasington R. Tight disease control in early RA. Rheum Dis Clin North Am. 2012;38(2):327-43. [PMID: 22819087]

Singh JA, Furst DE, Bharat A, et al. 2012 Update of the 2008 American College of Rheumatology recommendations for the use of disease-modifying antirheumatic drugs and biologic agents in the treatment of rheumatoid arthritis. Arthritis Care Res (Hoboken). 2012 May;64(5):625-39. [PMID: 22473917]

Vermeer M, Kuper HH, Bernelot Moens HJ, et al. Adherence to a treat-to-target strategy in early rheumatoid arthritis: results of the DREAM remission induction cohort. Arthritis Res Ther. 2012 Nov 23;14(6):R254. [PMID: 23176083]

Vermeer M, Kuper HH, Moens HJ, et al. Sustained beneficial effects of a protocolized treat-to-target strategy in very early rheumatoid arthritis: three year results of the DREAM remission induction cohort. Arthritis Care Res (Hoboken). 2013 Aug;65(8):1219-26. [PMID: 23436821]

Yarilina A, Xu K, Chan C, Ivashkiv LB. Regulation of inflammatory responses in tumor necrosis factor-activated and rheumatoid arthritis synovial macrophages by JAK inhibitors. Arthritis Rheum. 2012 Dec;64(12):3856-66. [PMID: 22941906]

Osteoarthritis

Fernandes L, Hagen KB, Bijlsma JWJ, et al. EULAR Recommendations for the non-pharmacological core management of hip and knee osteoarthritis. Ann Rheum Dis. 2013 Jul;72(7):1125-35. [PMID: 23595142]

Hochberg MC, Altman RD, April KT, et al. American College of Rheumatology 2012 recommendations for the use of nonpharmacologic and pharmacologic therapies in osteoarthritis of the hand, hip, and knee. Arthritis Care Res. 2012 Apr;64(4):465-74. [PMID: 22563589]

Kwok WY, Kloppenburg M, Rosendaal FR, van Meurs JB, Hofman A, Bierma-Zeinstra SM. Erosive hand osteoarthritis: its prevalence and clinical impact in the general population and symptomatic hand osteoarthritis. Ann Rheum Dis. 2011 Jul;70(7):1238-42. [PMID: 21474485]

Rutjes AW, Jüni P, da Costa BR, Trelle S, Niiesch E, Reichenbach S. Viscosupplementation for osteoarthritis of the knee: a systematic review and meta-analysis. Ann Intem Med. 2012 Aug 7;157(3):180-91. [PMID: 22868835]

Westerveld LA, Van Ufford HM, Verlaan JJ, Oner FC. The prevalence of diffuse idiopathic skeletal hyperostosis in an outpatient population in the Netherlands. J Rheumatol. 2008 Aug;35(8):1635-8. [PMID: 18528963]

Fibromyalgia

Atzeni F, Cazzola M, Benucci M, Di Franco M, Salaffi F, Sarzi-Puttini P. Chronic widespread pain in the spectrum of rheumatological diseases. Best Pract Res Clin Rheumatol. 2011 Apr;25(2):165-71. [PMID: 22094193]

Choy E, Marshall D, Gabriel ZL, Mitchell SA, Gylee E, Dakin HA. Systematic review and mixed treatment comparison of the efficacy of pharmacological treatments for fibromyalgia. Semin Arthritis Rheum. 2011 Dec;41(3):335-45. [PMID: 21868065]

McBeth J, Mulvey MR. Fibromyalgia: mechanisms and potential impact of the ACR 2010 classification criteria. Nat Rev Rheumatol. 2012 Jan 24;8(2):108-16. [PMID: 22270077]

Spondyloarthritis

Arvikar SL, Fisher MC. Inflammatory bowel disease associated arthropathy. Curr Rev Musculoskelet Med. 2011 Sep;4(3):123-31. [PMID: 21710141]

Carter JD, Hudson AP. Reactive arthritis: clinical aspects and medical management. Rheum Dis Clin North Am. 2009 Feb;35(1):21-44. [PMID: 19480995]

de Vries MK, van Eijk IC, van der Horst-Bruinsma IE, et al. Erythrocyte sedimentation rate, C-reactive protein level, and serum amyloid a protein for patient selection and monitoring of anti-tumor necrosis factor treatment in ankylosing spondylitis. Arthritis Rheum. 2009 Nov 15;61(11):1484-90. [PMID: 19877087]

Hannu T. Reactive arthritis. Best Pract Res Clin Rheumatol. 2011 Jun;25(3):347-57. [PMID: 22100285]

McGonagle D, Ash Z, Dickie L, McDermott M, Aydin SZ. The early phase of psoriatic arthritis. Ann Rheum Dis. 2011 Mar;70(Suppl 1):i71-6. [PMID: 21339224]

Morris D, Inman RD. Reactive arthritis: developments and challenges in diagnosis and treatment. Curr Rheumatol Rep. 2012 Oct;14(5):390-4. [PMID: 22821199]

Ostergaard M, Lambert RG. Imaging in ankylosing spondylitis. Ther Adv Musculoskelet Dis. 2012 Aug;4(4):301-11. [PMID: 22859929]

Poddubnyy D, van der Heijde D. Therapeutic controversies in spondyloarthritis: nonsteroidal anti-inflammatory drugs. Rheum Dis Clin North Am. 2012 Aug;38(3):601-11. [PMID: 23083758]

Robinson PC, Brown MA. The genetics of ankylosing spondylitis and axial spondyloarthritis. Rheum Dis Clin North Am. 2012 Aug;38(3):539-53. [PMID: 23083754]

Rohekar S, Pope J. Epidemiologic approaches to infection and immunity: the case of reactive arthritis. Curr Opin Rheumatol. 2009 Jul;21(4):386-90. [PMID: 19373091]

Rudwaleit M, Taylor WJ. Classification criteria for psoriatic arthritis and ankylosing spondylitis/axial spondyloarthritis. Best Pract Res Clin Rheumatol. 2010 Oct;24(5):589-604. [PMID: 21035082]

Rudwaleit M, van der Heijde D, Landewé R, et al. The Assessment of SpondyloArthritis International Society classification criteria for peripheral spondyloarthritis and for spondyloarthritis in general. Ann Rheum Dis. 2011 Jan;70(1):25-31. [PMID: 21109520]

Stolwijk C, Boonen A, van Tubergen A, Reveille JD. Epidemiology of spondyloarthritis. Rheum Dis Clin North Am. 2012 Aug;38(3):441-76. [PMID: 23083748]

Systemic Lupus Erythematosus

Barber C, Gold WL, Fortin PR. Infections in the lupus patient: perspectives on prevention. Curr Opin Rheumatol. 2011 Jul;23(4):358-65. [PMID: 21532484]

Dooley MA, Jayne D, Ginzler EM, et al. Mycophenolate versus azathioprine as maintenance therapy for lupus nephritis. N Engl J Med. 2011 Nov;365(20):1886-95. [PMID: 22087680]

Elkon KB, Wiedeman A. Type I IFN system in the development and manifestations of SLE. Curr Opin Rheumatol. 2012 Sept;24(5):499-505. [PMID: 22832823]

Giannakopoulos B, Krilis SA. The pathogenesis of the antiphospholipid syndrome. N Engl J Med. 2013 Mar;368(11):1033-44. [PMID: 23484830]

Hahn BH, McMahon MA, Wilkinson A, et al. American College of Rheumatology guidelines for screening, treatment, and management of lupus nephritis. Arthritis Care Res. 2012 Jun;64(6):797-808. [PMID: 22556106]

Hochberg MC. Updating the American College of Rheumatology revised criteria for the classification of systemic lupus erythematosus. Arthritis Rheum. 1997 Sep;40(9):1725. [PMID: 9324032]

Izmirly PM, Costedoat-Chalumeau N, Pisoni CN, et al. Maternal use of hydroxychloroquine is associated with a reduced risk of recurrent anti-SSA/Ro-antibody-associated cardiac manifestations of neonatal lupus. Circulation. 2012 Jul 3;126(1):76-82. [PMID: 22626746]

Lateef A, Petri M. Management of pregnancy in systemic lupus erythematosus. Nat Rev Rheumatol. 2012 Dec;8(12):710-8. [PMID: 22907290]

Lee SJ, Silverman E, Bargman JM. The role of antimalarial agents in the treatment of SLE and lupus nephritis. Nat Rev Nephrol. 2011 Oct 18;7(12):718-29. [PMID: 22009248]

Tsokos GC. Systemic lupus erythematosus. N Engl J Med. 2011 Dec 1;365(22):2110-21. [PMID: 22129255]

Wu H, Birmingham DJ, Rovin B, et al. D-dimer level and the risk for thrombosis in systemic lupus erythematosus. Clin J Am Soc Nephrol. 2008 Nov;3(6):1628-36. [PMID: 18945994]

Sjögren Syndrome

Delaleu N, Jonsson MV, Appel S, Jonsson R. New concepts in the pathogenesis of Sjögren's syndrome. Rheum Dis Clin North Am. 2008 Nov;34(4):833-45. [PMID: 18984407]

Helmick CG, Felson DT, Lawrence RC, et al; National Arthritis Data Workgroup. Estimates of the prevalence of arthritis and other rheumatic conditions in the United States. Part I. Arthritis Rheum. 2008 Jan;58(1):15-25. [PMID: 18163481]

Shiboski SC, Shiboski CH, Criswell L, et al; Sjögren's International Collaborative Clinical Alliance (SICCA) Research Groups. American College of Rheumatology classification criteria for Sjögren's syndrome: a data-driven, expert consensus approach in the Sjögren's International Collaborative Clinical Alliance cohort. Arthritis Care Res (Hoboken) 2012 Apr;64(4):475-87. [PMID: 22563590]

Solans-Laqué R, López-Hernandez A, Bosch-Gil JA, Palacios A, Campillo M, Vilardell-Tarres M. Risk, predictors, and clinical characteristics of lymphoma development in primary Sjögren's syndrome. Semin Arthritis Rheum. 2011 Dec;41(3):415-23. [PMID: 21665245]

Theander E, Henriksson G, Ljungberg O, Mandl T, Manthorpe R, Jacobsson LT. Lymphoma and other malignancies in primary Sjögren's syndrome: a cohort study on cancer incidence and lymphoma predictors. Ann Rheum Dis. 2006 Jun;65(6):796-803. [PMID: 16284097]

Theander E, Manthorpe R, Jacobsson LT. Mortality and causes of death in primary Sjögren's syndrome: a prospective cohort study. Arthritis Rheum. 2004 Apr;50(4):1262-9. [PMID: 15077310]

Mixed Connective Tissue Disease

Hajas A, Szodoray P, Nakken B, et al. Clinical course, prognosis, and causes of death in mixed connective tissue disease. J Rheumatol. 2013 Jul;40(7):1134-42. [PMID: 23637328]

Swanton J, Isenberg D. Mixed connective tissue disease: still crazy after all these years. Rheum Dis Clin North Am. 2005 Aug;31:421-36. [PMID: 16084316]

Crystal Arthropathies

Hamburger M, Baraf HS, Adamson TC 3rd, et al; European League Against Rheumatism. 2011 recommendations for the diagnosis and management of gout and hyperuricemia. Postgrad Med. 2011 Nov;123(6 suppl 1):3-36. [PMID: 22156509]

Khanna D, Fitzgerald JD, Khanna PP, et al; American College of Rheumatology. 2012 American College of Rheumatology guidelines for management of gout. Part 1: systematic nonpharmacologic and pharmacologic therapeutic approaches to hyperuricemia. Arthritis Care Res (Hoboken). 2012 Oct;64(10):1431-46. [PMID: 23024028]

Khanna D, Khanna PP, Fitzgerald JD, et al; American College of Rheumatology. 2012 American College of Rheumatology guidelines for management of gout. Part 2: therapy and antiinflammatory prophylaxis of acute gouty arthritis. Arthritis Care Res (Hoboken). 2012 Oct;64(10):1447-61. [PMID: 23024029]

Martinon F, Pétrilli V, Mayor A, Tardivel A, Tschopp J. Gout-associated uric acid crystals activate the NALP3 inflammasome. Nature. 2006 Mar 9;440(7081): 237-41. [PMID: 16407889]

Pascual E, Sivera F, Andrés M. Synovial fluid analysis for crystals. Curr Opin Rheumatol. 2011 Mar;23(2):161-9. [PMID: 21285711]

Terkeltaub RA, Furst DE, Digiacinto JL, Kook KA, Davis MW. Novel evidence-based colchicine dose-reduction algorithm to predict and prevent colchicine toxicity in the presence of cytochrome P450 3A4/P-glycoprotein inhibitors. Arthritis Rheum. 2011 Aug;63(8):2226-37. [PMID: 21480191]

Zhang W, Doherty M, Bardin T, et al. European League Against Rheumatism recommendations for calcium pyrophosphate deposition. Part I: terminology and diagnosis. Ann Rheum Dis. 2011 Apr;70(4):563-70. [PMID: 21216817]

Zhang W, Doherty M, Pascual E, et al. EULAR recommendations for calcium pyrophosphate deposition. Part II: management. Ann Rheum Dis. 2011 Apr;70(4):571-5. [PMID: 21257614]

Zhu Y, Pandya BJ, Choi HK: Prevalence of gout and hyperuricemia in the US general population: the National Health and Nutrition Examination Survey 2007-2008. Arthritis Rheum. 2011 Oct;63(10):3136-41. [PMID: 21800283]

Infectious Arthritis

Kohli R, Hadley S. Fungal arthritis and osteomyelitis. Infect Dis Clin North Am. 2005 Dec;19(4):831-51. [PMID: 16297735]

Mathews CJ, Weston VC, Jones A, Field M, Coakley G. Bacterial septic arthritis in adults. Lancet. 2010 Mar 6;375(9717):846-55. [PMID: 20206778]

Osmon DR, Berbari EF, Berendt AR, et al; Infectious Diseases Society of America. Diagnosis and management of prosthetic joint infection: clinical practice guidelines by the Infectious Diseases Society of America. Clin Infect Dis. 2013 Jan;56(1):e1-e25. [PMID: 23223583]

Peto HM, Pratt RH, Harrington TA, LoBue PA, Armstrong LR. Epidemiology of extrapulmonary tuberculosis in the United States, 1993-2006. Clin Infect Dis. 2009 Nov 1;49(9):1350-7. [PMID: 19793000]

Rice PA. Gonococcal arthritis (disseminated gonococcal infection). Infect Dis Clin North Am. 2005 Dec;19(4):853-61. [PMID: 16297736]

Wormser GP, Dattwyler RJ, Shapiro ED, et al. The clinical assessment, treatment, and prevention of lyme disease, human granulocytic anaplasmosis, and babesiosis: clinical practice guidelines by the Infectious Diseases Society of America. Clin Infect Dis. 2006 Nov 1;43(9):1089-34. [PMID: 17029130]

Idiopathic Inflammatory Myopathies

Airio A, Kautiainen H, Hakala M. Prognosis and mortality of polymyositis and dermatomyositis patients. Clin Rheum. 2006 Mar;25(2):234-9. [PMID: 16477398]

Bernatsky S, Joseph L, Pineau CA, et al. Estimating the prevalence of polymyositis and dermatomyositis from administrative data: age, sex and regional differences. Ann Rheum Dis. 2009 Jul;68(7):1192. [PMID: 18713785]

Buchbinder R, Forbes A, Hall S, Dennett X, Giles G. Incidence of malignant disease in biopsy-proven inflammatory myopathy. A population based cohort study. Ann Intern Med. 2001 Jun 19;134(12):1087. [PMID: 11412048]

Callen JP. Cutaneous manifestations of dermatomyositis and their management. Curr Rheum Rep. 2010 Jun;12(3):192. [PMID: 20425525]

Dalakas MC, Hohlfeld R. Polymyositis and dermatomyositis. Lancet. 2003 Sep 20;362(9388):971-82. [PMID: 14511932]

Marie I, Hachulla E, Hatron PY, et al. Polymyositis and dermatomyositis: short term and long term outcome, and predictive factors of prognosis. J Rheum. 2001 Oct;28(10):2230-7. [PMID: 11669162]

Oddis CV, Reed AM, Aggarwal R, et al; RIM Study Group. Rituximab in the treatment of refractory adult and juvenile dermatomyositis and adult polymyositis: a randomized, placebo-phase trial. Arthritis Rheum. 2013 Feb;65(2):314-24. [PMID: 23124935]

Patwa HS, Chaudhry V, Katzberg H, Rae-Grant AD, So YT. Evidence-based guideline: intravenous immunoglobulin in the treatment of neuromuscular disorders. Neurology. 2012 Mar 27;78(13):1009-15. [PMID: 22454268]

Targoff IN. Myositis specific antibodies. Curr Rheumatol Rep. 2006 Jun;8(3):196-203. [PMID: 16901077]

Systemic Vasculitis

Cacoub P, Terrier B, Saadoun D. Hepatitis C virus-induced vasculitis: therapeutic options. Ann Rheum Dis. 2014 Jan;73(1):24-30.[PMID: 23921995]

de Menthon M, Mahr A. Treating polyarteritis nodosa: current state of the art. Clin Exp Rheumatol. 2011 Jan-Feb;29(1 Suppl 64):S110-6. [PMID: 21586205]

Marzano AV, Vezzoli P, Berti E. Skin involvement in cutaneous and systemic vasculitis. Autoimmun Rev. 2013 Feb;(12)4:467-76. [PMID: 22959234]

Saulsbury FT. Henoch-Schonlein purpura. Curr Opin Rheumatol. 2010 Sep;22(5):598-602. [PMID: 20473173]

Scuccimarri R. Kawasaki disease. Pediatr Clin North Am. 2012 Apr;59(2):425-45. [PMID: 22560578]

Specks U, Merkel PA Seo P, et al; RAVE-ITN Research Group. Efficacy of remission-induction regimens for ANCA-associated vasculitis. N Engl J Med. 2013 Aug 1;369(5);417-27. [PMID: 23902481]

Unizony S, Arias-Urdaneta L, Miloslavsky E, et al. Tocilizumab for the treatment of large-vessel vasculitis (giant cell arteritis, Takayasu arteritis) and polymyalgia rheumatica. Arthritis Care Res. 2012 Nov;64(11):1720-9. [PMID: 22674883]

Systemic Sclerosis

Chifflot H, Fautrel B, Sordet C, Chatelus E, Sibilia J. Incidence and prevalence of systemic sclerosis: a systematic literature review. Semin Arthritis Rheum. 2008 Feb;37(4):223-35. [PMID: 17692364]

Gelber AC, Manno RL, Shah AA, et al. Race and association with disease manifestations and mortality in scleroderma: a 20-year experience at the Johns Hopkins scleroderma center and review of the literature. Medicine (Baltimore). 2013 Jul;92(4):191-205. [PMID: 23793108]

Hudson M, Baron M, Lo E, Weinfeld J, Furst DE, Khanna D. An International, Web-Based, Prospective Cohort Study to Determine Whether the Use of ACE Inhibitors prior to the Onset of Scleroderma Renal Crisis is Associated With Worse Outcomes-Methodology and Preliminary Results. Int J Rheumatol. 2010 doi: 10.1155/2010/347402. [PMID: 20936135]

Johnson SR, Fransen J, Khanna D, et al. Validation of potential classification criteria for systemic sclerosis. Arthritis Care Res (Hoboken). 2012 Mar;64(3):358-67. [PMID: 22052658]

Kumar U, Gokhle SS, Sreenivas V, Kaur S, Misra D. Prospective, open-label, uncontrolled pilot study to study safety and efficacy of sildenafil in systemic sclerosis-related pulmonary artery hypertension and cutaneous vascular complications. Rheumatol Int. 2013 Apr;33(4):1047-52. [PMID: 22833239]

Shanmugam VK, Steen VD. Renal disease in scleroderma: an update on evaluation, risk stratification, pathogenesis and management. Curr Opin Rheumatol. 2012 Nov;24(6):669-76. [PMID: 22955019]

Shenoy PD, Kumar S, Jha LK, et al. Efficacy of tadalafil in secondary Raynaud's phenomenon resistant to vasodilator therapy: a double-blind randomized cross-over trial. Rheumatology (Oxford). 2010 Dec;49(12):2420-8. [PMID: 20837499]

Spiera RF, Gordon JK, Mersten JN, et al. Imatinib mesylate (Gleevac) in the treatment of diffuse cutaneous systemic sclerosis: results of a 1-year, phase IIa, single-arm, open-label clinical trial. Annals of rheumatic disease. 2011 Jun;70(6):1003-9. [PMID: 21398330]

Tashkin DP, Elashoff R, Clements PJ, et al; Scleroderma Lung Study Research Group. Cyclophosphamide versus placebo in scleroderma lung disease. N Engl J Med. 2006 Jun 22;354:2655-66. [PMID: 16790698]

Walker KM, Pope J; participating members of the Scleroderma Clinical Trials Consortium (SCTC); Canadian Scleroderma Research Group (CSRG). Treatment of systemic sclerosis complications: what to use when first-line treatment fails—a consensus of systemic sclerosis experts. Semin Arthritis Rheum. 2012 Aug;42(1):42-55. [PMID: 22464314]

Other Rheumatologic Diseases

Chopra R, Chaudhary N, Kay J. Relapsing polychondritis. Rheum Dis Clin N Am. 2013 May;39(2):263-76. [PMID: 23597963]

Dalvi SR, Yildirim R, Yazici Y. Behcet's Syndrome. Drugs 2012 Dec 3;72(17):2223-41. [PMID: 23153327]

Gattorno M, Martini A. Beyond the NLRP3 inflammasome: autoinflammatory diseases reach adolescence. Arthritis Rheum 2013 May;65(5):1137-47. [PMID: 23400910]

Grahame R, Hakim AJ. Arachnodactyly—a key to diagnosing disorders of connective tissue. J Nat Rev. Rheumatol 2013 Jun;9(6):358-64. [PMID: 23478494]

McAdam LP, O'Hanlan MA, Bluestone R, Pearson CM. Relapsing polychondritis: prospective study of 23 patients and a review of the literature. Medicine (Baltimore). 1976 May;55(3):193-215. [PMID: 775252]

O'Regan A, Berman JS. Sarcoidosis. Ann Intern Med. 2012 May 1;156(9):ITC5-1-16. [PMID: 22547486]

Pouchot J, Arlet JB. Biologic treatment in adult-onset Still's disease. Best Pract Res Clin Rheumatol. 2012 Aug;26(4):477-87. [PMID: 23040362]

Stone JH, Zen Y, Deshpande V. IgG4-related disease. N Engl J Med. 2012 Feb 9;366(6):539-51. [PMID: 22316447]

Rheumatology Self-Assessment Test

This self-assessment test contains one-best-answer multiple-choice questions. Please read these directions carefully before answering the questions. Answers, critiques, and bibliographies immediately follow these multiple-choice questions. The American College of Physicians is accredited by the Accreditation Council for Continuing Medical Education (ACCME) to provide continuing medical education for physicians.

The American College of Physicians designates MKSAP 17 **Rheumatology** for a maximum of **16** *AMA PRA Category 1 Credits*™. Physicians should claim only the credit commensurate with the extent of their participation in the activity.

Earn "Instantaneous" CME Credits Online

Print subscribers can enter their answers online to earn Continuing Medical Education (CME) credits instantaneously. You can submit your answers using online answer sheets that are provided at mksap.acponline.org, where a record of your MKSAP 17 credits will be available. To earn CME credits, you need to answer all of the questions in a test and earn a score of at least 50% correct (number of correct answers divided by the total number of questions). Take any of the following approaches:

➢ Use the printed answer sheet at the back of this book to record your answers. Go to mksap.acponline.org, access the appropriate online answer sheet, transcribe your answers, and submit your test for instantaneous CME credits. There is no additional fee for this service.

➢ Go to mksap.acponline.org, access the appropriate online answer sheet, directly enter your answers, and submit your test for instantaneous CME credits. There is no additional fee for this service.

➢ Pay a $15 processing fee per answer sheet and submit the printed answer sheet at the back of this book by mail or fax, as instructed on the answer sheet. Make sure you calculate your score and fax the answer sheet to 215-351-2799 or mail the answer sheet to Member and Customer Service, American College of Physicians, 190 N. Independence Mall West, Philadelphia, PA 19106-1572, using the courtesy envelope provided in your MKSAP 17 slipcase. You will need your 10-digit order number and 8-digit ACP ID number, which are printed on your packing slip. Please allow 4 to 6 weeks for your score report to be emailed back to you. Be sure to include your email address for a response.

If you do not have a 10-digit order number and 8-digit ACP ID number or if you need help creating a user name and password to access the MKSAP 17 online answer sheets, go to mksap.acponline.org or email custserv@acponline.org.

CME credit is available from the publication date of July 31, 2015, until July 31, 2018. You may submit your answer sheets at any time during this period.

Directions

*Each of the numbered items is followed by lettered answers. Select the **ONE** lettered answer that is **BEST** in each case.*

Self-Assessment Test

Item 1

A 59-year-old man is evaluated for a 6-month history of gout. He was doing well on colchicine and allopurinol but developed hypersensitivity to allopurinol, which resolved with cessation of the agent. He then began to have more frequent gout flares; two flares occurred in the past month and were treated with prednisone. History is also significant for hypertension, chronic kidney disease, and dyslipidemia. Current medications are colchicine, lisinopril, metoprolol, and simvastatin.

On physical examination, temperature is 37.2 °C (98.9 °F), blood pressure is 142/86 mm Hg, pulse rate is 64/min, and respiration rate is 12/min. BMI is 30. The remainder of the examination is normal.

Laboratory studies reveal a serum creatinine level of 2.3 mg/dL (203.3 μmol/L), a serum urate level of 9.2 mg/dL (0.54 mmol/L), and normal liver chemistry studies; estimated glomerular filtration rate is 48 mL/min/1.73 m².

Which of the following is the most appropriate next step in management?

(A) Discontinue colchicine
(B) Start febuxostat
(C) Start pegloticase
(D) Start probenecid

Item 2

A 32-year-old woman undergoes a new patient evaluation. She was diagnosed with systemic lupus erythematosus 10 years ago; manifestations have included arthritis, pericarditis, leukopenia, and rash. She reports increasing difficulty using her hands due to joint deformities. Medications are hydroxychloroquine and prednisone.

On physical examination, temperature is 36.8 °C (98.2 °F), blood pressure is 130/85 mm Hg, pulse rate is 80/min, and respiration rate is 16/min. BMI is 24. Examination of the hands reveals subluxation and ulnar deviation of the metacarpophalangeal joints on both hands, swan neck deformity of fingers on both hands, flexion and subluxation of the metacarpophalangeal joint of both thumbs, and hallux valgus of the first metatarsophalangeal joints bilaterally.

Hand radiographs demonstrate no deformities or evidence of erosions.

Which of the following is the most likely diagnosis?

(A) Hypermobility syndrome
(B) Jaccoud arthropathy
(C) Mixed connective tissue disease
(D) Rheumatoid arthritis

Item 3

A 30-year-old woman is evaluated for a 4-month history of increasing foot pain. She also has a 2-month history of increasing pain and swelling in her fingers and right wrist as well as morning stiffness for more than 1 hour. She has no other pertinent medical history and does not take any medications.

On physical examination, vital signs are normal. There are tenderness and swelling of the second and fifth proximal interphalangeal joints and the second and third metacarpophalangeal joints of the feet bilaterally, and tenderness with movement and swelling of the right wrist.

Radiographs of the hands and wrists are normal.

Which of the following combination of tests is most helpful in confirming the diagnosis?

(A) Anti–cyclic citrullinated peptide antibodies and anti-nuclear antibodies
(B) Anti–cyclic citrullinated peptide antibodies and C-reactive protein
(C) Anti–cyclic citrullinated peptide antibodies and rheumatoid factor
(D) Antinuclear antibodies and rheumatoid factor

Item 4

A 46-year-old woman is evaluated for a 3-month history of a rash during the summertime. She is otherwise well and takes no medications.

On physical examination, vital signs are normal. BMI is 23. Examination of the skin reveals eyelid swelling and a periorbital violaceous rash, erythema and poikiloderma of the anterior chest and upper back, and an erythematous papular rash on the hands; there is no malar eruption, skin thickening, or digital ulcers. Muscle strength and reflexes are normal.

The appearance of the hands is shown.

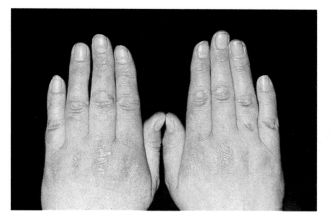

Laboratory studies:

Complete blood count	Normal
Chemistry panel	Normal
Aldolase	5.1 U/L (normal range, 1.0–8.0 U/L)
Creatine kinase	100 U/L
Antinuclear antibodies	Titer of 1:640
Anti-Jo-1 antibodies	Negative
Urinalysis	Normal

Electromyogram and chest radiograph are normal.

Which of the following is the most likely diagnosis?

(A) Amyopathic dermatomyositis

(B) Polymorphous light eruption

(C) Rosacea

(D) Systemic lupus erythematosus

Item 5

A 62-year-old woman is evaluated for a 2-year history of progressively frequent and severe pain in the right knee. She has osteoarthritis with good control of her other joint symptoms with her current therapy that includes medication and a daily exercise regimen. She notes about 20 minutes of morning stiffness in the right knee with significant pain with use after rest; her activities are increasingly limited due to these symptoms. History is otherwise unremarkable. Medications are acetaminophen and celecoxib.

On physical examination, blood pressure is 135/82 mm Hg. BMI is 32. There are Heberden nodes of the second and fifth distal interphalangeal joints bilaterally and Bouchard nodes of the second and third proximal interphalangeal joints bilaterally. Bony hypertrophy of the knees is present. There is a positive bulge sign for effusion of the right knee with slight warmth but no erythema.

Standing radiographs of the knees show right (greater than left) medial joint-space narrowing, bilateral osteophytes, and bilateral peaking of the tibial spines.

Aspiration of the right knee is performed; synovial fluid analysis shows a leukocyte count of 250/μL (0.25 × 10^9/L) and no evidence of crystals.

Which of the following is the most appropriate next step in management?

(A) Administer intra-articular glucocorticoids

(B) Administer intra-articular hyaluronic acid

(C) Refer for arthroscopic lavage

(D) Substitute indomethacin for celecoxib

Item 6

A 72-year-old man is evaluated in the emergency department for acute onset of pain and swelling of the left knee. He was diagnosed with community-acquired pneumonia 4 days ago, and a 7-day course of clarithromycin was started at that time. He reports marked improvement of his respiratory symptoms. History is also significant for gout, with attacks occurring approximately once a year; hypertension; diet-controlled diabetes mellitus; and chronic kidney disease. Other medications are nifedipine and hydrochlorothiazide.

On physical examination, temperature is 37.1 °C (98.8 °F), blood pressure is 117/86 mm Hg, pulse rate is 76/min, and respiration rate is 14/min. BMI is 32. Mildly decreased breath sounds in the right lung midfield are noted. The left knee is swollen, red, warm, tender, and fluctuant with limited range of motion.

Laboratory studies are significant for a leukocyte count of 7200/μL (7.2 × 10^9/L) and a serum creatinine level of 1.7 mg/dL (150.3 μmol/L).

A radiograph of the left knee is normal.

Aspiration of the left knee is performed; synovial fluid analysis reveals a leukocyte count of 20,000/μL (20 × 10^9/L), extracellular and intracellular urate crystals, and a negative Gram stain.

Which of the following is the most appropriate treatment?

(A) Acetaminophen

(B) Colchicine

(C) Indomethacin

(D) Intra-articular glucocorticoids

Item 7

A 65-year-old man is evaluated for severe abdominal pain, joint pain, and a rash. He states that he had an upper respiratory infection about 10 days ago. Three days ago he noted a rash on his lower extremities. One day later, he experienced pain in his knees and ankles, along with abdominal pain that worsened over the past two days. He reports no visual symptoms, numbness, weakness, or other symptoms.

On physical examination, the patient appears uncomfortable. The chest and cardiac examinations are unremarkable. Decreased bowel sounds and diffuse abdominal tenderness without rebound are noted. The knees and ankles are tender and mildly swollen. Palpable purpuric lesions are present on the lower extremities, including the soles of the feet. The remainder of the physical examination reveals no abnormalities.

Laboratory studies show a normal complete blood count, an erythrocyte sedimentation rate of 88 mm/h, a serum creatinine level of 1.7 mg/dL (150.3 μmol/L), and a urinalysis showing 3+ protein, 20-30 erythrocytes/hpf, 20-30 leukocytes/hpf, and mixed granular and cellular casts. A stool test is positive for occult blood.

An abdominal ultrasound reveals thickening and edema of the ileum. A biopsy of an affected skin lesion demonstrates the presence of small-vessel, leukocytoclastic vasculitis accompanied by deposition of IgA.

Which of the following is the most appropriate therapy at this time?

(A) Cyclophosphamide

(B) Dapsone

(C) Ibuprofen

(D) Prednisone

Item 8

A 28-year-old woman is evaluated for a 6-month history of joint pain and swelling. She was diagnosed with rheumatoid arthritis 5 years ago; current medications are etanercept, sulfasalazine, and etodolac. She was initially treated with methotrexate, which was stopped due to gastrointestinal intolerance, and she refuses to retry it.

On physical examination, temperature is 36.7 °C (98.0 °F), blood pressure is 126/74 mm Hg, pulse rate is 68/min, and respiration rate is 14/min. BMI is 24. Two proximal interphalangeal (PIP) joints of the left hand and one metacarpophalangeal (MCP) joint bilaterally are swollen and tender. Examination of the elbows, wrists, knees, and feet is normal. The remainder of the examination, including cardiopulmonary examination, is normal.

Laboratory studies, including complete blood count, chemistry panel, and liver chemistries, are normal; erythrocyte sedimentation rate is 35 mm/h, and C-reactive protein level is 1.1 mg/dL (11 mg/L).

Which of the following is the most appropriate next step in the management of this patient's disease activity?

(A) Add abatacept
(B) Add anakinra
(C) Add leflunomide
(D) Add rituximab

Item 9

A 42-year-old woman is evaluated for a 4-year history of diffuse muscle and joint pain, most notably of her shoulders, low back, hips, and knees. The pain is present in the morning and throughout the day. She wakes unrefreshed and reports problems with her memory. She also describes diarrhea alternating with constipation with no blood or mucus in the stool. She reports no weight loss. She quit working 2 years ago due to her symptoms, which were made worse by her work as a baker. She has been to multiple medical providers who have not established a diagnosis despite numerous tests.

On physical examination, temperature is 37.2 °C (99.0 °F), blood pressure is 134/88 mm Hg, pulse rate is 92/min, and respiration rate is 16/min. BMI is 36. Muscles are generally tender to light palpation but without weakness on muscle strength testing. The remainder of the examination is normal.

Laboratory studies, including complete blood count, chemistry panel, erythrocyte sedimentation rate, serum creatine kinase, and thyroid-stimulating hormone, are normal.

Which of the following is the most likely diagnosis?

(A) Adrenal insufficiency
(B) Fibromyalgia
(C) Hypothyroidism
(D) Polymyositis

Item 10

A 28-year-old woman seeks preconception counseling. She has a 4-year history of systemic lupus erythematosus (SLE) with manifestations of photosensitive rash, arthritis, and pericarditis; she has been treated with hydroxychloroquine and low-dose prednisone with good control of her symptoms for 18 months. She has never been pregnant. She also takes vitamin D and calcium.

The physical examination and vital signs are normal.

Laboratory studies indicate that the patient's SLE is quiescent. A recent urinalysis is normal, and a previously checked antiphospholipid panel and lupus anticoagulant were negative.

SLE antinuclear antibody profile:

Antinuclear antibodies	Positive (titer: 1:320), speckled pattern
Anti-Ro/SSA antibodies	Positive
Anti–double-stranded DNA antibodies	Negative
Anti–U1-ribonucleoprotein antibodies	Negative
Anti-Smith antibodies	Negative

The increased risk of preeclampsia and preterm delivery in SLE as well as avoidance of NSAIDs prior to conception and in the later stages of pregnancy is discussed.

Which of the following also needs to be discussed with this patient based on her antibody profile?

(A) Need to discontinue hydroxychloroquine
(B) Risk of congenital heart block in her child
(C) Risk of developing lupus nephritis
(D) Risk of developing subacute cutaneous lupus

Item 11

A 50-year-old man is evaluated for an 8-year history of joint pain, particularly in the hands, and progressively worsening fatigue. Medical history is otherwise unremarkable. He takes ibuprofen as needed.

On physical examination, vital signs are normal. BMI is 32. There are swelling and tenderness of the second and third metacarpophalangeal (MCP) joints bilaterally, and tenderness but no swelling of the fourth and fifth MCP joints bilaterally. There is bony hypertrophy of the first MCP joints and knees bilaterally. The proximal interphalangeal joints and wrists are normal.

Laboratory studies are notable for an alanine aminotransferase level of 53 U/L and an aspartate aminotransferase level of 55 U/L; rheumatoid factor is negative.

A radiograph of the hand is shown (see top of next page).

Which of the following is the most appropriate diagnostic test to perform next?

(A) Anti–cyclic citrullinated peptide antibody assay
(B) Hepatitis C antibody assay
(C) Serum α-fetoprotein measurement
(D) Transferrin saturation measurement

Item 12

A 25-year-old man is evaluated for a 3-year history of low back and bilateral buttock pain that has gradually increased over the past year. The pain is worse in the morning and after inactivity; he feels better after stretching his back. He has 90 minutes of morning stiffness in his back. Ibuprofen provides moderate relief of symptoms. He reports no other arthritic symptoms, rash, or gastrointestinal symptoms. Family history is notable for his paternal uncle with long-standing back problems.

On physical examination, vital signs are normal. There is painful and diminished forward flexion and extension of the lumbar spine. Tenderness to palpation over both buttocks is noted.

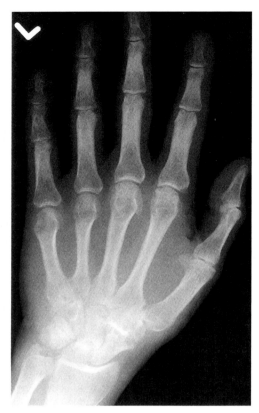

ITEM 11

Laboratory studies reveal an erythrocyte sedimentation rate of 35 mm/h; HLA-B27 testing is negative.

Plain radiographs of the lumbar spine and sacroiliac joints are normal.

Which of the following is the most appropriate diagnostic test to perform next?

(A) CT of the sacroiliac joints
(B) MRI of the sacroiliac joints
(C) Technetium bone scan
(D) Ultrasonography of the sacroiliac joints

Item 13

A 52-year-old woman is evaluated for an 8-week history of fatigue and shortness of breath. She has gastroesophageal reflux disease, hypertension, and a 3-year history of limited cutaneous systemic sclerosis. Medications are omeprazole, nifedipine, lisinopril, and aspirin.

On physical examination, temperature is 36.4 °C (97.6 °F), blood pressure is 126/72 mm Hg, pulse rate is 114/min, and respiration rate is 20/min. BMI is 24. Oxygen saturation is 88% on ambient air. A prominent single S_2 is heard. The chest is clear on auscultation. Sclerodactyly and multiple healed digital pits are noted. There is no rash.

Chest radiograph is normal.

Which of the following is the most appropriate diagnostic test to perform next?

(A) Bronchoscopy with bronchoalveolar lavage
(B) Doppler echocardiography
(C) N-terminal proBNP (B-type natriuretic peptide) measurement
(D) Right heart catheterization

Item 14

A 34-year-old woman is evaluated during a follow-up visit for polymyositis. She was diagnosed 1 year ago and has responded well to therapy. She reports no weakness, chest pain, or shortness of breath on exertion. Current medications are prednisone and azathioprine.

On physical examination, temperature is normal, blood pressure is 106/72 mm Hg, pulse rate is 84/min, and respiration rate is 26/min. BMI is 23. Oxygen saturation is 98% on ambient air. Cardiac and pulmonary examinations are normal. Strength is normal in proximal and distal muscles. Slight hyperkeratosis and cracking of the palmar surface of the hands are present. There are no other rashes, skin thickening, or digital ulcers.

Laboratory studies are notable for a serum creatine kinase level of 100 U/L, an antinuclear antibody titer of 1:1280, and anti–Jo-1 antibody positivity.

Electrocardiogram is normal.

Which of the following is the most appropriate diagnostic test to perform next?

(A) 6-Minute walk test
(B) Cardiac MRI
(C) Chest radiography
(D) Exercise stress testing
(E) No additional testing

Item 15

A 52-year-old woman is evaluated during a follow-up visit for a 6-year history of rheumatoid arthritis. She has not responded to combination therapy with methotrexate and etanercept, abatacept, or rituximab. Current medications are methotrexate and tofacitinib, which was initiated 1 month ago.

On physical examination, vital signs are normal. Examination of the joints shows mild swelling and tenderness of the proximal interphalangeal and metacarpophalangeal joints and wrists bilaterally.

Which of the following laboratory studies should be monitored in this patient?

(A) Alkaline phosphatase
(B) Bilirubin
(C) Glucose
(D) Lipid profile

Item 16

A 56-year-old man is evaluated during a follow-up visit. He was diagnosed with gout 4 months ago based on recurrent episodes of podagra and a serum urate level of 7.2 mg/dL (0.42 mmol/L). Colchicine and allopurinol were initiated at that time and have been maintained at their initial doses. History is also significant for chronic kidney disease and hypertension, for which he takes losartan.

On physical examination, temperature is 37.1 °C (98.8 °F), blood pressure is 130/85 mm Hg, pulse rate is 75/min, and respiration rate is 15/min. BMI is 27. There is no swelling of the joints. The remainder of the examination is unremarkable.

Current laboratory studies reveal a serum urate level of 6.4 mg/dL (0.38 mmol/L) and a serum creatinine level of 2.1 mg/dL (185.6 μmol/L).

Which of the following is the most appropriate management?

(A) Discontinue colchicine
(B) Discontinue losartan
(C) Increase allopurinol
(D) No change in therapy

Item 17

An 82-year-old woman is evaluated for a 2-week history of left-sided headaches with pain on chewing, accompanied by achiness in the shoulders and hips. She has no other pertinent personal or family history. She takes no medications.

On physical examination, temperature is 38.1 °C (100.6 °F), blood pressure is 132/86 mm Hg, pulse rate is 88/min, and respiration rate is 18/min. BMI is 25. Eye examination is normal. There are tenderness and swelling over the left temporal area. Moderate to severe pain on range of motion of the shoulders and hips is noted. There is no pain over the temporomandibular joints on palpation.

Laboratory studies, including basic metabolic panel, complete blood count, and liver chemistries, are normal; erythrocyte sedimentation rate is 85 mm/h.

Which of the following is the most appropriate immediate next step in management?

(A) Initiate prednisone, 15 mg/d
(B) Initiate prednisone, 60 mg/d
(C) Obtain MRI of the head
(D) Obtain temporal artery biopsy

Item 18

A 25-year-old woman is evaluated for a 2-month history of increasing joint pain and swelling. She was diagnosed with rheumatoid arthritis 1 year ago and initially treated with methotrexate with good response but recently has had more pain and swelling. With an increase of the methotrexate dosage and the addition of sulfasalazine and hydroxychloroquine, there was improvement but incomplete control of the disease. She also takes naproxen daily.

On physical examination, vital signs are normal. BMI is 23. Two metacarpophalangeal joints of both hands are tender and swollen. There is palpable warmth and tenderness of both wrists. The remainder of the examination is normal.

Laboratory studies, including complete blood count, chemistry panel, and liver chemistries, are normal; erythro-

cyte sedimentation rate is 45 mm/h, C-reactive protein level is 1.8 mg/dL (18 mg/L), and rheumatoid factor is 112 U/mL (112 kU/L). Hepatitis B and C serologies are negative.

The decision is made to start treatment with adalimumab.

Which of the following is the most appropriate screening test to perform before initiating adalimumab?

(A) Chest radiography
(B) Immunoglobulin level measurement
(C) Interferon-γ release assay
(D) Radiography of hands and feet

Item 19

A 30-year-old man is evaluated for a 1-year history of low back pain. The pain frequently spreads to the buttocks but does not radiate to the legs. The pain is worse in the morning and is associated with stiffness but improves 2 hours later after he starts working. Symptoms are worse at the end of the day and during the night. He takes ibuprofen with good relief of the pain. He is otherwise healthy and reports no other joint pain, rash, diarrhea, or dysuria.

On physical examination, vital signs are normal. Eye examination is normal. There is mild pain with normal range of motion in all directions of the lumbar spine. Tenderness over the buttocks is noted. There is no joint swelling or tenderness in the upper or lower extremities. There is no rash or nail pitting.

Laboratory studies are significant for an erythrocyte sedimentation rate of 40 mm/h, and HLA-B27 testing is positive.

Plain radiographs of the lumbar spine and sacroiliac joints are normal.

Which of the following is the most likely diagnosis?

(A) Ankylosing spondylitis
(B) Lumbar degenerative disk disease
(C) Psoriatic arthritis
(D) Reactive arthritis

Item 20

A 52-year-old woman is evaluated for a 6-year history of Sjögren syndrome. During the past 3 months, she has had low-grade fevers up to 37.5 °C (99.5 °F), weight loss of 6.8 kg (15 lb), and increased fatigue and sicca symptoms. She recently noted a rash on her legs. She reports no current joint pain. Medications are hydroxychloroquine and acetaminophen as needed.

On physical examination, temperature is 37.2 °C (99.0 °F), blood pressure is 135/85 mm Hg, and pulse rate is 82/min. BMI is 28. The oral mucosa is dry. Bilateral parotid fullness is present. There is bilateral cervical adenopathy. The tip of the spleen is palpable. There are a few scattered palpable purpura on the lower legs. The remainder of the physical examination is unremarkable.

Laboratory studies show a normal complete blood count except for a hemoglobin level of 11 g/dL (110 g/L); serum C3 and C4 levels are low, and serum and urine protein electrophoresis reveals M-component.

Chest radiograph and echocardiogram are normal. CT scan of the abdomen shows numerous enlarged retroperitoneal lymph nodes and splenomegaly.

Which of the following is the most appropriate next step in the management of this patient?

(A) Obtain a lymph node biopsy
(B) Obtain a skin biopsy
(C) Order heterophile antibody testing
(D) Start prednisone
(E) Start prednisone and cyclophosphamide

Item 21

A 30-year-old man is evaluated for a 6-month history of pain behind his right heel. The pain is worse after immobility, and he has morning stiffness in the foot lasting 1 hour. He has tried acetaminophen without much relief. History is also significant for a 3-year history of intermittent left eye uveitis treated with a prednisolone ophthalmic solution. He has no other symptoms.

On physical examination, vital signs are normal. There is no tenderness of the lumbar spine or sacroiliac joints; full range of motion of the lumbar spine is noted. Mild swelling and tenderness at the insertion of the Achilles tendon are noted. The remainder of the examination is normal.

Radiographs of the sacroiliac joints are normal. Radiographs of the right heel show soft-tissue swelling and an erosion at the insertion of the Achilles tendon.

Which of the following is the most appropriate diagnostic test to perform next?

(A) Anti–cyclic citrullinated peptide antibody assay
(B) Antineutrophil cytoplasmic antibody assay
(C) Antinuclear antibody assay
(D) HLA–B27 testing

Item 22

A 22-year-old woman is evaluated for a 2-year history of recurrent abdominal pain often accompanied by fever; episodes occur every 3 to 4 months and last 1 to 3 days and resolve completely. She went to the emergency department during an episode 6 weeks ago. She was noted to be mildly febrile, and laboratory studies showed an erythrocyte sedimentation rate of 84 mm/h and a leukocyte count of 16,000/µL (16×10^9/L) with neutrophilia. She was diagnosed with viral gastroenteritis and recovered completely with supportive treatment. She has been treated on several occasions for cellulitis that occurs on her foot or lower extremity, but the reason for repeated infection or a responsible organism has not been identified. On two occasions, she had pain and swelling in the knee that lasted several weeks and was not associated with the abdominal pain. She has tried naproxen without relief. She currently feels well and has no complaints.

On physical examination today, temperature is 36.6 °C (97.9 °F), blood pressure is 120/74 mm Hg, pulse rate is 74/min, and respiration rate is 14/min. BMI is 23.

The cardiopulmonary and abdominal examinations are normal. There is no joint swelling.

Current laboratory studies, including complete blood count, chemistry panel, and erythrocyte sedimentation rate, are normal.

Which of the following is the most appropriate treatment?

(A) Anakinra
(B) Colchicine
(C) Indomethacin
(D) Prednisone

Item 23

A 75-year-old woman is evaluated for progressive left knee pain. She has a 20-year history of bilateral knee osteoarthritis. There is no recent history of injury. She was recently discharged from the hospital for gastrointestinal bleeding related to her use of ibuprofen. She experienced only transient relief from previous glucocorticoid and hyaluronic acid injections. She is enrolled in physical therapy and exercises to increase her quadriceps strength. History is also significant for hypertension, coronary artery disease, hypercholesterolemia, and osteoporosis. Other medications are omeprazole, aspirin, lisinopril, propranolol, rosuvastatin, and alendronate.

On physical examination, vital signs are normal. BMI is 24. Mild weakness on muscle group testing and atrophy are noted in the quadriceps. There is marked bony hypertrophy of the left knee (greater than the right) without warmth, erythema, or effusion.

Which of the following is the most appropriate management for this patient?

(A) Celecoxib
(B) Duloxetine
(C) Fentanyl
(D) Prednisone

Item 24

A 45-year-old woman is evaluated in the emergency department for progressive shortness of breath and fatigue for the past 6 weeks. She also has a 5-year history of diffuse cutaneous systemic sclerosis. Medications are nifedipine, lisinopril, omeprazole, and aspirin.

On physical examination, the patient is alert but short of breath. Temperature is 37.2 °C (99.0 °F), blood pressure is 126/92 mm Hg, pulse rate is 124/min, and respiration rate is 26/min. BMI is 25. Oxygen saturation is 98% on 2 L of oxygen. Cardiac examination is normal. Velcro-like crackles are heard throughout the chest. Diffuse skin thickening of the face, anterior chest, arms stopping at the elbows, and legs is present; sclerodactyly of the fingers is also noted. There is no rash. Pedal edema is present.

Chest radiograph shows bilateral reticulonodular infiltrates and ground glass opacities with normal cardiac silhouette. High-resolution CT scan is consistent with active nonspecific interstitial pneumonitis. An open lung biopsy confirms the diagnosis of nonspecific interstitial pneumonitis.

Which of the following is the most appropriate treatment?

CONT. (A) Cyclophosphamide

(B) D-penicillamine

(C) Infliximab

(D) Methotrexate

Item 25

A 72-year-old man is evaluated in the emergency department for acute swelling, severe pain, and warmth of the right knee that woke him from sleep. He does not recall any inciting injury to the knee. Three months ago, he had an acutely swollen great toe that improved within 3 days, for which he did not seek treatment. History is also significant for hypertension and diabetes mellitus. Medications are hydrochlorothiazide and metformin.

On physical examination, temperature is 37.8 °C (100.1 °F), blood pressure is 130/75 mm Hg, pulse rate is 90/min, and respiration rate is 12/min. BMI is 33. The right knee is warm and swollen without overlying erythema; tenderness to palpation and decreased range of motion due to pain are noted. There is no skin breakdown or abrasions over the right knee. Examination of the other joints is unremarkable.

Which of the following is the most appropriate next step in management?

(A) Obtain a knee MRI

(B) Obtain a serum urate level

(C) Perform joint aspiration

(D) Start empiric colchicine

Item 26

A 40-year-old woman is evaluated for a 6-month history of pain and swelling in her left thumb, left fifth finger, and left foot. She also has morning stiffness lasting 2 to 3 hours. She has a 4-year history of lumbar and thoracic back pain that is worse with bending and lifting and is better with rest. Naproxen is only mildly helpful for the pain.

On physical examination, vital signs are normal. Patches of erythema and scaling behind the right ear and on the scalp at the occiput are noted. Fusiform swelling of the left thumb and left fifth finger is present. Tenderness and swelling at the left third metatarsophalangeal joint are noted. There is mild lumbar tenderness, and full range of motion of the lumbar spine and cervical spine is noted. No other joint swelling or tenderness is present.

Nail findings are shown (see top of next column).

Laboratory studies, including complete blood count with differential, comprehensive metabolic panel, rheumatoid factor, and urinalysis, are normal; HLA-B27 testing is positive.

Which of the following is the most likely diagnosis?

(A) Ankylosing spondylitis

(B) Inflammatory bowel disease–associated arthritis

(C) Psoriatic arthritis

(D) Reactive arthritis

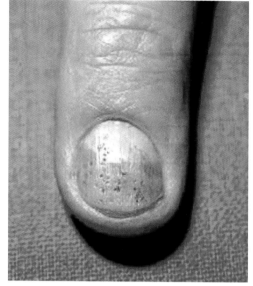

ITEM 26

Item 27

A 42-year-old man is evaluated in the hospital for a 2-week history of progressive shortness of breath, with hemoptysis developing in the past 48 hours. During the past week he has also noted weakness of the left foot, numbness in the right hand, and the onset of a rash. He has a 7-year history of asthma. His only medication is an as-needed albuterol metered-dose inhaler.

On physical examination, temperature is 38.0 °C (100.4 °F), blood pressure is 142/87 mm Hg, pulse rate is 72/min, and respiration rate is 26/min. Diffuse crackles are heard in the lung fields. Diminished sensation in the right hand and weakness on dorsiflexion in the left foot are noted. There is palpable purpura on the arms and legs. The remainder of the physical examination is normal.

Laboratory studies:

Erythrocyte sedimentation rate	98 mm/h
Leukocyte count	16,000/µL (16×10^9/L), 22% eosinophils
Creatinine	0.8 mg/dL (70.7 µmol/L)
IgE	Elevated
ANCA	Negative
Antimyeloperoxidase antibodies	Negative
Antiproteinase 3 antibodies	Negative
Urinalysis	Normal

Chest radiograph shows diffuse pulmonary infiltrates.

Which of the following is the most likely diagnosis?

(A) Cryoglobulinemia

(B) Eosinophilic granulomatosis with polyangiitis

(C) Granulomatosis with polyangiitis

(D) Microscopic polyangiitis

Item 28

A 42-year-old woman is evaluated for a 3-month history of symmetric proximal muscle weakness. She takes no medications.

On physical examination, vital signs are normal. Symmetric weakness of the arm and thigh muscles is noted. There are no skin findings.

Laboratory studies are significant for a serum creatine kinase level of 2000 U/L and a normal thyroid-stimulating hormone level.

Electromyogram shows increased insertional activity, spontaneous fibrillations, and polyphasic motor unit potentials in the proximal muscles. MRI of the thighs shows inflammatory changes in the quadriceps.

A muscle biopsy is recommended, but the patient refuses.

Which of the following is the most appropriate treatment at this time?

(A) Adalimumab
(B) Cyclosporine
(C) Leflunomide
(D) Prednisone

Item 29

A 71-year-old man is evaluated for long-standing stiffness, decreased range of motion, and pain of the neck, mid back, and low back. He has no history of falls or injuries. The stiffness and pain do not improve with activity and are not noticeably worse in bed or with inactivity. Acetaminophen provides minimal relief. He has no other medical problems.

On physical examination, vital signs and BMI are normal. Skin examination is normal. Bony hypertrophy of the second through fifth distal interphalangeal joints and the second and fifth proximal interphalangeal joints is present. Marked reduction in thoracic lateral bending and reduction of spinal flexion and extension are noted.

Plain radiographs of the thoracic spine show flowing osteophytes involving the anterolateral aspect of the thoracic spine at five contiguous vertebrae; there is normal disk height, the apophyseal joints are without osteophytes or bony sclerosis, and the sacroiliac joints are without erosions.

Which of the following is the most likely diagnosis?

(A) Ankylosing spondylitis
(B) Degenerative disk disease
(C) Diffuse idiopathic skeletal hyperostosis
(D) Psoriatic arthritis

Item 30

A 46-year-old woman is evaluated for a 1-week history of symmetric polyarthritis of the hands, wrists, and knees, accompanied by a rash. She is a home health aide. She has no other pertinent history and takes no medications.

On physical examination, temperature is 37.7 °C (99.8 °F), blood pressure is 118/72 mm Hg, pulse rate is 78/min, and respiration rate is 13/min. BMI is 22. There are symmetric tenderness, warmth, erythema, and swelling of the wrists, proximal interphalangeal and metacarpophalangeal joints, and knees bilaterally. Bilateral knee effusions are noted. There is mild right upper quadrant pain. A maculopapular rash over the trunk and legs is present.

Laboratory studies:

Erythrocyte sedimentation rate	63 mm/h
Alanine aminotransferase	1050 U/L
Aspartate aminotransferase	800 U/L
Creatinine	Normal

Which of the following is the most likely diagnosis?

(A) Autoimmune hepatitis
(B) Hemochromatosis
(C) Hepatitis B virus–associated arthritis
(D) Primary biliary cirrhosis

Item 31

A 65-year-old woman is seen at the request of her ophthalmologist. Two days ago, she was diagnosed with scleritis and began using an ophthalmic prednisolone solution. She notes progressive fatigue and intermittent episodes of sinus congestion during the past 5 weeks. She has a 10-year history of joint pain in her hands and low back pain that has not recently changed. History is also significant for hypertension diagnosed 3 months ago, for which she takes hydrochlorothiazide. She reports no dyspnea, cough, rash, diarrhea, or abdominal pain.

On physical examination, vital signs are normal. The ears are normal. Right eye scleral injection is present. There is mild redness and crusting of the nasal mucosa. There are no oral ulcerations. There is bony enlargement with tenderness over the distal interphalangeal joints bilaterally and squaring with tenderness over the first carpometacarpal joints bilaterally. Mild lumbar and paraspinal muscle tenderness is present; full range of motion of the lumbar spine is noted. There is no sacroiliac joint tenderness. The remainder of the physical examination is normal.

Laboratory studies:

Comprehensive metabolic panel	Normal
Erythrocyte sedimentation rate	55 mm/h
Hemoglobin	11 g/dL (110 g/L)
Leukocyte count	5000/µL (5.0 × 10⁹/L)
Platelet count	550,000/µL (550 × 10⁹/L)
Urinalysis	2+ protein; trace blood; no leukocytes; 1 erythrocyte cast

Chest radiograph is normal.

Which of the following is the most likely diagnosis?

(A) Ankylosing spondylitis
(B) Behçet syndrome
(C) Granulomatosis with polyangiitis
(D) Sarcoidosis

Item 32

An 80-year-old man is evaluated for severe right knee pain that began yesterday. He has a 10-year history of gout that has affected his great toes and knees; his last attack was 2 years ago in the right great toe. Medications are allopurinol and ibuprofen as needed.

On physical examination, temperature is 37.8 °C (100.0 °F), blood pressure is 150/85 mm Hg, pulse rate is 80/min, and respiration rate is 16/min. BMI is 31. The right knee is warm, swollen, slightly erythematous, and tender; range of motion is limited to 90 degrees of flexion and associated with pain. There is no inflammation in the remainder of the joints.

Aspiration of the right knee yields 30 mL of cloudy yellow fluid. Synovial fluid leukocyte count is 55,000/µL (55×10^9/L), with 95% polymorphonuclear cells. Extracellular negatively birefringent needle-shaped crystals are seen under polarized light. Synovial fluid Gram stain is negative. Synovial fluid cultures are pending.

Which of the following is the most appropriate treatment?

(A) Add probenecid
(B) Increase allopurinol
(C) Perform an intra-articular glucocorticoid injection
(D) Start antibiotics
(E) Start prednisone

Item 33

A 25-year-old woman is evaluated during a follow-up visit for an 18-month history of ankylosing spondylitis. She has minimal lower back pain with morning stiffness lasting 20 minutes. She is able to pursue her activities of daily living without any restrictions. She has been taking etanercept for 1 year with good results.

On physical examination, vital signs are normal. Full range of motion of the thoracic and cervical spine without tenderness is noted. There is no lumbar or sacroiliac tenderness. The Schober test increases by 5 cm (same as at the time of diagnosis).

Laboratory studies are notable for a normal erythrocyte sedimentation rate and a normal C-reactive protein level.

At the time of diagnosis, radiographs showed normal thoracic and lumbar spine and sacroiliac joints, and an MRI showed edema of the sacroiliac joints and in the lumbar and thoracic spine.

Which of the following should be performed next?

(A) Bone scan
(B) CT of the sacroiliac joints
(C) MRI of the sacroiliac joints
(D) Plain radiography of the sacroiliac joints
(E) No new imaging

Item 34

A 35-year-old man is evaluated for a 2-month history of abrupt left knee swelling. He notes prominent stiffness of both joints but no significant pain. He previously felt well. He lives in Vermont and goes hiking during the summer. He

has not had any episodes of diarrhea or abdominal pain and reports no trauma to the knee, fever, rash, or known insect bites. He does not have a history of sexually transmitted infections. He has no history of injection drug use and does not take any medications.

On physical examination, temperature is 37.1 °C (98.8 °F), blood pressure is 115/70 mm Hg, pulse rate is 82/min, and respiration rate is 12/min. BMI is 20. There is a large effusion over the left knee with warmth and mild tenderness but no overlying erythema; range of motion is limited by swelling, but stability is intact. There is no heart murmur. Lung and abdominal examinations are normal. There are no skin lesions.

Laboratory studies reveal an erythrocyte sedimentation rate of 12 mm/h and a leukocyte count of 6000/µL (6.0×10^9/L).

Radiograph of the left knee shows a large effusion but is otherwise unremarkable.

Which of the following is most likely to provide the diagnosis?

(A) Blood cultures
(B) Lyme serologic testing
(C) MRI of the knee
(D) Synovial fluid cultures

Item 35

A 21-year-old woman is evaluated for a 3-week history of painful nodules and a rash in the lower extremities, along with pain and swelling of the wrists, knees, and ankles. She reports a low-grade fever and a 2.7-kg (6.0-lb) weight loss since the onset of symptoms. She has taken naproxen with some relief. History is significant for gastroesophageal reflux disease and acne. Medications are over-the-counter famotidine as needed and minocycline.

On physical examination, temperature is 38.2 °C (100.8 °F), blood pressure is 110/60 mm Hg, pulse rate is 92/min, and respiration rate is 16/min. BMI is 24. Mild swelling of the wrists, knees, and ankles is noted. There are scattered 1- to 2-cm painful erythematous nodules as well as livedo reticularis in the lower extremities beginning at the thighs. The remainder of the examination is normal.

Laboratory studies:

Antinuclear antibodies	Positive (titer: 1:320)
Anti–double-stranded DNA antibodies	Negative
Anti-Smith antibodies	Negative
Anti-U1-ribonucleoprotein antibodies	Negative
Anti-Ro/SSA antibodies	Negative
Anti-La/SSB antibodies	Negative
Antihistone antibodies	Negative
ANCA	Positive (titer: 1:320) in a perinuclear pattern; negative for myeloperoxidase
Urinalysis	Normal

Chest radiograph is normal.

Which of the following is the most appropriate next step in management?

(A) Start azathioprine

(B) Start high-dose prednisone

(C) Discontinue famotidine

(D) Discontinue minocycline

Item 36

A 61-year-old man is evaluated for a 10-month history of generalized weakness. He reports no pain or myalgia. History is significant for hypercholesterolemia treated with a stable dose of simvastatin for the past 3 years.

On physical examination, temperature is normal, blood pressure is 138/74 mm Hg, pulse rate is 70/min, and respiration rate is 16/min. BMI is 27. There is symmetric weakness of the arm and thigh muscles with slightly reduced grip and power of the finger flexors. No muscle tenderness is noted. There is no rash, skin thickening, or digital ulcers. Reflexes and the remainder of the physical examination are normal.

Laboratory studies are notable for a normal complete blood count, an erythrocyte sedimentation rate of 23 mm/h, and a serum creatine kinase level of 365 U/L.

Chest radiograph is normal. Electromyogram and nerve conduction studies show myopathic changes in the proximal and distal muscles of the extremities as well as some neurogenic changes.

Which of the following is the most likely diagnosis?

(A) Amyotrophic lateral sclerosis

(B) Inclusion body myositis

(C) Myasthenia gravis

(D) Statin-induced myopathy

Item 37

A 72-year-old man is evaluated for a 1-year history of progressive worsening of bilateral knee pain and stiffness. He has had no locking, popping, or giving way in either knee. He has pain in both knees at rest and at night, which awakens him from sleep. He has no history of injury. Acetaminophen and over-the-counter ibuprofen improve his pain temporarily.

On physical examination, vital signs are normal. BMI is 35. Bilateral bony hypertrophy and valgus deformity of the knees are noted. There is no warmth, erythema, swelling, or effusion. Anterior drawer sign is negative, and there is no compromise in stability.

Which of the following studies of the knees is the most appropriate diagnostic test to perform next?

(A) Bone scintigraphy

(B) MRI

(C) Standing plain radiography

(D) Ultrasonography

Item 38

A 60-year-old woman is evaluated during a follow-up visit for Sjögren syndrome. She reports persistent eye discomfort described as a sandy or gritty sensation. She has had recurrent corneal abrasions and erosions. She has been using artificial tears with minimal improvement. She saw her ophthalmologist who inserted punctal plugs, but they caused excessive tearing and were removed. She otherwise feels well and reports no fever, chills, weight loss, rash, joint pain, chest pain, or dyspnea.

On physical examination, temperature is 36.7 °C (98.0 °F), blood pressure is 135/80 mm Hg, pulse rate is 75/min, and respiration rate is 18/min. The oral mucosa is dry. Moderately injected sclerae are noted. There is no cervical or supraclavicular adenopathy and no parotid gland swelling. Lung, heart, musculoskeletal, and skin examinations are normal.

Which of the following is the most appropriate treatment?

(A) Certolizumab pegol

(B) Cyclosporine drops

(C) Hydroxychloroquine

(D) Olopatadine drops

(E) Prednisone

Item 39

A 25-year-old man undergoes a new patient evaluation. He has Marfan syndrome. His clinical course has been unremarkable. History is significant for inguinal hernia repair; family history is notable for his father who has Marfan syndrome. The patient takes no medications.

On physical examination, temperature is 37.4 °C (99.3 °F), blood pressure is 134/89 mm Hg, pulse rate is 80/min, and respiration rate is 14/min. BMI is 22. Tall stature and pectus excavatum are noted. Oral examination demonstrates a high arched palate. Arachnodactyly is noted. Scoliosis is present on forward bending. Examination of the feet reveals bilateral pes planus without obvious osteoarthritic mid-foot changes.

Which of the following is the most appropriate periodic imaging test for this patient?

(A) Abdominal ultrasonography

(B) Chest radiography

(C) Echocardiography

(D) Spine radiography

Item 40

A 32-year-old woman is evaluated for a new rash on her legs. She was diagnosed with pyelonephritis 4 days ago and was started on a 7-day regimen of trimethoprim-sulfamethoxazole based on urine culture and sensitivity data; her urinary symptoms have improved. Medical history includes Hashimoto thyroiditis treated with levothyroxine; her dose was increased 4 weeks ago based on thyroid function studies. Medical history is otherwise unremarkable.

On physical examination, temperature is normal, blood pressure is 124/82 mm Hg, pulse rate is 66/min, and respiration rate is 13/min. BMI is 21. Cardiopulmonary examination is unremarkable. The abdomen is soft and nontender. Musculoskeletal examination shows no evidence of joint swelling, warmth, or tenderness. The remainder of the examination is normal.

The appearance of the legs is shown.

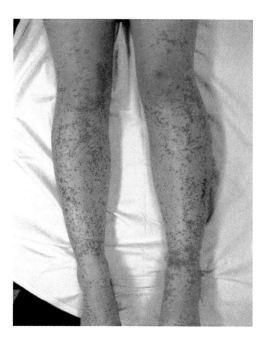

Which of the following is the most appropriate next step in management?

(A) Discontinue trimethoprim-sulfamethoxazole
(B) Initiate prednisone
(C) Measure antihistone antibodies
(D) Obtain skin biopsy

Item 41

A 30-year-old woman is evaluated during a follow-up visit for systemic lupus erythematosus. She was diagnosed 3 months ago after presenting with pericarditis and arthritis. She was initially treated with prednisone, 40 mg/d, with improvement of her presenting symptoms. The prednisone has been tapered over 3 months to her current dose of 10 mg/d with no recurrence. She also takes vitamin D and a calcium supplement.

On physical examination, vital signs are normal. BMI is 25. Cardiac examination is normal. There is no evidence of arthritis. The remainder of the examination is normal.

Which of the following is the most appropriate next step in treating this patient?

(A) Add azathioprine
(B) Add hydroxychloroquine
(C) Add mycophenolate mofetil
(D) Add a scheduled NSAID

Item 42

A 65-year-old man is evaluated during a follow-up visit for gout. He initially presented 6 months ago with acute pain and swelling of the right great toe and a serum urate level of 7.2 mg/dL (0.42 mmol/L); symptoms resolved with naproxen. He then presented last week with recurrent symptoms of great toe pain, redness, and swelling that began during sleep. Colchicine was initiated, and symptoms resolved. History is also significant for hypertension, coronary artery disease, hyperlipidemia, and urolithiasis. Current medications are colchicine, metoprolol, simvastatin, and low-dose aspirin.

On physical examination, temperature is 37.1 °C (98.8 °F), blood pressure is 138/80 mm Hg, pulse rate is 60/min, and respiration rate is 15/min. BMI is 30. Examination of the joints reveals no swelling.

Laboratory studies reveal a serum urate level of 7.6 mg/dL (0.45 mmol/L) and normal kidney and liver chemistries.

Which of the following is the most appropriate treatment for this patient?

(A) Discontinue aspirin
(B) Discontinue colchicine
(C) Start allopurinol
(D) Start probenecid

Item 43

A 50-year-old woman is evaluated for slowly worsening joint pain in her fingers for the past 5 years. She notes swelling, morning stiffness lasting 10 minutes, and pain that is worse after housework or typing. She has no other joint pain and otherwise feels well. She reports no fevers, weight loss, rashes, alopecia, oral ulcers, dyspnea, chest pain, or abdominal pain. The patient takes no medications.

On physical examination, vital signs are normal. There is squaring, crepitus, and tenderness of the first carpometacarpal joints. Bony enlargement and tenderness over all distal interphalangeal (DIP) joints are present. Limited range of motion of the thumbs and DIP joints is noted. There is no joint warmth, redness, or effusions. The remainder of the joint examination is normal.

Which of the following is the most appropriate next step in management?

(A) Anti–double-stranded DNA antibody testing
(B) Antinuclear antibody testing
(C) Radiography of the hands
(D) Rheumatoid factor testing
(E) No further testing

Item 44

A 74-year-old man is evaluated for a 2-month history of progressively worsening bilateral shoulder and hip pain. He currently has difficulty rising from a chair and reaching overhead because of the pain. He also reports fatigue, malaise, and 4.5-kg (10-lb) weight loss during this period. He reports no other symptoms. He takes acetaminophen as needed for pain with little or no relief.

On physical examination, the patient appears depressed. Temperature is 37.9 °C (100.2 °F), blood pressure is 126/66 mm Hg, pulse rate is 72/min, and respiration rate is 18/min. BMI is 26. There is markedly limited range of motion of the shoulders and hips due to pain; strength cannot be adequately assessed. The remainder of the physical examination is normal.

Laboratory studies, including basic metabolic panel, complete blood count, liver chemistries, and thyroid-stimulating hormone level, are normal. Erythrocyte sedimentation rate is 68 mm/h.

Which of the following is the most appropriate treatment?

(A) Aspirin, 81 mg/d
(B) Aspirin, 650 mg three times daily
(C) Duloxetine, 60 mg/d
(D) Prednisone, 15 mg/d
(E) Prednisone, 60 mg/d

Item 45

A 45-year-old man is evaluated for a 2-week history of progressive pain and swelling of the third and fourth toes of the right foot. He has a rash on the soles of his feet that appeared 4 weeks ago. He reports no fever, back pain, chest pain, dyspnea, dysuria, diarrhea, ocular problems, oral ulcers, Raynaud phenomenon, psoriasis, or photosensitivity. He is sexually active. He takes no medications.

On physical examination, vital signs are normal. There is no nail pitting. Dactylitis and diffuse swelling of the right third and fourth toes are noted. The soles of the feet have yellow-brown vesicles and hyperkeratotic nodules with overlying keratotic crust. The remainder of the examination is normal.

Laboratory studies reveal an erythrocyte sedimentation rate of 35 mm/h; complete blood count with differential and urinalysis are normal.

Radiographs of the toes reveal diffuse soft-tissue swelling of the right third and fourth toes but are otherwise normal.

Which of the following is the most appropriate diagnostic test to perform next?

(A) Anti–cyclic citrullinated peptide antibody assay
(B) Antinuclear antibody assay
(C) DNA amplification urine test for *Chlamydia trachomatis*
(D) HLA–B27 testing

Item 46

A 52-year-old man is evaluated during a follow-up visit for a 2-year history of progressively symptomatic rheumatoid arthritis. He reports increased difficulty with his job due to persistent pain and swelling in the first proximal interphalangeal joints, second and third metacarpophalangeal joints, and bilateral wrists. He also has increased difficulty climbing stairs due to persistent pain and swelling in the right knee. Medications are methotrexate, 25 mg weekly; prednisone, 10 mg/d; naproxen; and folic acid.

On physical examination, vital signs are normal. There is 1+ tenderness to palpation and 1+ swelling of the affected joints.

Plain radiographs of the hands and wrists show periarticular osteopenia, multiple erosions, and carpal joint-space narrowing. Plain radiographs of the knees show medial and lateral joint-space narrowing.

Which of the following is the most appropriate next step in management?

(A) Add etanercept
(B) Add rituximab
(C) Increase methotrexate
(D) Increase prednisone

Item 47

A 39-year-old man is evaluated for a lower extremity rash of 3 weeks' duration. He has no recent history of a cold, flu, or other infection. He takes no medications.

On physical examination, temperature is 37.3 °C (99.2 °F), blood pressure is 136/86 mm Hg, pulse rate is 66/min, and respiration rate is 12/min. BMI is 24. Small vascular infarctions are observed on the ears and fingertips. There are scattered palpable purpuric lesions on the bilateral lower extremities, which are less prominent on the soles. Strength is reduced in the right wrist.

Laboratory studies:

Erythrocyte sedimentation rate	66 mm/h
C3	Normal
C4	Decreased
Creatinine	2.1 mg/dL (185.6 µmol/L)
Rheumatoid factor	Positive
Hepatitis C antibodies	Positive, genotype 2
Serum protein electrophoresis	Monoclonal spike in IgG band
Urinalysis	Positive for erythrocytes, leukocytes, erythrocyte casts

Which of the following is most likely to establish the diagnosis?

(A) Anti–cyclic citrullinated peptide antibody levels
(B) Anti–glomerular basement membrane antibody levels
(C) Antinuclear antibody levels
(D) p–ANCA levels
(E) Serum cryoglobulin levels

Item 48

A 71-year-old woman is evaluated during an office visit. Four months ago, she fell on an outstretched hand. During the next several weeks, she noted gradual pain, stiffness, and swelling of her right shoulder; the pain occurs with movement and at night. History is significant for knee osteoarthritis, gout, and hypertension. Medications are acetaminophen, colchicine, allopurinol, and lisinopril.

On physical examination, vital signs are normal. BMI is 25. The right shoulder has a large effusion without warmth or overlying erythema; range of motion is limited by pain and swelling, and prominent crepitus is palpable with motion.

Erythrocyte sedimentation rate, leukocyte count, C-reactive protein level, and serum urate level are within normal limits.

A radiograph of the shoulder is shown.

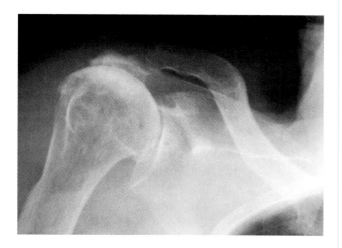

Aspiration of the right shoulder shows blood-tinged synovial fluid with a leukocyte count of 8300/μL (8.3×10⁹/L); Gram stain is negative, and there are no crystals.

Which of the following is the most likely diagnosis?

(A) Acute calcium pyrophosphate crystal arthritis
(B) Acute gouty arthritis
(C) Basic calcium phosphate deposition
(D) Infectious arthritis

Item 49

A 23-year-old woman is evaluated for a 1-week history of fevers, malaise, aches of her elbows and left knee, and pain of her wrists, hands, and ankles that is worse with movement. She has noticed transient skin lesions resembling pustules. She reports no urinary symptoms or vaginal discharge. She has no history of illicit drug use; she drinks alcohol socially and is sexually active. She has not traveled recently. Her only medication is an oral contraceptive.

On physical examination, the patient appears uncomfortable. Temperature is 38.3 °C (100.9 °F), blood pressure is 115/75 mm Hg, pulse rate is 95/min, and respiration rate is 12/min. BMI is 23. Ulnar deviation of the wrists while holding the thumbs down elicits pain over the radial side of the wrists (positive Finkelstein test). There is generalized swelling of several fingers with tenderness to palpation diffusely. The left knee is warm, with a small effusion and pain with range of motion. The ankles have tenderness to palpation over the posterior aspects, with erythema along the Achilles tendons and pain with range of motion bilaterally. There are a few scattered vesiculopustular lesions over the palmar aspect of the hands and upper extremities.

Laboratory studies reveal a leukocyte count of 13,500/μL (13.5×10⁹/L) and normal kidney and liver chemistries.

Which of the following is most likely to provide the diagnosis?

(A) Cervical culture
(B) Hepatitis B serologies
(C) Rapid streptococcal antigen testing
(D) Synovial fluid analysis

Item 50

A 26-year-old woman seeks preconception counseling. She has a 3-year history of rheumatoid arthritis. Medications are methotrexate, hydroxychloroquine, low-dose prednisone, and folic acid. Currently her disease is under excellent control.

On physical examination, vital signs are normal. There is no warmth, erythema, swelling, or tenderness of the joints.

Which of the following is the most appropriate next step in management?

(A) Discontinue hydroxychloroquine
(B) Discontinue methotrexate
(C) Discontinue prednisone
(D) Discontinue prednisone, methotrexate, and hydroxychloroquine

Item 51

A 52-year-old man is evaluated for a 4-month history of slowly progressive unilateral proptosis. He reports enlargement of the glands under his jaw on both sides. He generally feels well and has no other medical problems. He takes no medications.

On physical examination, vital signs are normal. Marked proptosis of the left eye is noted; there is no inflammation of the sclerae or conjunctivae. There is bilateral enlargement of the lacrimal, parotid, and submandibular glands. There is an enlarged lymph node at the angle of the jaw on the right. The remainder of the examination is normal.

Laboratory studies include a normal complete blood count with differential, chemistry panel, liver chemistries, antinuclear antibody panel, and urinalysis.

MRI of the head and orbits demonstrates a homogeneous enhancing mass behind the left eye and enlargement of the parotid and submandibular glands. Biopsy of the ocular mass demonstrates a lymphoplasmacytic infiltrate with storiform fibrosis and obliterative phlebitis, rare neutrophils, and no granulomas; a monoclonal population of cells is not identified.

Which of the following is the most likely diagnosis?

(A) Hodgkin lymphoma
(B) IgG4-related disease
(C) Sarcoidosis
(D) Sjögren syndrome

Item 52

A 58-year-old woman is evaluated for a 2-year history of hand pain and increasing difficulty using her hands. She reports worsening grip strength as well as increasing pain in the distal interphalangeal (DIP) and proximal interphalangeal (PIP) joints. She has intermittent erythema and swelling in some of these joints (such as the fifth DIP joint and the right second PIP and left third PIP joints) sometimes lasting for weeks at a time. She takes naproxen twice daily.

On physical examination, vital signs are normal. BMI is 29. Bony hypertrophy and malalignment of the DIP joints are noted; there is mild erythema over the right fifth DIP joint. There are bony hypertrophy of the PIP joints and swelling and tenderness of the right second PIP joint and the left third PIP joint. There is bony hypertrophy of the first carpometacarpal (CMC) joint bilaterally.

Laboratory studies, including a complete blood count, erythrocyte sedimentation rate, C-reactive protein, serum creatinine, rheumatoid factor, anti–cyclic citrullinated antibodies, and urinalysis, are normal.

Plain hand radiographs show central erosions and collapse of the subchondral bone in the right second PIP joint and the left third PIP joint; osteophytes at the second, third, and fifth DIP joints bilaterally; and joint-space narrowing at the first CMC joint bilaterally. There is no periarticular osteopenia or marginal erosions.

Which of the following is the most likely diagnosis?

(A) Erosive osteoarthritis

(B) Reactive arthritis

(C) Rheumatoid arthritis

(D) Tophaceous gout

Item 53

A 44-year-old man is evaluated for a 2-month history of color change in the hands when exposed to the cold, finger skin tightness with palpable nodules, fatigue, and pruritus. He has no other medical problems and takes no medications or nutritional supplements.

On physical examination, vital signs are normal. BMI is 23. Skin thickening of the face and fingers is noted. There are a few firm, gritty nodules on the palmar aspect of the digits. There is no rash or digital pits.

The appearance of the hands is shown.

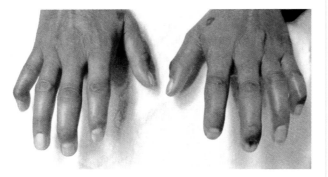

Which of the following is the most likely diagnosis?

(A) Eosinophilia myalgia syndrome

(B) Limited cutaneous systemic sclerosis

(C) Morphea

(D) Primary biliary cirrhosis

Item 54

A 42-year-old woman is evaluated for a 6-month history of pain and swelling of several small hand joints, an elbow, and an ankle. She gets modest relief with naproxen. She has no other medical problems and takes no additional medications.

On physical examination, vital signs are normal. There are tenderness to palpation and swelling of the second and third proximal interphalangeal joints bilaterally, second and fifth metacarpophalangeal joints bilaterally, left wrist, right elbow, and right ankle. The remainder of the physical examination is normal.

Laboratory studies are significant for a rheumatoid factor of 85 U/mL (85 kU/L) and positive anti–cyclic citrullinated peptide antibodies.

Radiographs of the hands and wrists show periarticular osteopenia at the metacarpophalangeal joints and a marginal erosion at the right second metacarpal head.

Which of the following is the most appropriate initial treatment?

(A) Hydroxychloroquine

(B) Methotrexate

(C) Rituximab

(D) Tofacitinib

Item 55

A 40-year-old woman is evaluated for a 7-year history of color changes associated with pain that occurs in her fingers. Her second and third fingertips turn white in the cold, then become blue, and eventually become dark red and painful. These symptoms last approximately 15 minutes before resolving. She also reports a 3-month history of pain and swelling in the second and third metacarpophalangeal joints. History is also significant for dry eyes and dry mouth of 5 years' duration as well as recent onset of diffusely puffy hands and increasing fatigue. She reports no gastrointestinal symptoms, including gastroesophageal reflux disease. She takes no medications.

On physical examination, vital signs are normal. No rash or oral ulcers are noted. Slightly cool, diffusely edematous fingers are noted. Scattered palmar telangiectasias are present. There is swelling and tenderness of the second and fourth metacarpophalangeal joints.

Laboratory studies:

C3	Normal
C4	Normal
Creatine kinase	596 U/L
Creatinine	Normal
Antinuclear antibodies	Positive (titer: 1:320)
Anti–double-stranded DNA antibodies	Negative
Anti-Ro/SSA antibodies	Negative
Anti-La/SSB antibodies	Negative
Anti-Scl-70 antibodies	Negative
Anti-Smith antibodies	Negative
Anti-U1-ribonucleoprotein antibodies	Positive
Urinalysis	Negative

Which of the following is the most likely diagnosis?

(A) Mixed connective tissue disease
(B) Polymyositis
(C) Systemic lupus erythematosus
(D) Systemic sclerosis
(E) Undifferentiated connective tissue disease

Item 56

A 28-year-old woman is evaluated in the emergency department for a 1-day history of progressive shortness of breath, cough, and hemoptysis. She reports a fever but no chills. She has a 2-year history of systemic lupus erythematosus. Medications are mycophenolate mofetil, hydroxychloroquine, prednisone, naproxen as needed, vitamin D, and calcium.

On physical examination, temperature is 38.9 °C (102.0 °F), blood pressure is 100/60 mm Hg, pulse rate is 110/min, and respiration rate is 24/min. Oxygen saturation is 88% on ambient air. BMI is 29. Diffuse hair thinning is noted. A malar rash is present. There is symmetric swelling of metacarpophalangeal and proximal interphalangeal joints as well as both wrists and knees. There are no cardiac rubs or murmurs. Diffuse crackles are heard on lung auscultation.

Laboratory studies:
Hematocrit   22% (30% in office 1 week ago)
Leukocyte count   3200/μL (3.2 × 10⁹/L)
Platelet count   90,000/μL (90 × 10⁹/L)
Creatinine   1.3 mg/dL (115 μmol/L)
Urinalysis   3+ blood; 2+ protein; erythrocyte casts

Chest radiograph reveals diffuse bilateral pulmonary infiltrates with sparing of the apices.

Which of the following is most likely to establish a diagnosis?

(A) Bronchoalveolar lavage and biopsy
(B) Chest CT
(C) MRI of the chest
(D) Pulmonary angiography

Item 57

A 24-year-old woman is evaluated for a 1-week history of tender nodules over the legs about 2 to 3 cm in size along with pain and stiffness in the ankles. She also notes a nonproductive cough of 3 days' duration. Her only medication is an oral contraceptive.

On physical examination, temperature is 38.4 °C (101.1 °F), blood pressure is 110/65 mm Hg, pulse rate is 85/min, and respiration rate is 18/min. BMI is 24. There are four 3-cm erythematous tender nodules on the left anterior lower leg and three on the right. Swelling of both ankles with tenderness at the right Achilles tendon insertion into the calcaneus is noted; no other joints are swollen. Cardiopulmonary examination is normal.

Laboratory studies reveal an erythrocyte sedimentation rate of 38 mm/h and a hematocrit of 35%; leukocyte and platelet counts are normal.

A chest radiograph is shown.

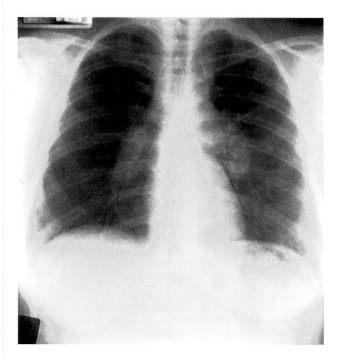

Which of the following is the most appropriate treatment?

(A) Adalimumab
(B) High-dose prednisone
(C) Methotrexate
(D) Naproxen

Item 58

A 35-year-old man is evaluated for a 4-week history of persistent pain and swelling in the left knee and right ankle. Symptoms are worse in the morning and associated with stiffness lasting 1 hour. Ibuprofen is beneficial. Seven weeks ago he had diarrhea that lasted one week and resolved without treatment. One week ago he was diagnosed with anterior uveitis, which is resolving with a prednisolone ophthalmic solution. He reports no current gastrointestinal or genitourinary symptoms, rash, or cardiorespiratory symptoms.

On physical examination, vital signs are normal. Slightly injected sclera of the right eye is noted. There are swelling, warmth, and tenderness of the right knee joint. Tenderness and swelling at the right Achilles tendon insertion to the calcaneus are noted. There is no rash or nail pitting. The remainder of the physical examination is normal.

Laboratory studies done at the time of the visit:

Complete blood count with differential	Normal
Erythrocyte sedimentation rate	30 mm/h
Stool cultures	Negative
Urinalysis	Normal
DNA amplification urine test for *Chlamydia trachomatis*	Negative

Aspiration of the left knee is performed; synovial fluid analysis reveals a leukocyte count of 15,000/μL (15 × 10⁹/L) with 70% monocytes and no crystals. Gram stain is negative, and cultures are pending.

Radiographs of the knee and ankle are normal.

Which of the following is the most likely diagnosis?

(A) Infectious arthritis
(B) Psoriatic arthritis
(C) Reactive arthritis
(D) Rheumatoid arthritis

Item 59

A 68-year-old man is evaluated during a follow-up visit for long-standing tophaceous gout that caused almost monthly gout flares. Five months ago, colchicine and allopurinol were initiated. He reached his serum urate goal (<6.0 mg/dL [0.35 mmol/L]) within 3 months of starting therapy, and he has not had a gout flare since reaching this target. He has not developed any new tophi; his original tophi on his hands and elbows have begun to shrink in size. History is also significant for hypertension, for which he takes losartan.

On physical examination, temperature is 37.2 °C (98.9 °F), blood pressure is 133/79 mm Hg, pulse rate is 79/min, and respiration rate is 12/min. BMI is 28. A moderate-sized tophus is visible on the right elbow as well as two small tophi on different distal interphalangeal joints. There is no swelling or tenderness to palpation of any joints.

Current laboratory studies reveal a serum urate level of 5.4 mg/dL (0.32 mmol/L) and normal kidney and liver chemistries.

Which of the following is the most appropriate next step in management?

(A) Add probenecid
(B) Change allopurinol to febuxostat
(C) Continue colchicine and allopurinol
(D) Discontinue colchicine

Item 60

A 27-year-old man is evaluated for a 2-year history of ankylosing spondylitis. Symptoms were initially responsive to physical therapy and naproxen; however, for the past 6 months he has experienced increasing back and buttock pain and stiffness, with difficulty bending downward. One month ago naproxen was discontinued, and indomethacin was initiated but with no improvement.

On physical examination, vital signs are normal. BMI is 25. Tenderness to palpation over the sacroiliac joints and lower lumbar spine is noted. There is limited range of motion of the lumbar spine manifested by an increase of 1 cm of change on forward flexion.

Laboratory studies reveal an erythrocyte sedimentation rate of 40 mm/h.

In addition to continuing physical therapy, which of the following is the most appropriate treatment?

(A) Adalimumab
(B) Methotrexate

(C) Rituximab
(D) Sulfasalazine

Item 61

A 28-year-old woman is evaluated for a 2-week history of left hip pain that occurs at night and with walking. She has a 1-year history of systemic lupus erythematosus with class IV nephritis. Treatment has included prednisone as high as 60 mg/d and cyclophosphamide. Current medications are mycophenolate mofetil, hydroxychloroquine, prednisone, furosemide, lisinopril, calcium, and vitamin D.

On physical examination, vital signs are normal. BMI is 26. She has a cushingoid appearance. There is pain on internal rotation of the left hip. There is no pain on hip adduction or with pressure over the lateral hip. The remainder of the examination is normal.

Laboratory studies reveal an erythrocyte sedimentation rate of 18 mm/h, normal complement (C3 and C4) levels, and stable anti–double-stranded DNA antibodies.

Anterior-posterior pelvis and lateral left hip radiographs are normal.

Which of the following is the most appropriate diagnostic test to perform next?

(A) CT of the left hip
(B) MRI of the left hip
(C) Repeat plain radiography in 1 month
(D) Ultrasonography of the left hip

Item 62

A 58-year-old woman is evaluated in the hospital for a 3-month history of fatigue and a 4.5-kg (10-lb) weight loss. She also has dermatomyositis that was diagnosed 1 year ago, at which time she underwent detailed evaluation for myopathy and age-appropriate malignancy screening. She has also noticed worsening muscle weakness and rash in the past 2 weeks.

On physical examination, temperature is normal, blood pressure is 148/94 mm Hg, pulse rate is 90/min, and respiration rate is 16/min. BMI is 27. Cardiac and pulmonary examinations are normal. Abdominal examination reveals ascites without organomegaly. There is symmetric weakness of the arm and thigh muscles. A violaceous rash is present on the extensor surface of the metacarpophalangeal joints. A few areas of palpable purpura on the lower extremities are noted.

Laboratory studies:

Complete blood count	Normal
Chemistry panel	Normal
Aldolase	31 U/L (normal range, 1.0–8.0 U/L)
Aspartate aminotransferase	98 U/L
Creatine kinase	1400 U/L
Antinuclear antibodies	Titer of 1:640
Urinalysis	Normal

Which of the following is the most appropriate diagnostic test to perform next?

(A) Chest CT with contrast
(B) Liver biopsy

(C) PET scan

(D) Thigh muscle MRI

(E) Transvaginal pelvic ultrasonography

Item 63

A 52-year-old man is evaluated in the hospital for fever, malaise, arthralgia, left foot drop, abdominal pain that is worse after eating, and a 4.5-kg (10-lb) weight loss, all of which gradually developed over the past 2 months.

On physical examination, temperature is 38.4 °C (101.1 °F), blood pressure is 154/92 mm Hg, pulse rate is 76/min, and respiration rate is 18/min. BMI is 29. There is no temporal or sinus tenderness. The nasal passages and oropharynx are normal. The chest is clear. An abdominal bruit is heard on the right, inferior to the costal margin. The abdomen is otherwise normal. The testicles are tender to palpation. The joints are tender to palpation without synovitis. Weakness of the left foot to dorsiflexion is noted.

The appearance of the trunk and thighs is shown.

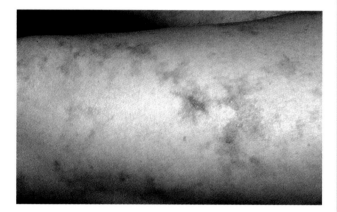

Laboratory studies:

Erythrocyte sedimentation rate	72 mm/h
Complements (C3 and C4)	Normal
Creatinine	2.2 mg/dL (194.5 µmol/L)
IgA	Normal
Hepatitis B surface antigen	Positive
Hepatitis B surface antibodies	Negative
Hepatitis C antibodies	Negative
ANCA	Negative
Urinalysis	Negative

Chest radiograph is unremarkable. Abdominal angiogram shows aneurysms and stenoses of the mesenteric and renal arteries.

Which of the following is the most likely diagnosis?

(A) Goodpasture syndrome

(B) Granulomatosis with polyangiitis

(C) Henoch-Schönlein purpura

(D) Polyarteritis nodosa

Item 64

A 34-year-old man is evaluated for progressive left knee pain. The pain causes difficulty with his work as a mail carrier, particularly when walking. His occupation does not require repetitive bending. He played football in college and experienced left knee trauma during sports participation; he underwent left meniscectomy and stopped playing sports. His mother has osteoarthritis of the hands that developed at age 65 years.

On physical examination, vital signs are normal. BMI is 27. Bone hypertrophy of the left knee is noted. There is crepitus but no warmth, erythema, swelling, or effusion of the knees.

Plain radiographs (anteroposterior views) show medial joint-space narrowing of both knees but greater on the left as well as osteophytes and bony sclerosis of the tibial plateau of the left knee; there is no periarticular osteopenia or erosive or destructive changes.

Which of the following is the most likely cause of this patient's left knee osteoarthritis?

(A) BMI

(B) Family history

(C) Meniscectomy

(D) Occupation

Item 65

A 62-year-old woman is evaluated in the emergency department for right knee pain. Three days ago she developed increasing pain, swelling, warmth, and erythema of the right knee as well as fevers and chills. She underwent total knee replacement of her right knee 2 months ago.

On physical examination, temperature is 38.4 °C (101.2 °F), blood pressure is 110/75 mm Hg, pulse rate is 98/min, and respiration rate is 12/min. BMI is 23. The right knee has a well-healed surgical scar, but there are significant knee joint swelling, warmth, tenderness to palpation, mild overlying erythema, and decreased range of motion. The remainder of the examination is normal.

Laboratory studies reveal a leukocyte count of 15,500/µL (15.5 × 10⁹/L) with 89% neutrophils, a C-reactive protein level of 6.8 mg/dL (68 mg/L), and an erythrocyte sedimentation rate of 45 mm/h.

Radiograph of the right knee shows only an effusion.

Which of the following is the most appropriate next step in management?

(A) Begin vancomycin and cefepime

(B) Obtain blood and synovial fluid cultures

(C) Obtain a bone scan

(D) Obtain a CT of the knee

Item 66

A 76-year-old man seeks advice regarding dietary modifications to help prevent gout flares. He recently experienced his first episode of podagra. At his initial visit, serum urate level was 7.2 mg/dL (0.42 mmol/L). History is also significant for hypertension, for which he takes losartan.

On physical examination, temperature is 37.1 °C (98.8 °F), blood pressure is 135/80 mm Hg, pulse rate is 80/min, and respiration rate is 15/min. BMI is 27. The remainder of the examination is unremarkable.

In addition to meat restriction, increased intake of which of the following may help to decrease this patient's risk of gout flares?

(A) Leafy green vegetables

(B) Low-fat dairy products

(C) Red wine

(D) Shellfish

Item 67

A 29-year-old woman is evaluated for increasing fatigue and diffuse pain of 6 months' duration. The pain becomes more severe for several days if she "overdoes it." She reports chronically poor sleep and has difficulty concentrating at work. History is also significant for hypothyroidism, for which she takes levothyroxine. She takes ibuprofen as needed for the pain, which provides minimal benefit.

On physical examination, vital signs are normal. BMI is 25. Tenderness to palpation of multiple muscle groups is noted. Muscle strength is normal. There is no joint swelling or rash. The remainder of the examination is normal.

Laboratory studies, including complete blood count, chemistry panel, erythrocyte sedimentation rate, and thyroid-stimulating hormone, are normal.

Which of the following is the most appropriate next step in management?

(A) Begin scheduled ibuprofen

(B) Increase levothyroxine

(C) Obtain an antinuclear antibody panel

(D) Start an aerobic exercise program

Item 68

A 75-year-old man is evaluated for gradual progression of right knee pain. He has a 10-year history of right knee osteoarthritis, which was previously controlled with acetaminophen. He recently discontinued the acetaminophen because of continued pain and began over-the-counter oral naproxen, with good results. He can walk again without pain or difficulty. He has no other medical problems and takes no other medications.

On physical examination, blood pressure is 124/82 mm Hg. The right knee demonstrates evidence of bony enlargement and crepitus on flexion and extension; no warmth, tenderness, or effusion is noted.

Which of the following is the most appropriate next step in management?

(A) Continue oral naproxen

(B) Discontinue oral naproxen; begin celecoxib

(C) Discontinue oral naproxen; begin a topical NSAID

(D) Refer for knee joint replacement

Item 69

A 52-year-old man is evaluated for a 6-month history of increasingly swollen and painful joints of the fingers of both hands, both wrists, and the left ankle associated with 90 minutes of morning stiffness. He has tried over-the-counter ibuprofen and naproxen without sustained benefit. He has no other symptoms.

On physical examination, vital signs are normal. There are swelling and tenderness of the second, third, and fifth proximal interphalangeal joints; first, second, and third metacarpophalangeal joints; both wrists; and left ankle. Decreased range of motion of the right wrist is noted. The remainder of the physical examination is normal.

Laboratory studies reveal an erythrocyte sedimentation rate of 45 mm/h and a C-reactive protein level of 5.2 mg/dL (52 mg/L); rheumatoid factor and anti–cyclic citrullinated peptide antibody tests are negative.

Hand radiographs show an erosion of the second right metacarpal head with mild symmetric joint-space narrowing and mild periarticular osteopenia of the metacarpophalangeal joints; there is no bony sclerosis or osteophytes.

Which of the following is the most likely diagnosis?

(A) Osteoarthritis

(B) Rheumatoid arthritis

(C) Sarcoidosis

(D) Systemic lupus erythematosus

Item 70

A 41-year-old man is evaluated for a 1-month history of daily fever as high as 39.0 °C (102.2 °F), a 4.5-kg (10.0-lb) weight loss, myalgia, and swollen lymph nodes. He reports joint pain and stiffness in the shoulders, hands, wrists, and knees. He has also noted a pink rash over the trunk and extremities associated with the fever.

On physical examination, temperature is 38.4 °C (101.1 °F), blood pressure is 128/78 mm Hg, pulse rate is 100/min, and respiration rate is 18/min. BMI is 28. Multiple enlarged lymph nodes in the anterior cervical chain are present. Splenomegaly is noted. There is an erythematous maculopapular rash on the trunk and extremities. Swelling of the wrists and knees is present. The remainder of the examination is normal.

Laboratory studies:

Erythrocyte sedimentation rate	100 mm/h
Hematocrit	31%
Leukocyte count	30,000/μL (30 × 10⁹/L), with 80% neutrophils; no blasts
Platelet count	350,000/μL (350 × 10⁹/L)
Alanine aminotransferase	68 U/L
Aspartate aminotransferase	75 U/L
C-reactive protein	30 mg/dL (300 mg/L)
Creatinine	0.9 mg/dL (79.6 μmol/L)
Ferritin	20,000 ng/mL (20,000 μg/L)
Urinalysis	Normal

Chest radiograph is normal.

Which of the following is the most likely diagnosis?

(A) Acute myeloid leukemia
(B) Adult-onset Still disease
(C) Granulomatosis with polyangiitis
(D) Systemic lupus erythematosus

Item 71

A 29-year-old man is evaluated for pain and photophobia in the left eye that began 3 days ago. He reports a 6-month history of recurrent painful oral and genital ulcers that last 1 to 2 weeks and then resolve, as well as waxing and waning knee, ankle, and wrist pain during this time. Medical history had been unremarkable until the onset of these symptoms, and he takes no medications.

On physical examination, temperature is 38.2 °C (100.7 °F), blood pressure is 134/82 mm Hg, pulse rate is 90/min, and respiration rate is 14/min. BMI is 22. The left eye is diffusely erythematous, and a small amount of white fluid on the bottom of the anterior chamber is noted. There is an ulcer on the right side of the tongue.

The genital ulcers are shown.

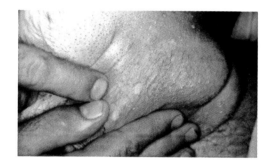

Laboratory studies show an erythrocyte sedimentation rate of 76 mm/h as well as a normal complete blood count and metabolic profile.

The patient is urgently referred to an ophthalmologist.

Which of the following is the most likely diagnosis?

(A) Behçet syndrome
(B) Cytomegalovirus infection
(C) Herpes simplex virus type 1 infection
(D) Reactive arthritis

Item 72

A 66-year-old man is evaluated for a 2-month history of right knee pain. The pain is worse with walking and is accompanied by approximately 5 minutes of morning stiffness. Medical history is significant for chronic kidney disease, hypertension, and mild gastroesophageal reflux disease. Medications are lisinopril, hydrochlorothiazide, and ranitidine as needed for heartburn.

On physical examination, vital signs are normal. BMI is 29. Medial joint line tenderness and mild crepitus are noted in the right knee. There is no redness, warmth, or instability of the affected joint; minimal swelling is noted.

Laboratory studies reveal a serum creatinine level of 1.6 mg/dL (141.4 µmol/L).

Radiographs of the right knee show mild medial joint-space narrowing, subchondral sclerosis of the same region, and small osteophytes at the medial femoral and tibial joint margins.

In addition to an exercise program, which of the following is the most appropriate initial treatment?

(A) Acetaminophen
(B) Celecoxib
(C) Colchicine
(D) Ibuprofen

Item 73

A 24-year-old woman is evaluated for a 6-month history of color change in her hands and feet, which is worse during stress. She is a nonsmoker. Family history is negative.

On physical examination, temperature is normal, blood pressure is 116/72 mm Hg, pulse rate is 64/min, and respiration rate is 12/min. BMI is 22. There is mild reversible discoloration of the fingertips upon exposure to cold. Cool tips of the fingers without digital pits are noted. Cardiopulmonary examination is normal. Muscle strength and reflexes are normal. There is no rash. The remainder of the examination is normal.

Laboratory studies, including complete blood count and chemistry panel, are normal. Nailfold capillary examination is normal.

Which of the following is the most appropriate next step in management?

(A) Measure antinuclear and anti-U1-ribonucleoprotein antibodies
(B) Measure antiphospholipid antibody panel and cryoglobulins
(C) Obtain digital arteriography
(D) Clinical observation

Item 74

A 64-year-old man is evaluated in the emergency department for progressively deteriorating mental status. His wife states that he has been experiencing episodic headaches during the past several months, and his mental status has changed progressively over the past several days. History is significant for atherosclerosis, hypertension, and coronary artery disease. He has a 40-pack-year history of smoking. Medications are atorvastatin, lisinopril, and low-dose aspirin.

On physical examination, the patient is alert and oriented to self but not to place or year. Vital signs are normal. BMI is 26. On the Mini–Mental State Examination, he is unable to do serial sevens, is able to recall only one object out of three, and cannot draw a geometric figure that is shown to him. The remainder of the examination, including the neurologic assessment, is within normal limits.

Laboratory studies, including complete blood count, basic metabolic panel, liver chemistries, and urinalysis, are normal; erythrocyte sedimentation rate is 22 mm/h.

Lumbar puncture is performed; cerebrospinal fluid analysis reveals a leukocyte count of 15/μL (15×10^6/L), 90% lymphocytes, and a protein level of 45 mg/dL (450 mg/L).

Chest radiograph is unremarkable. A brain MRI shows scattered lesions, mainly in the white matter, and an MR angiogram shows possible narrowing of the intracerebral arteries.

Which of the following is the most appropriate next step in management?

(A) Initiate azathioprine

(B) Initiate cyclophosphamide and glucocorticoids

(C) Obtain functional MRI

(D) Obtain intracerebral angiography and brain biopsy

Item 75

A 45-year-old woman is evaluated for a 2-week history of nausea, right upper quadrant abdominal pain and fullness, and malaise. She has rheumatoid arthritis that was diagnosed 2 years ago. Initial treatment with methotrexate lost its efficacy after 6 months, and she was switched to leflunomide. She had partial response to leflunomide and was started on etanercept in combination. Other medications are sulfasalazine and naproxen. In the past 6 months, she has had no active swollen or tender joints.

On physical examination, vital signs are normal. BMI is 28. Icterus is noted. The liver is palpable with slight tenderness. Murphy sign is negative. The remainder of the examination is normal.

Laboratory studies:

Hemoglobin	11.1 g/dL (111 g/L)
Leukocyte count	12,500/μL (12.5×10^9/L)
Alkaline phosphatase	162 U/L
Alanine aminotransferase	73 U/L
Aspartate aminotransferase	81 U/L
Total bilirubin	2.6 mg/dL (44.5 μmol/L)
Hepatitis B serologies	Negative
Hepatitis C serologies	Negative

Abdominal ultrasound shows multiple gallstones, no thickening of the gallbladder, and normal extrahepatic bile ducts.

Which of the following is the most appropriate next step in management?

(A) Discontinue etanercept

(B) Discontinue leflunomide

(C) Schedule a cholecystectomy

(D) Schedule a liver biopsy

Item 76

A 55-year-old man is evaluated during a follow-up visit for gout. Two years ago, he had been treated with allopurinol and developed a hypersensitivity reaction. Over the past several months, he has had recurrent attacks of acute, episodic swelling of the first metatarsophalangeal joints with increasing involvement of other joints, including the ankles and knees. Laboratory studies showed significant hyperuricemia. History is also significant for Crohn

disease, hypertension, chronic kidney disease (estimated glomerular filtration rate of 55 mL/min/1.73 m²), and non-alcoholic fatty liver disease. Current medications are diltiazem and azathioprine, which he has been taking for the past 9 months.

On physical examination, temperature is 37.1 °C (98.8 °F), blood pressure is 125/70 mm Hg, pulse rate is 80/min, and respiration rate is 12/min. BMI is 28. The examination is unremarkable, including no joint abnormalities.

Which of the following is a contraindication to the use of febuxostat in this patient?

(A) Azathioprine

(B) Diltiazem

(C) Mild to moderate chronic kidney disease

(D) Nonalcoholic fatty liver disease

Item 77

A 28-year-old woman is evaluated in the emergency department for a 3-week history of progressively worsening pain in the left arm. The pain worsens with use of the arm. She also notes fatigue, malaise, and the inability to walk long distances due to discomfort in her legs. She reports no cough, nausea, vomiting, or burning on urination. She takes no medications.

On physical examination, temperature is 38.1 °C (100.5 °F), blood pressure is 166/95 mm Hg in the right arm and 115/56 mm Hg in the left arm, pulse rate is 72/min, and respiration rate is 14/min. BMI is 27. Pallor of the fingertips and delayed capillary refill of the nail beds are noted in the left hand. A diminished radial pulse of the left arm and decreased dorsalis pedis pulses bilaterally are noted. A bruit is heard over the mid abdomen. There is no rash.

Laboratory studies:

Erythrocyte sedimentation rate	115 mm/h
Creatinine	1.3 mg/dL (115 μmol/L)
Partial thromboplastin time	Normal
Prothrombin time	Normal
D-dimer	Negative
Urinalysis	Normal

Which of the following is the most appropriate diagnostic test to perform next?

(A) Antimyeloperoxidase antibody assay

(B) Antiphospholipid antibody assay

(C) Aortic arteriography

(D) Temporal artery biopsy

Item 78

A 28-year-old woman seeks preconception counseling. She has a 5-year history of systemic lupus erythematosus, which initially presented with nephritis, rash, and arthritis. Her disease has been well controlled for 1 year with hydroxychloroquine, mycophenolate mofetil, and prednisone, 5 mg/d.

On physical examination, vital signs are normal. BMI is 28. There is a discoid rash on the ear pinna, unchanged since the last examination. No other rashes or ulcers are noted.

The remainder of the examination, including cardiopulmonary examination, is normal.

Laboratory studies, including complete blood count, chemistry panel, liver chemistries, complement levels, and urinalysis, are normal.

Which of the following is the most appropriate next step in management?

(A) Discontinue hydroxychloroquine
(B) Discontinue mycophenolate mofetil
(C) Discontinue prednisone
(D) Continue current regimen
(E) Stop all medications

Item 79

A 42-year-old woman is evaluated for a 4-month history of progressive right hip pain. Plain radiographs obtained 2 months ago showed early osteoarthritis. Her symptoms have steadily worsened and are now limiting mobility. She reports no recent trauma or injuries, fevers, or pain of other joints. She is originally from India. She has lived in the United States for 15 years but visits her family abroad occasionally. She reports no injection drug use and is not sexually active. She was found to be positive for latent tuberculosis infection several years ago and underwent standard treatment at that time. History is significant for rheumatoid arthritis, for which she takes methotrexate and folic acid; she also started etanercept 3 months ago.

On physical examination, temperature is 37.1 °C (98.8 °F), blood pressure is 135/80 mm Hg, pulse rate is 75/min, and respiration rate is 12/min. BMI is 23. Range of motion of the right hip is limited by pain without overlying erythema or warmth. There are no visible joint or skin abnormalities. There are no heart murmurs, and the lungs are clear.

Laboratory studies reveal an erythrocyte sedimentation rate of 40 mm/h; complete blood count and kidney and liver chemistries are normal.

Radiograph of the right hip reveals an effusion and new erosive changes.

Arthrocentesis of the right hip is performed.

Which of the following is the most likely cause of this patient's hip pain?

(A) Gout
(B) *Mycobacterium tuberculosis* infection
(C) *Neisseria gonorrhea* infection
(D) Rheumatoid arthritis

Item 80

A 35-year-old woman is evaluated for weakness in the right foot and left wrist with paresthesia in the right leg, right foot, left forearm, and left hand. She also reports facial erythema and joint stiffness. She has a 6-year history of systemic lupus erythematosus (SLE). Medications are hydroxychloroquine, prednisone, vitamin D, and calcium.

On physical examination, vital signs are normal. There is a new malar rash. Swelling of the second through fourth metacarpophalangeal joints of the hands is present. There is dorsiflexion weakness of the right ankle and a left wrist

drop. Reflexes are normal. The remainder of the examination is normal.

Laboratory studies indicate that her SLE appears to be active with an elevation of erythrocyte sedimentation rate compared with baseline, leukopenia, and anemia typical of her previous SLE flares.

Which of the following is the most appropriate next step in management?

(A) Discontinue hydroxychloroquine
(B) Obtain electromyography/nerve conduction studies
(C) Obtain MRI of the cervical spine
(D) Obtain skin biopsy for small-fiber neuropathy

Item 81

A 40-year-old man has a 15-year history of well-controlled chronic plaque psoriasis and psoriatic arthritis and is now evaluated for a severe flare of both the skin and joint disease. One month ago, he developed severe pain and swelling of the hands, elbows, knees, ankles, and toes; symptoms have been unresponsive to ibuprofen. He also developed sudden worsening of psoriasis over the trunk and extremities. He notes increased fatigue and intermittent lymphadenopathy in the neck for the past 3 months. He has no other symptoms. His only medication is sulfasalazine.

On physical examination, temperature is 37.8 °C (100.0 °F), blood pressure is 130/85 mm Hg, and pulse rate is 80/min. Swelling and tenderness of the bilateral elbows, wrists, proximal interphalangeal joints, knees, ankles, and metatarsophalangeal joints are noted. Oropharyngeal candidiasis is present. Cervical lymphadenopathy is noted bilaterally. Except for the skin, the remainder of the physical examination is normal.

The appearance of the skin is shown.

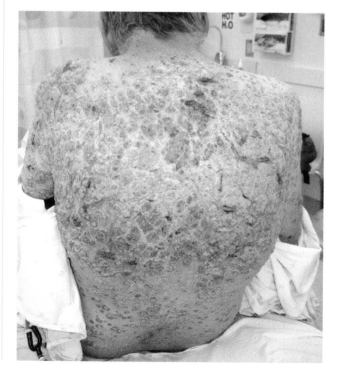

Which of the following is the most appropriate diagnostic test to perform next?

(A) Heterophile antibody testing

(B) HIV antibody testing

(C) HLA–B27 testing

(D) Lyme antibody testing

(E) Rapid streptococcal testing

Item 82

A 28-year-old woman is evaluated for a 1-week history of pain and morning stiffness in her hands. Three weeks ago, she had muscle aches, malaise, fevers, and coryza, all of which have resolved. She is an elementary school teacher; prior to her initial illness, several children in her class had similar symptoms accompanied by an erythematous rash on the cheeks. She does not have other pertinent personal or family history, and she takes no medications.

On physical examination, temperature is 37.3 °C (99.2 °F), blood pressure is 120/78 mm Hg, pulse rate is 66/min, and respiration rate is 13/min. BMI is 22. Symmetric wrist, metacarpophalangeal, and proximal interphalangeal joint tenderness and pain with motion are noted without significant joint swelling. The remainder of the examination is normal.

Laboratory studies are significant for an erythrocyte sedimentation rate of 38 mm/h.

Which of the following is the most appropriate initial treatment?

(A) Azithromycin

(B) Ibuprofen

(C) Interferon alfa

(D) Prednisone

Item 83

A 52-year-old man is evaluated in the hospital for several episodes of hemoptysis that developed over the past day. He reports feeling well until about 3 weeks ago when he developed myalgia, arthralgia, occasional epistaxis, and diminished hearing. One week ago he developed a rash and weakness in his right hand. History is otherwise unremarkable, and he takes no medications.

On physical examination, temperature is 38.0 °C (100.4 °F), blood pressure is 152/100 mm Hg, pulse rate is 72/min, and respiration rate is 24/min. Conjunctivitis is present in both eyes. Decreased hearing in both ears is noted. Bilateral maxillary sinus tenderness is present. Chest examination reveals diffuse rhonchi. The right hand has decreased grip strength. Palpable purpura of the bilateral lower extremities is present.

Laboratory studies:

Erythrocyte sedimentation rate	84 mm/h
Leukocyte count	12,300/µL (12.3 × 10⁹/L), eosinophils <2%
Complements (C3, C4)	Normal
Creatinine	2.1 mg/dL (185.6 µmol/L)
Urinalysis	3+ protein; 50 erythrocytes/hpf; 20 leukocytes/hpf; several mixed cellular casts

Sinus radiograph shows bony erosion of the septum and turbinates. Chest radiograph shows diffuse infiltrates.

Which of the following is most likely to establish the diagnosis?

(A) Anti–double-stranded DNA antibody levels

(B) Antimyeloperoxidase antibody levels

(C) Antiproteinase 3 antibody levels

(D) Serum cryoglobulin levels

Item 84

A 31-year-old woman is evaluated during a follow-up visit for systemic lupus erythematosus. She was diagnosed 6 months ago after presenting with a malar rash, pericarditis, and arthritis. She was initially treated with prednisone, 40 mg/d, and hydroxychloroquine with good control of symptoms. The prednisone was subsequently tapered to the current dose of 5 mg/d.

On physical examination, temperature is normal, blood pressure is 130/92 mm Hg, pulse rate is 90/min, and respiration rate is 16/min. BMI is 27. There is edema of the lower extremities to just above the ankles. There are no cardiac or pleural rubs. No rash is present.

Laboratory studies:

	One month ago	Today
C3	Normal	Decreased
C4	Normal	Decreased
Creatinine	0.7 mg/dL (61.9 µmol/L)	1.3 mg/dL (115 µmol/L)
Anti–double-stranded DNA antibodies	225 U/mL	721 U/mL
Urinalysis	Trace erythrocytes; trace protein	1+ erythrocytes; 2+ protein; 1 erythrocyte cast; no bacteria
Spot urine protein-creatinine ratio	300 mg/g	1200 mg/g

In addition to an increase in prednisone, which of the following is the most appropriate next step in management?

(A) Add methotrexate

(B) Repeat laboratory testing in 1 month

(C) Schedule kidney biopsy

(D) Schedule renal artery Doppler examination

Item 85

A 55-year-old man is diagnosed with hypertension. Other than a single episode of podagra 6 months ago, his medical history is unremarkable. He takes no medications. Family history is notable for his father and brother who have gout and hypertension.

On physical examination, temperature is 36.6 °C (97.9 °F), blood pressure is 152/100 mm Hg, pulse rate is 82/min, and respiration rate is 14/min. BMI is 24. The remainder of the physical examination is unremarkable.

Laboratory studies are significant for normal blood urea nitrogen, serum creatinine, and electrolyte levels; the serum urate level is 7.9 mg/dL (0.47 mmol/L).

Which of the following antihypertensive drugs is the most appropriate for this patient?

(A) Hydrochlorothiazide

(B) Lisinopril

(C) Losartan

(D) Metoprolol

Item 86

A 71-year-old man is evaluated for severe tophaceous gout. Colchicine has been effective in reducing flares to approximately two in the past year. On initial evaluation 1 year ago, serum urate level was 10.2 mg/dL (0.60 mmol/L). Allopurinol was initiated but subsequently discontinued because of gastrointestinal intolerance. He was switched to febuxostat, which was increased to maximum dose without success in reaching the serum urate goal of less than 6.0 mg/dL (0.35 mmol/L). He recently had a gout flare of his right great toe, which has nearly resolved.

On physical examination, temperature is 36.6 °C (97.9 °F), blood pressure is 140/80 mm Hg, pulse rate is 89/min, and respiration rate is 15/min. BMI is 32. Bulky tophi are present over bilateral elbows, hands, and feet with drainage of pasty material from a large tophus over the second metacarpophalangeal joint of the left hand. There are mild swelling and tenderness to palpation over the right first metatarsophalangeal joint.

Laboratory studies reveal a serum urate level of 10.9 mg/dL (0.64 mmol/L), an estimated glomerular filtration rate of 42 mL/min/1.73 m², and a normal glucose-6-phosphate dehydrogenase level.

Which of the following is the most appropriate next step in management?

(A) Add pegloticase

(B) Start prednisone

(C) Switch colchicine to anakinra

(D) Switch febuxostat to pegloticase

Item 87

A 25-year-old woman is evaluated during a follow-up visit for systemic lupus erythematosus. She was feeling well until 2 weeks ago when she developed increased fatigue and diffuse arthralgia. Medications are hydroxychloroquine and ibuprofen as needed.

On physical examination, temperature is 37.2 °C (99.0 °F), blood pressure is 140/80 mm Hg, pulse rate is 80/min, and respiration rate is 16/min. There is diffuse alopecia of the scalp. Malar erythema is noted. Heart sounds are normal, and the chest is clear. Examination of the abdomen is normal. Tenderness with minimal swelling of the proximal interphalangeal joints is present bilaterally. Small effusions on both knees with pain on range of motion are noted.

Laboratory studies:

Leukocyte count	3000/μL (3.0 × 10⁹/L), with 900 lymphocytes
Creatinine	Normal
Electrolytes	Normal
Urinalysis	2+ protein; trace blood

Which of the following tests should be obtained next?

(A) Anti–double-stranded DNA antibodies

(B) Antinuclear antibodies

(C) Anti-Ro/SSA and anti-La/SSB antibodies

(D) Anti-Smith antibodies

(E) Anti-U1-ribonucleoprotein antibodies

Item 88

A 31-year-old woman is evaluated in the hospital for headache, blurred vision, and nausea occurring for the past 12 hours. She has a 2-year history of diffuse cutaneous systemic sclerosis with recent worsening of Raynaud phenomenon that is treated with nifedipine.

On physical examination, the patient is alert but is somnolent and has altered sensorium. Temperature is normal, blood pressure is 150/92 mm Hg, pulse rate is 104/min, and respiration rate is 16/min. BMI is 22. Oxygen saturation is 95% on ambient air. Cardiopulmonary examination is normal. Examination of the skin reveals diffuse skin thickening of the face, anterior chest, and distal extremities; sclerodactyly; and multiple healed digital pits. Neurologic examination is nonfocal.

Laboratory studies:

Complete blood count	Normal
Albumin	3.0 g/dL (30 g/L)
Bicarbonate	32 mEq/L (32 mmol/L)
Creatinine	4.2 mg/dL (371.3 μmol/L); baseline, 0.8 mg/dL (70.7 μmol/L)
Urinalysis	2+ protein; 3 erythrocytes/hpf; 5 leukocytes/hpf; few granular casts
Urine protein-creatinine ratio	1200 mg/g

Chest radiograph is normal. Noncontrast CT of the head is normal. MRI of the brain shows bilateral parietal lobe white matter prominence.

Which of the following is the most appropriate treatment?

(A) Captopril

(B) Cyclophosphamide

(C) Methylprednisolone

(D) Sildenafil

Item 89

A 55-year-old woman is evaluated for a 3-year history of gradual left knee pain. She reports increased difficulty with stair climbing and an increase in pain over the past 6 months. She has no history of injury. She was prescribed acetaminophen, 1000 mg three times daily, and an exercise program 3 months ago but continues to have activity-limiting symptoms. Family history is notable for her mother who had a total knee replacement at the age of 65 years.

On physical examination, vital signs are normal. BMI is 31. There is bony hypertrophy of the left knee and the first metacarpophalangeal joints without warmth, erythema, swelling, or effusion.

Laboratory studies, including an erythrocyte sedimentation rate and serum creatinine, are normal.

Knee radiographs (including standing views) show medial joint-space narrowing and small osteophytes of the left knee; there is no periarticular osteopenia or marginal erosions.

Which of the following is the most appropriate next treatment?

(A) Capsaicin
(B) Diclofenac
(C) Duloxetine
(D) Hyaluronic acid
(E) Hydrocodone

Item 90

A 56-year-old man is evaluated for painless intermittent bloody urine of 6 weeks' duration. History is significant for granulomatosis with polyangiitis (formerly known as Wegener granulomatosis) diagnosed 10 years ago, which is now in remission; he was treated with prednisone for 3 years and oral cyclophosphamide for 1 year. He also has hypertension and hyperlipidemia. Current medications are metoprolol and atorvastatin.

On physical examination, temperature is 36.7 °C (98.0 °F), blood pressure is 146/94 mm Hg, pulse rate is 68/min, and respiration rate is 14/min. BMI is 28. There are no rashes or ulcers. Genitalia are normal. The remainder of the examination, including cardiopulmonary examination, is normal.

Laboratory studies:

Chemistry panel and kidney function tests	Normal
Hemoglobin	12.1 g/dL (121 g/L)
Erythrocyte sedimentation rate	35 mm/h
p-ANCA	Negative
Antimyeloperoxidase antibodies	Negative
Antiproteinase 3 antibodies	Negative
Urinalysis	Trace protein; 10-20 erythrocytes/hpf; 0-2 leukocytes/hpf; no casts
Urine cultures	Negative

A chest radiograph is normal.

Which of the following is the most appropriate diagnostic test to perform next?

(A) CT of the abdomen and pelvis with contrast
(B) Cystoscopy
(C) Kidney and bladder ultrasonography
(D) Urine eosinophil measurement
(E) Urine protein-creatinine ratio

Item 91

A 35-year-old woman is evaluated in the hospital for a 6-month history of worsening fatigue and a 3-week history of progressive shortness of breath. Over the past 2 weeks she has developed orthopnea and leg edema. Medical history is significant for diffuse cutaneous systemic sclerosis and gastroesophageal reflux disease. Her only medication is omeprazole.

On physical examination, the patient is alert but in respiratory distress. Temperature is 37.2 °C (99.0 °F), blood pressure is 106/74 mm Hg, pulse rate is 108/min, and respiration rate is 24/min. BMI is 31. Oxygen saturation is 92% on ambient air. An S_3 and elevated jugular venous pressure are noted. Crackles are noted at the lung bases. Diffuse skin thickening of the face, anterior chest, arms stopping at the elbows, and legs is noted; there is sclerodactyly of the hands. There is lower extremity edema to the knees.

Laboratory studies are normal except for a serum creatinine level of 2.2 mg/dL (194.5 μmol/L).

Chest radiograph shows bilateral pleural effusions and diffuse alveolar infiltrates. Echocardiogram shows generalized myocardial hypokinesis and a left ventricular ejection fraction of 20%. Electrocardiogram shows nonspecific T-wave changes.

Which of the following is the most likely cause of this patient's clinical presentation?

(A) Cardiomyopathy
(B) Constrictive pericarditis
(C) Pulmonary arterial hypertension
(D) Scleroderma renal crisis

Item 92

A 32-year-old woman is evaluated for a 2-month history of weight loss, abdominal cramping, and loose stools. Her stools are malodorous, but she has not noted any blood associated with her bowel movements. Although her appetite is good, she has lost 3.2 kg (7.0 lb). She has an 8-year history of diffuse cutaneous systemic sclerosis.

On physical examination, temperature is normal, blood pressure is 146/92 mm Hg, pulse rate is 94/min, and respiration rate is 16/min. BMI is 19. Cardiopulmonary examination is normal. The abdomen is soft and nontender with normal bowel sounds. Diffuse skin thickening of the face, anterior chest, and distal extremities is noted as well as sclerodactyly and multiple healed digital pits. There is no rash. Muscle strength and reflexes are normal.

Laboratory studies:

Hematocrit	30%
Albumin	2.6 g/dL (26 g/L)
Alanine aminotransferase	Normal
Aspartate aminotransferase	Normal
Total bilirubin	Normal
Lipase	Normal
Urinalysis	Normal

Which of the following is the most appropriate diagnostic test to perform next?

(A) Colonoscopy
(B) CT of the abdomen and pelvis with contrast

(C) Endoscopic retrograde cholangiopancreatography

(D) Glucose hydrogen breath test

Item 93

A 65-year-old woman is evaluated for bilateral hand and wrist pain that worsens with activity. She reports no swelling or redness but has morning stiffness lasting less than 30 minutes. History is also significant for hypertension and diabetes mellitus. There is no personal or family history of psoriasis. Medications are hydrochlorothiazide and metformin.

On physical examination, vital signs are normal. BMI is 29. The right wrist has a mild effusion and slightly reduced range of motion. There is mild pain with range of motion of both wrists. The hands have bony hypertrophy of the proximal and distal interphalangeal joints, with mild tenderness to palpation but no swelling. Bilateral crepitus of the knees is noted. There are no rashes or nail changes.

Laboratory studies reveal a negative rheumatoid factor, and erythrocyte sedimentation rate, C-reactive protein, and serum urate levels are within normal limits.

A radiograph of the wrist is shown.

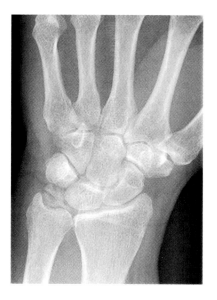

Aspiration of the wrist is performed, and results are pending.

Which of the following is the most likely diagnosis?

(A) Chronic gouty arthropathy

(B) Osteoarthritis with calcium pyrophosphate deposition

(C) Psoriatic arthritis

(D) Rheumatoid arthritis

Item 94

A 74-year-old woman is evaluated during a follow-up visit for polymyalgia rheumatica diagnosed 8 weeks ago after developing shoulder and hip girdle pain and morning stiffness. Symptoms resolved on prednisone, 15 mg/d. She feels well and reports no headache, jaw claudication, visual changes, or recurrence of myalgia or stiffness. History is significant for type 2 diabetes mellitus and hypertension. Medications are metformin, lisinopril, and prednisone, which has been tapered to 10 mg/d.

On physical examination, temperature is normal, blood pressure is 140/80 mm Hg, pulse rate is 70/min, and respiration rate is 14/min. BMI is 31. There is no temporal tenderness or induration. No carotid or subclavian bruits are present. Good range of motion without pain in the shoulders and hips is noted. Proximal strength is normal.

Laboratory studies:

	Initial	Current
Erythrocyte sedimentation rate	90 mm/h	42 mm/h
Hemoglobin	11.5 g/dL (115 g/L)	12 g/dL (120 g/L)

Which of the following is the most appropriate management at this time?

(A) Increase prednisone

(B) Increase prednisone and add methotrexate

(C) Schedule temporal artery biopsy

(D) Continue current treatment

Item 95

A 47-year-old woman is evaluated in the emergency department for sharp mid-chest pain that developed abruptly. The pain is exacerbated by lying down, deep inspiration, or coughing but improves when she sits up.

On physical examination, temperature is 37.8 °C (100.0 °F), blood pressure is 140/88 mm Hg, pulse rate is 100/min, and respiration rate is 22/min. A friction rub at the left sternal border is heard. The lungs are clear. There are swelling and tenderness of the second and third proximal interphalangeal and metacarpophalangeal joints.

Electrocardiogram shows diffuse ST-segment elevations in all leads except aVR and V_1 and PR-segment depression in leads V_2 to V_6.

Which of the following is the most likely cause of this patient's pericarditis?

(A) Ankylosing spondylitis

(B) Polymyalgia rheumatica

(C) Psoriatic arthritis

(D) Rheumatoid arthritis

Item 96

An 80-year-old woman was hospitalized 2 days ago for upper gastrointestinal bleeding due to peptic ulcer disease. She was placed on omeprazole and given intravenous normal saline for hydration. Today she has developed right knee pain and swelling. History is also significant for osteoarthritis of the hands and knees. Her only medication prior to admission was ibuprofen as needed.

H
CONT.

On physical examination, temperature is 37.8 °C (100.0 °F); the remainder of the vital signs is normal. Hand findings are consistent with osteoarthritis. The right knee is warm with a large effusion, is tender to palpation, and has limited flexion to 90 degrees.

Aspiration of the right knee is performed; the synovial fluid is yellow and cloudy, and the leukocyte count is 15,000/μL (15×10^9/L).

Which of the following synovial fluid tests will be most helpful in establishing a diagnosis?

(A) Antinuclear antibody measurement

(B) Glucose measurement

(C) Gram stain, culture, and crystal analysis

(D) Protein measurement

Answers and Critiques

Item 1   Answer: B

Educational Objective: Treat hyperuricemia with febuxostat in a patient with an adverse reaction to allopurinol.

Febuxostat is indicated for this patient with frequent gout attacks. He had been taking allopurinol, a first-line agent for serum urate reduction in patients with gout. Urate-lowering therapy is indicated for patients with gout who experience repeated attacks (≥2 per year), have one attack in the setting of chronic kidney disease (CKD) of stage 2 or worse, have tophaceous deposits found on examination or imaging, or have a history of urolithiasis. This patient developed an adverse reaction to allopurinol but still needs urate-lowing therapy. Febuxostat is a newer non-purine, non-competitive xanthine oxidase inhibitor, which is a viable alternative to allopurinol. It can be used in patients with mild to moderate CKD and is safe to try after an adverse reaction or failure of allopurinol.

Anti-inflammatory prophylaxis to prevent gout attacks is recommended when urate-lowering therapy is initiated because of the paradoxical increased risk of acute gout attacks when serum urate levels are rapidly decreased by medication. Prophylaxis should be continued in the presence of any active disease (tophi or flares). Colchicine is a first-line option for gout prophylaxis and should not be discontinued in this patient who requires flare prophylaxis during urate-lowering therapy.

Pegloticase is an intravenous synthetic uricase replacement approved for treatment-failure gout. Pegloticase is immunogenic, and the development of antibodies eventually occurs in most patients taking the drug, which leads to reduced effectiveness and increases the risk of hypersensitivity reactions.

The uricosuric drugs probenecid and sulfinpyrazone promote kidney clearance of uric acid by inhibiting urate-anion exchangers in the proximal tubule responsible for urate reabsorption. These agents are relatively contraindicated in patients with impaired kidney function or those at risk for kidney stones.

KEY POINT

- In patients with gout who require urate-lowering therapy, febuxostat is a viable alternative for those who have an adverse reaction to allopurinol.

Bibliography

Khanna D, Fitzgerald JD, Khanna PP, et al; American College of Rheumatology. 2012 American College of Rheumatology guidelines for management of gout. Part 1: systematic nonpharmacologic and pharmacologic therapeutic approaches to hyperuricemia. Arthritis Care Res (Hoboken). 2012 Oct;64(10):1431–46. [PMID: 23024028]

Item 2   Answer: B

Educational Objective: Diagnose Jaccoud arthropathy in a patient with systemic lupus erythematosus.

The most likely diagnosis is Jaccoud arthropathy, which is most commonly caused by systemic lupus erythematosus (SLE). SLE arthritis is nonerosive, but persistent periarticular inflammation that affects the structural integrity of the joint capsule/supporting joint ligaments can result in Jaccoud arthropathy, or reversible hand deformities, which is characterized by reducible subluxation of the digits, swan neck deformities, and ulnar deviation of the fingers due to attenuation of the joint-supporting structures. It is reported to occur in 5% of patients with SLE and can be confused with rheumatoid arthritis. Jaccoud arthropathy can be seen in other inflammatory illnesses, including scleroderma, mixed connective tissue disease, and Sjögren syndrome, and was first described in patients with recurrent episodes of rheumatic fever. This patient with SLE demonstrates the classic features of Jaccoud arthropathy, including subluxation, ulnar deviation, and swan neck deformities, with radiographs that do not show evidence of erosions.

Joint hypermobility refers to the ability to painlessly move a joint beyond normal range of movement. Hypermobility syndrome describes a disorder characterized by musculoskeletal pain and generalized joint hypermobility occurring in otherwise healthy individuals. Patients with joint hypermobility can rarely have swan neck deformities but do not generally have deformities of the severity seen in this patient. In addition, the presence of another disease that can cause joint hypermobility (SLE in this patient) excludes hypermobility syndrome.

Mixed connective tissue disease (MCTD) is characterized by features of systemic sclerosis, polymyositis, and SLE and is by definition associated with high titers of anti-U1-ribonucleoprotein antibodies. This patient does not have any of the characteristic symptoms of MCTD, including Raynaud phenomenon, hand edema, puffy fingers, and/or prominent synovitis.

Rheumatoid arthritis generally causes nonreducible hand deformities; furthermore, severe hand changes associated with rheumatoid arthritis typically show erosions on radiograph and periarticular osteopenia, which are not present in this patient.

KEY POINT

- Jaccoud arthropathy is a nonerosive arthritis most commonly caused by systemic lupus erythematosus and is characterized by reducible subluxation of the digits, swan neck deformities, and ulnar deviation of the fingers due to attenuation of the joint-supporting structures.

Answers and Critiques

Bibliography

Skare TL, Godoi AL, Ferreira V. Jaccoud arthropathy in systemic lupus ery-thematosus: clinical and serologic findings. Rev Assoc Med Bras. 2012 Jul-Aug;58(4):489–92. [PMID: 22930030]

Item 3   Answer: C

Educational Objective: Diagnose rheumatoid arthritis with appropriate laboratory testing.

This patient most likely has rheumatoid arthritis (RA), and testing for both anti–cyclic citrullinated peptide (CCP) antibodies and rheumatoid factor will be most helpful in confirming the diagnosis. RA is an autoimmune disorder that typically presents as a symmetric inflammatory polyarthritis affecting the proximal interphalangeal and metacarpophalangeal joints of the fingers, the wrists, and the analogous joints of the feet. Prolonged morning stiffness is common. Anti-CCP antibody testing has the greatest specificity (95%) for the diagnosis of RA. Although no single laboratory test will diagnose RA, the combination of a compatible clinical presentation and a positive rheumatoid factor and positive anti-CCP antibodies is more specific for the diagnosis than any other combination of tests. Approximately 75% of patients with RA are rheumatoid factor positive, but specificity is only around 80%. Rheumatoid factor positivity frequently occurs in other autoimmune disorders and chronic infections, most notably chronic active hepatitis C virus infection.

Testing for antinuclear antibodies (ANA) is usually performed in patients with suspected systemic lupus erythematosus (SLE). A new onset of polyarticular inflammatory arthritis as seen in this patient can be indicative of SLE; however, she has no other signs or symptoms suggestive of SLE such as alopecia, aphthous ulcers, malar rash, pericardial and pleural serositis, or cytopenias. Furthermore, an ANA test may be positive in 40% of patients with RA and would not distinguish between RA and SLE with as much specificity as the combination of anti-CCP antibodies and rheumatoid factor.

Although an elevated C-reactive protein may provide laboratory evidence of inflammation that can complement the physical examination findings of inflammatory synovitis, this inflammatory marker lacks diagnostic specificity and does not distinguish RA from other forms of inflammatory arthritis.

KEY POINT

- The combination of anti–cyclic citrullinated peptide antibodies and rheumatoid factor has the greatest specificity for the diagnosis of rheumatoid arthritis.

Bibliography

Pincus T, Sokka T. Laboratory tests to assess patients with rheumatoid arthritis: advantages and limitations. Rheum Dis Clin N Am. 2009 Nov;35(4):731–4. [PMID: 19962617]

Item 4   Answer: A

Educational Objective: Diagnose amyopathic dermatomyositis.

The most likely diagnosis is amyopathic dermatomyositis. This patient has a clinical presentation of heliotrope eruption in the form of a violaceous periorbital rash, Gottron papules over the extensor surface of small joints of the hands, and photodistributed violaceous poikiloderma (V sign and Shawl sign) without muscle weakness. These are findings of skin involvement seen in dermatomyositis without any clinical, serum, or electromyogram (EMG) findings of muscle involvement or myositis, suggesting the diagnosis of amyopathic dermatomyositis. Amyopathic dermatomyositis is seen in about 20% to 25% of patients with dermatomyositis, but some of these patients have evidence of myositis on one of the evaluation studies (muscle enzymes, EMG, or muscle biopsy) in the absence of muscle weakness. To qualify for the diagnosis of amyopathic dermatomyositis, the patient should have the characteristic rash but no clinical, laboratory, or muscle evaluation findings of myositis. Amyopathic dermatomyositis may be triggered by sunlight exposure and also is associated with an underlying malignancy. Treatment is usually with glucocorticoids and immunosuppressive agents.

Polymorphous light eruption (PMLE) is another dermatologic condition in which patients develop skin lesions after exposure to sunlight; these lesions last several days and resolve spontaneously in the absence of reexposure. A variety of skin lesions may be seen in PMLE, including urticarial wheals, papules, plaques, and vesicles. PMLE usually develops early in the spring, with the first few exposures to sunlight, and can be triggered by intense exposures. These lesions occur in photodistributed areas but lack characteristic heliotrope or Gottron eruptions. A diagnosis of PMLE is unlikely in this patient.

Rosacea is a chronic, inflammatory condition that causes an acneiform eruption and flushing on the mid-face. There are two types, vascular and papular pustular (inflammatory) rosacea. Vascular rosacea presents as persistent flushing, especially of the central face, with prominent telangiectasias. Pustules and papules are seen in the inflammatory variant, but in contrast to acne, rosacea pustules are not follicular based. The patient's findings are not consistent with rosacea.

Although this patient has positive antinuclear antibodies, she lacks the associated findings of systemic lupus erythematosus (SLE), including malar/discoid rash, arthritis, organ involvement, and kidney disease. SLE can cause a rash on the hands similar to Gottron papules, but it more typically involves skin located between the joints.

KEY POINT

- Amyopathic dermatomyositis refers to dermatomyositis with cutaneous involvement in the absence of clinical, laboratory, electromyogram, or biopsy evidence of myositis.

Bibliography

Gerami P, Schope JM, McDonald L, Walling HW, Sontheimer RD. A systematic review of adult-onset clinically amyopathic dermatomyositis (dermatomyositis sinémyositis): a missing link within the spectrum of the idiopathic inflammatory myopathies. J Am Acad Dermatol. 2006 Apr;54(4):597-613. [PMID: 16546580]

Item 5   Answer: A

Educational Objective: Treat inadequately controlled osteoarthritis with intra-articular glucocorticoids.

Intra-articular glucocorticoids are appropriate for this patient. She has osteoarthritis in multiple joints based on her history, physical examination, and plain radiographs. Although her overall osteoarthritis symptoms appear to be well controlled, the right knee is clearly more affected than any other joint. Therefore, therapy targeted toward this joint is indicated, and intra-articular glucocorticoids are the most appropriate choice for this patient to address her localized symptoms. Meta-analyses of clinical trials evaluating the use of glucocorticoid injection in osteoarthritis suggest that the technique may be particularly helpful. Individual studies have shown that the presence of an effusion, withdrawal of fluid from the knee, severity of disease, absence of synovitis, injection delivery under ultrasound guidance, and greater symptoms at baseline may all improve the likelihood of response.

Hyaluronic acid injections have shown only a minimal degree of benefit in the treatment of knee osteoarthritis. They generally require a series of three weekly injections and are more invasive, considerably more expensive, and less predictably efficacious than glucocorticoid injections.

Arthroscopic lavage for knee osteoarthritis is a technique in which fluid is instilled and aspirated from the joint through an arthroscope with the intention of removing the debris often present in these joints. Although observational studies originally suggested that the technique might be of benefit, more recent studies and meta-analyses have suggested otherwise. No differences in pain measured by visual analogue scale or function measured by the Western Ontario McMaster University Index have been identified in controlled trials using sham procedures.

The patient's symptoms are reasonably well controlled on her current NSAID. Therefore, there is no clear benefit to switching to another medication within this class.

KEY POINT

- Targeted therapy with an intra-articular glucocorticoid injection is appropriate in patients with osteoarthritis who have one symptomatic joint.

Bibliography

Maricar N, Callaghan MJ, Felson DT, O'Neill TW. Predictors of response to intra-articular steroid injections in knee osteoarthritis--a systematic review. Rheumatology (Oxford). 2013 Jun;52(6):1022-32. [PMID: 23264554]

Item 6   Answer: D

Educational Objective: Treat an acute monoarticular gouty attack with intra-articular glucocorticoids.

Intra-articular glucocorticoid therapy is appropriate for this patient. Intra-articular glucocorticoid injections are a good treatment strategy when only one or two joints are affected, the presence of joint infection has been ruled out, and oral therapies have potential adverse events. This patient has a history of gout and currently presents with evidence of an acute gouty attack in the knee. Given the synovial fluid leukocyte count (<50,000/μL [50×10^9/L]), the documented presence of intracellular crystals, and the negative synovial fluid Gram stain, the probability of a joint infection is very low. The onset of gout in this patient was preceded by community-acquired pneumonia, which may have promoted the gout attack by causing fever and dehydration. Treatment for acute gout should focus on anti-inflammatory therapy, typically using colchicine, an NSAID, or a glucocorticoid. Although all three would effectively treat this patient's gout, the best choice would be an intra-articular glucocorticoid because of potential adverse effects of the other anti-inflammatories. Although both systemic and local glucocorticoid therapy are effective in treating acute gout, intra-articular glucocorticoids are preferred in this patient to avoid systemic immunosuppressive effects in the setting of resolving pneumonia and the possible adverse impact of systemic glucocorticoids in a patient with diabetes mellitus.

Acetaminophen is analgesic but not anti-inflammatory and does not promote the resolution of a gouty attack.

Colchicine effectively treats acute gout, especially in the early phases of an attack. However, colchicine is metabolized by the hepatic CYP3A4 enzyme, which clarithromycin strongly inhibits; coadministration raises the risk of colchicine toxicity and even death, and colchicine should be avoided while this patient is taking clarithromycin.

The presence of significant kidney disease makes the use of an NSAID such as indomethacin undesirable because cyclooxygenase inhibition adversely affects the kidneys.

KEY POINT

- Intra-articular glucocorticoid injections are a good treatment strategy when only one or two joints are affected, the presence of joint infection has been ruled out, and oral therapies have potential adverse events.

Bibliography

Khanna D, Khanna PP, Fitzgerald JD, et al; American College of Rheumatology. 2012 American College of Rheumatology guidelines for management of gout. Part 2: therapy and antiinflammatory prophylaxis of acute gouty arthritis. Arthritis Care Res (Hoboken). 2012 Oct;64(10):1447-61. [PMID: 23024029]

Item 7   Answer: D

Educational Objective: Treat an adult with severe Henoch-Schönlein purpura using prednisone.

Prednisone is appropriate for this patient. His findings demonstrate the presence of a small-vessel vasculitis affecting the skin, joints, kidneys, and gastrointestinal tract. Deposition of IgA in the skin confirms the diagnosis of adult-onset Henoch-Schönlein purpura (HSP). In children, HSP is generally a benign, self-limited condition, and treatment is most commonly supportive pending spontaneous remission. HSP in adults is less common and typically is more severe. Although adult HSP also tends to run a self-limited course, adults with HSP are more likely to experience severe disease and to accumulate irreversible organ damage before the acute disease resolves. In this case, the involvement of multiple organ systems, including the gastrointestinal tract, probably warrants prednisone treatment based upon expert consensus recommendation.

Cyclophosphamide is an alkylating agent and potent immunosuppressant. It is commonly used for treatment of severe autoimmune disease such as systemic lupus erythematosus and ANCA-associated vasculitis. Its use in adult-onset HSP is less well established; although it is sometimes used in conjunction with prednisone for severe HSP nephritis, it would not be a first-choice therapy in the absence of prednisone use.

Dapsone is an antibiotic that has antileukocyte activity and is occasionally used to treat the leukocytoclastic vasculitides, including HSP. However, given the severity of this patient's condition, dapsone is less likely to be effective, and prednisone use is warranted.

Like all NSAIDs, ibuprofen may help alleviate joint pain and swelling and may have some modest effect on reducing the inflammation of small-vessel vasculitis. However, ibuprofen is unlikely to be adequately effective in a serious case such as this. Moreover, the nephrotoxic and antiplatelet effects of an NSAID would be undesirable in this patient who already has acute kidney injury and intestinal bleeding.

KEY POINT

- Treatment with prednisone should be considered for patients who have severe Henoch-Schönlein purpura with involvement of multiple organ systems.

Bibliography

Reamy BV, Williams PM, Lindsay TJ. Henoch-Schönlein purpura. Am Fam Physician. 2009 Oct 1;80(7):697–704. [PMID: 19817340]

Item 8   Answer: C

Educational Objective: Avoid combining biologic agents when treating rheumatologic disease.

Addition of the nonbiologic disease-modifying antirheumatic drug (DMARD) leflunomide is indicated for this patient. She has chronic moderate to severe rheumatoid arthritis with one or more poor prognostic markers, which may include young age, involvement of more than three joints, seropositivity, elevated inflammatory markers, and radiographic changes. She has continued to have active disease despite treatment with sulfasalazine and the biologic agent etanercept as suggested by continued synovitis of four joints and elevated inflammatory markers. A "treat to target" approach has been found to

improve the outcomes in patients such as in this case, and additional therapy is needed to achieve a low disease activity or remission. A combination of a biologic agent (preferably a tumor factor necrosis α inhibitor) and a nonbiologic DMARD is thought to be the best option to achieve this goal. Because of her side-effect history with methotrexate, the addition of the alternative nonbiologic DMARD leflunomide at this point would be the next best strategy.

Biologic agents are frequently used in combination with a nonbiologic DMARD. However, concurrent use of two or more biologic agents is not recommended because infection rates are significantly increased with minimal, if any, added efficacy. Therefore, the addition of abatacept, anakinra, or rituximab is inappropriate.

KEY POINT

- Concurrent use of two or more biologic agents is not recommended because infection rates are significantly increased with minimal, if any, added efficacy.

Bibliography

Singh JA, Furst DE, Bharat A, et al. 2012 update of the 2008 American College of Rheumatology recommendations for the use of disease-modifying antirheumatic drugs and biologic agents in the treatment of rheumatoid arthritis. Arthritis Care Res (Hoboken). 2012 May;64(5):625–39. [PMID: 22473917]

Item 9   Answer: B

Educational Objective: Diagnose fibromyalgia.

The most likely diagnosis is fibromyalgia, which is characterized by chronic widespread pain, tenderness of skin and muscles to pressure (allodynia), fatigue, sleep disturbance, and exercise intolerance. Previous lack of response to multiple medications, including NSAIDs, also provides a diagnostic clue. Examination is generally unremarkable except for allodynia. An association with other pain syndromes, including irritable bowel syndrome, irritable bladder, pelvic pain, vulvodynia, headache, and temporomandibular jaw pain, is not uncommon. This patient fulfills the 2010 American College of Rheumatology diagnostic criteria for fibromyalgia (widespread pain, wakes unrefreshed, significant fatigue, and cognitive difficulties), with symptoms present for more than 3 months.

The clinical manifestations of adrenal insufficiency are often insidious, with fatigue and malaise being the dominant symptoms; a high degree of clinical suspicion may be needed to pursue the diagnosis in the presence of subtle systemic symptoms. The patient's 4-year history of symptoms and a normal chemistry panel makes adrenal insufficiency unlikely.

The numerous and largely nonspecific clinical manifestations of hypothyroidism include fatigue, reduced endurance, weight gain, cold intolerance, constipation, impaired concentration and short-term memory, dry skin, edema, mood changes, depression, psychomotor retardation, muscle cramps, myalgia, menorrhagia, and reduced fertility. Some patients with mild hypothyroidism will exhibit few or none of these symptoms. A normal thyroid-stimulating hormone level makes hypothyroidism very unlikely.

The classic findings of polymyositis are symmetric proximal muscle weakness with little or no pain and elevation in muscle-associated enzymes. This patient has pain, a normal serum creatine kinase level, and no true weakness on examination, making polymyositis an unlikely diagnosis.

KEY POINT

- Current criteria for the diagnosis of fibromyalgia include chronic widespread pain, fatigue, waking unrefreshed, and cognitive symptoms, with symptoms present for more than 3 months.

Bibliography

Wolfe F, Clauw DJ, Fitzcharles MA, et al. The American College of Rheumatology preliminary diagnostic criteria for fibromyalgia and measurement of symptom severity. Arthritis Care Res (Hoboken). 2010 May;62(5):600-10. [PMID: 20461783]

Item 10   Answer: B

Educational Objective: Provide preconception counseling to a patient with systemic lupus erythematosus who has positive anti-Ro/SSA antibodies.

Preconception counseling regarding congenital heart block in her child is appropriate for this patient with systemic lupus erythematosus (SLE) who is positive for anti-Ro/SSA antibodies. Patients with SLE experience miscarriage, stillbirth, preeclampsia and premature delivery two to five times more often than patients without the disease. This patient has mild SLE, and her disease has been quiescent for 18 months; therefore, this is an appropriate time to attempt pregnancy. Expert opinion recommends conception when SLE has been quiescent for at least 6 months. A major risk to her child would be congenital heart block, which affects approximately 2% of pregnancies in which the mother is positive for anti-Ro/SSA or anti-La/SSB antibodies. Some of these newborns require pacing from birth if there is complete heart block at delivery. Pregnancies in mothers who are positive for anti-Ro/SSA or anti-La/SSB antibodies should be monitored closely and should include input from high-risk obstetrics and neonatology because these antibodies can pass the placenta and affect the developing cardiac conduction system. If the mother has had a previously affected child, subsequent pregnancies carry a 12% risk of congenital heart block. Positivity for anti-Ro/SSA or anti-La/SSB antibodies also confers a risk for neonatal lupus erythematosus, which is characterized by rash as well as hematologic and hepatic abnormalities that generally resolve when the antibody dissipates. The use of phototherapy for neonatal hyperbilirubinemia may cause the rash to develop because the antibody is associated with photosensitivity.

Hydroxychloroquine is thought to be safe in pregnancy and has been shown to reduce the risk of congenital heart block in newborns whose mothers are positive for anti-Ro/SSA or anti-La/SSB antibodies. It should therefore not be discontinued in this patient.

This patient is not at an increased risk of lupus nephritis because it has not been a feature of her disease to date, and she is negative for anti–double-stranded DNA antibodies.

Although anti-Ro/SSA antibodies increase the risk of developing subacute cutaneous lupus, pregnancy does not increase this risk further and does not need to be part of preconception counseling. Because a photosensitive rash has been one of the features of this patient's illness, she is aware of the hazard of sun exposure.

KEY POINT

- Neonatal congenital heart block affects approximately 2% of pregnancies in which the mother is positive for anti-Ro/SSA or anti-La/SSB antibodies.

Bibliography

Lateef A, Petri M. Management of pregnancy in systemic lupus erythematosus. Nat Rev Rheumatol. 2012 Dec;8(12):710-8. [PMID: 22907290]

Item 11   Answer: D

Educational Objective: Diagnose hemochromatosis as a cause of secondary osteoarthritis.

Measurement of transferrin saturation is the most appropriate diagnostic test to perform next in this patient. He has signs and symptoms suggestive of hemochromatosis, an autosomal recessive disorder characterized by increased absorption of iron from the gut. Approximately 40% to 60% of patients with hemochromatosis develop arthropathy that is osteoarthritis-like, but characteristically involves the second and third metacarpophalangeal (MCP) or wrist joints. Transferrin saturation and serum ferritin levels are usually elevated in patients with arthropathy due to hemochromatosis. Although a variety of more specific diagnostic maneuvers may be undertaken, including liver biopsy and genetic testing for homozygosity for the C282Y mutation of the *HFE* gene, the most appropriate and cost-effective next step is measurement of transferrin saturation. A consensus does not exist for transferrin saturation cut-off levels for diagnosis of hemochromatosis, with some guidelines recommending a value of greater than 60% in men or greater than 50% in women, and others suggesting a level of greater than 55% for all patients. Measurement of ferritin levels is indicated in patients with an elevated transferrin saturation; a markedly elevated level further supports the diagnosis and predicts the development of symptoms. The presence of clinical MCP involvement with radiographic evidence of hook-shaped osteophytes is most characteristic of hemochromatosis.

Anti–cyclic citrullinated peptide antibodies are never associated with hemochromatosis, and rheumatoid factor is generally negative in patients with hemochromatosis as seen in this patient. These autoantibodies have specificity for rheumatoid arthritis.

Arthritis may occur in up to 20% of patients with hepatitis C virus infection and may mimic rheumatoid arthritis clinically and radiographically. However, the characteristic findings of hemochromatosis on this patient's radiographs and the lack of more typical findings of erosions or bony decalcification adjacent to the involved joints make a diagnosis of hepatitis C–associated arthritis less likely.

Serum α-fetoprotein is elevated in liver disease such as acute or chronic viral hepatitis infection as well as in hepatocellular and numerous other cancers. It would have little diagnostic specificity in this clinical setting.

KEY POINT

- Secondary osteoarthritis may occur in the setting of hemochromatosis, which is associated with an arthropathy that is osteoarthritis-like, but characteristically involves the metacarpophalangeal and wrist joints.

Bibliography

Husar-Memmer E, Stadlmayr A, Datz C, Zwerina J. HFE-Related hemochromatosis: an update for the rheumatologist. Curr Rheumatol Rep. 2014 Jan;16(1):393. [PMID: 24264720]

Item 12   Answer: B

Educational Objective: Diagnose spondyloarthritis using MRI.

MRI of the sacroiliac joints and/or spine is the most appropriate diagnostic test to perform next in this patient with suspected spondyloarthritis, considered in patients with chronic inflammatory back pain beginning before the age of 45 years. It is important to establish the diagnosis of spondyloarthritis even if it will not change immediate management because it requires life-long monitoring for the development of cardiovascular and other major organ damage. A positive HLA-B27 can be supportive of this diagnosis, but a negative result does not rule it out. Conventional radiographs can demonstrate sacroiliitis (erosive changes and sclerosis) but may be normal in early disease. If there is high suspicion for axial inflammation and conventional radiographs are normal, MRI of the sacroiliac joints and/or spine should be considered to further evaluate for inflammation. MRI is the most sensitive imaging technique for detecting early inflammation in the spine and sacroiliac joints. Although his radiographs and HLA-B27 testing were negative, this 25-year-old patient has probable inflammatory back (morning stiffness lasting 90 minutes) and sacroiliac pain, making spondyloarthritis, specifically ankylosing spondylitis, a likely diagnosis. Advanced imaging is often needed to show sacroiliac joint abnormalities.

CT of the sacroiliac joints can provide evidence of erosive changes in the bone but has limited ability to detect soft-tissue inflammation of the spine and may be normal until bony changes are present.

When injected intravenously, technetium-99m binds to hydroxyapatite crystals. Increased uptake reflects increased bone turnover related to infection, cancer, trauma, and arthritis. Because of these characteristics, a positive scan is a sensitive but nonspecific indicator of bone, joint, and periarticular disorders and may be most useful when other

first-line imaging modalities are negative but the suspicion of disease remains high.

Ultrasonography is relatively inexpensive, poses no radiation hazard, can scan across three-dimensional structures, and may be used concurrently with physical examination to evaluate moving structures (for example, tendon evaluation). Musculoskeletal ultrasonography can be helpful in detecting evidence of peripheral enthesitis and arthritis but has not demonstrated usefulness in detecting axial involvement such as sacroiliitis.

KEY POINT

- MRI is the most sensitive imaging technique for detecting early inflammation in the spine and sacroiliac joints in patients with suspected spondyloarthritis.

Bibliography

Ostergaard M, Lambert RG. Imaging in ankylosing spondylitis. Ther Adv Musculoskelet Dis. 2012 Aug;4(4):301-11. [PMID: 22859929]

Item 13   Answer: B

Educational Objective: Diagnose pulmonary arterial hypertension in a patient with limited cutaneous systemic sclerosis.

Doppler echocardiography is the most appropriate test to perform next in this patient with a 3-year history of limited cutaneous systemic sclerosis (LcSSc) who now presents with shortness of breath and fatigue, a prominent single S_2, and a normal pulmonary examination and chest radiograph. LcSSc is characterized by isolated distal skin thickening (face, neck, and hands distal to wrists), is typically not accompanied by internal organ fibrosis, and is more likely to be associated with pulmonary arterial hypertension (PAH). The initial screening test for those with systemic sclerosis who have suspected PAH is echocardiography, which can rapidly and noninvasively estimate elevated pulmonary pressure as well as rule out some etiologies in the differential diagnosis such as intracardiac shunts, valvular heart disease, or heart failure. A moderate to high tricuspid gradient correlates well with PAH confirmed with gold standard right heart catheterization, which is 97% specific but may not be sensitive.

Bronchoscopy with lavage is often used in immunocompromised patients with rapidly deteriorating lung function to assess for infection and/or pulmonary hemorrhage. This test is not indicated in a patient with findings suggestive of PAH.

B-type natriuretic peptide (BNP) or N-terminal proBNP levels should be assessed in patients suspected of having heart failure. Preliminary data suggest that N-terminal proBNP may be helpful in the assessment of PAH and may provide prognostic information. BNP and N-terminal proBNP measurement cannot be recommended at this time until further studies validate their usefulness in patients with PAH.

In patients with echocardiographic findings suggesting PAH, an array of studies (such as imaging of the chest to assess parenchymal lung disease; V/Q scanning to assess potential chronic thromboembolic disease; pulmonary function testing with D_{LCO}; serologic studies for connective tissue disease, liver disease, and HIV; and sleep studies) are helpful in selected patients. All patients suspected of having PAH should be considered for right heart/pulmonary artery catheterization to confirm the diagnosis suggested by clinical presentation, echocardiography, and pulmonary function tests and to accurately measure the arterial pressure. It is also very useful in evaluating responsiveness to therapeutic medications and helps guide therapy. However, right heart catheterization follows these preliminary diagnostic tests and would not be done next.

KEY POINT

- Echocardiography can rapidly and noninvasively estimate elevated pulmonary pressure as well as rule out some etiologies in the differential diagnosis of pulmonary arterial hypertension.

Bibliography

Steen V. Advancements in diagnosis of pulmonary arterial hypertension in scleroderma. Arthritis Rheum. 2005 Dec;52(12):3698-700. [PMID: 16320319]

Item 14   Answer: C

Educational Objective: Recognize the risk of interstitial lung disease in patients with polymyositis.

Chest radiography is the most appropriate diagnostic test to perform next in this patient with polymyositis who has positive anti–Jo-1 antibodies and features of the antisynthetase syndrome. Pulmonary manifestations of dermatomyositis and polymyositis are common and may result from interstitial lung disease (ILD), hypoventilation (weakness of respiratory muscles), aspiration pneumonia, and, rarely, pulmonary arterial hypertension (PAH). Clinical manifestations of ILD range from being asymptomatic to severe progressive cough and dyspnea. ILD is strongly associated with the presence of positive autoantibodies to transfer RNA synthetases, including anti–Jo-1 antibodies. In clinical practice, chest radiography, high-resolution chest CT, and pulmonary function testing are used to evaluate for the presence of this manifestation, and periodic follow-up in an asymptomatic patient is appropriate. Various patterns of ILD occur, ranging from nonspecific interstitial pneumonitis (most common) to usual interstitial pneumonia or bronchiolitis obliterans organizing pneumonia. The pattern of involvement determines glucocorticoid responsiveness and, ultimately, prognosis.

6-Minute walk testing is an important test used in the evaluation and follow-up of patients with an established diagnosis of PAH, but there is no evidence that this patient has PAH.

Myocarditis has a highly variable presentation, including fatigue, chest pain, heart failure, cardiogenic shock, arrhythmias, and sudden death. This patient has no cardiovascular symptoms suggesting myocarditis, and a cardiac

MRI is not necessary in a patient with a low suspicion for this condition.

Coronary artery disease most classically presents with exertional substernal chest pain relieved with rest or nitroglycerin. Variant presentation may include dyspnea on exertion and exertional fatigue. Exercise stress testing would be indicated if there was a high level of suspicion for coronary artery disease, which is not the case here.

No additional testing is incorrect because ILD may be asymptomatic in some patients and can be missed without additional testing.

KEY POINT

- Interstitial lung disease is strongly associated with polymyositis and the presence of positive autoantibodies to transfer RNA synthetases, including anti–Jo-1 antibodies.

Bibliography

Connors GR, Christopher-Stine L, Oddis CV, Danoff SK. Interstitial lung disease associated with the idiopathic inflammatory myopathies: what progress has been made in the past 35 years? Chest. 2010 Dec;138(6):1464-74. [PMID: 21138882]

Item 15   Answer: D

Educational Objective: Identify the association of tofacitinib with a risk of causing an abnormal lipid profile.

The lipid profile should be monitored in this patient with rheumatoid arthritis who began taking tofacitinib 1 month ago. Elevation of all components of the lipid panel, including cholesterol, triglycerides, HDL cholesterol, and LDL cholesterol, has been found to occur as rapidly as 1 month after initiation of therapy with the biologic agent tofacitinib. Generally, these elevations remain stable over time. In the first 3 months of clinical trials evaluating the efficacy of tofacitinib, mean LDL cholesterol increased by 15%, and mean HDL cholesterol increased by 10%. In a subsequent clinical trial, statin therapy resulted in a return to pretreatment levels of LDL cholesterol. It is unknown to what extent these lipid abnormalities may impact the long-term risk of cardiovascular disease in patients treated with tofacitinib. Tofacitinib may initially raise then lower leukocyte counts. Furthermore, lymphopenia, neutropenia, and anemia may be seen with long-term use.

Elevated aminotransaminase levels may be seen with exposure to tofacitinib. However, abnormalities of bilirubin, glucose, and alkaline phosphatase would not be expected to result from exposure to 1 month of therapy with tofacitinib.

KEY POINT

- The biologic agent tofacitinib is associated with a risk of causing an abnormal lipid profile.

Bibliography

Fleischmann R, Kremer J, Cush J, et al. Placebo-controlled trial of tofacitinib monotherapy in rheumatoid arthritis. N Engl J Med. 2012 Aug 9;367(6):495-507. [PMID: 22873530]

Item 16   Answer: C

Educational Objective: Prevent gout by titrating allopurinol to achieve a target serum urate level.

The allopurinol dose should be increased for this patient with gout who has not yet reached the serum urate target goal of less than 6.0 mg/dL (0.35 mmol/L). Allopurinol is considered a first-line agent for serum urate reduction in patients with gout. Historically, concern has been expressed regarding allopurinol dosing and the risk of hypersensitivity reaction; however, it appears that gradual dose escalation with monitoring for side effects is a safe approach, even in patients with chronic kidney disease. Recent American College of Rheumatology recommendations advocate for a starting dose of 100 mg/d (or 50 mg/d in those with stage 4 or 5 chronic kidney disease) with titration upward every 2 to 5 weeks, aiming for a target serum urate level of less than 6.0 mg/dL (0.35 mmol/L). Despite the patient's kidney dysfunction, it is safe to up titrate the allopurinol gradually over several months to reach the target goal. If intolerance to allopurinol emerges, alternative urate-lowering therapy (such as the xanthine oxidase inhibitor febuxostat) should be pursued.

Gout flare prophylaxis such as colchicine should be maintained during urate-lowering therapy because patients are paradoxically at increased risk of gout flares during this time.

This patient is taking losartan to treat hypertension. This agent should not be discontinued because it has uricosuric effects and thus may be helping with efforts to lower his serum urate level.

This patient is not yet at the target serum urate goal; therefore, continuation of the same therapy is not appropriate.

KEY POINT

- Gradual dose escalation of allopurinol, with monitoring for side effects, is a safe approach for patients (even those with chronic kidney disease) with gout who have not reached a target serum urate level of less than 6.0 mg/dL (0.35 mmol/L).

Bibliography
Khanna D, Khanna PP, Fitzgerald JD, et al; American College of Rheumatology. 2012 American College of Rheumatology guidelines for management of gout. Part 2: therapy and antiinflammatory prophylaxis of acute gouty arthritis. Arthritis Care Res (Hoboken). 2012 Oct;64(10): 1447-61. [PMID: 23024029]

Item 17   Answer: B

Educational Objective: Treat giant cell arteritis with high-dose prednisone.

Treatment with prednisone, 60 mg/d (or 1 mg/kg/d), is indicated immediately for this patient. She has temporal artery pain and tenderness, along with jaw claudication in the setting of low-grade fever and a very high erythrocyte sedimentation rate. Given her age, these findings are most consistent with giant cell arteritis (GCA). The presence of shoulder and hip symptoms is consistent with polymyalgia rheumatica (PMR), which commonly co-occurs in patients with GCA (approximately 50% of cases). Despite a lack of visual symptoms to date, the patient is at risk of acute and potentially catastrophic visual loss. Immediate treatment is therefore warranted, the standard regimen being prednisone at a dose of 60 mg/d. (In the setting of severe visual loss, high-dose pulse glucocorticoids might be considered.) The addition of low-dose aspirin has been shown in limited studies to further reduce the risk of visual loss in patients with GCA already receiving prednisone and is favored by some experts.

Low-dose prednisone in the range of 10 to 20 mg/d is generally adequate treatment for isolated PMR but has not been shown to adequately treat GCA or to prevent visual complications.

MRI of the head permits the visualization of structures that could potentially be associated with headache and/or visual symptoms, including tumors, hydrocephalus, and/or large aneurysms. However, the presence of jaw claudication, as well as the presence of PMR symptoms, is not consistent with an intracranial lesion.

A temporal artery biopsy should be obtained as rapidly as possible to confirm the GCA diagnosis and to help direct long-term management; however, the histopathology of the disease will still be readable up to 1 to 2 weeks after initiation of treatment, and treatment should not be deferred pending biopsy.

KEY POINT

- Immediate treatment with prednisone, 60 mg/d (or 1 mg/kg/d), is indicated for patients with suspected giant cell arteritis to prevent visual complications.

Bibliography
Frazer JA, Weyand CM, Newman JN, Biousse V. The treatment of giant cell arteritis. Rev Neurol Dis. 2008 Summer;5(3):140-52. [PMID: 18838954]

Item 18   Answer: C

Educational Objective: Screen for tuberculosis prior to starting biologic therapy.

Screening for tuberculosis using an interferon-γ assay is indicated for this patient before initiation of a tumor necrosis factor (TNF)-α inhibitor. This patient with rheumatoid arthritis has active disease despite treatment with triple therapy using nonbiologic disease-modifying antirheumatic drugs. In addition, she has poor prognostic markers, including positive rheumatoid serology and high inflammatory markers. Appropriate therapy with a biologic agent is being planned. TNF-α inhibitors are the mainstay of initial biologic therapy for rheumatoid arthritis. Reactivation of tuberculosis is a significant risk for most biologic agents, and particularly with TNF-α inhibitors because they inhibit formation of granuloma. Prior to starting any biologic agent, appropriate testing for latent tuberculosis is needed by obtaining either a tuberculosis skin test or an interferon-γ release assay (IGRA). Either of these two tests can be used to screen for latent tuberculosis. IGRA is more costly but may be more sensitive in patients on immunosuppressive therapy.

Chest radiography will be needed if the patient is symptomatic with pulmonary symptoms or has positive testing for latent tuberculosis infection but is currently not necessary.

Common variable immunodeficiency (CVID) occurs in both adults and children. Serum IgG levels are markedly reduced, and serum IgA and/or IgM levels are frequently low. Patients with CVID frequently develop chronic lung diseases, autoimmune disorders such as rheumatoid arthritis, malabsorption, recurrent infections, and lymphoma. Recurrent sinopulmonary infections, ear infections, and conjunctivitis are common. Measuring immunoglobulin levels in this patient without evidence of recurrent infection is not indicated.

Radiographs of the hands and feet can confirm the presence of erosions in active rheumatoid disease but are not needed in this patient prior to starting a biologic because disease activity has already been established by physical examination and laboratory testing.

KEY POINT

- Screening for tuberculosis is indicated before initiation of any biologic agent.

Bibliography

Singh JA, Furst DE, Bharat A, et al. 2012 update of the 2008 American College of Rheumatology recommendations for the use of disease-modifying antirheumatic drugs and biologic agents in the treatment of rheumatoid arthritis. Arthritis Care Res (Hoboken). 2012 May;64(5):625-39. [PMID: 22473917]

Item 19   Answer: A

Educational Objective: **Diagnose ankylosing spondylitis.**

The most likely diagnosis is ankylosing spondylitis, which is characterized by inflammatory back pain that manifests as pain and stiffness in the spine that is worse after immobility and better with use. Symptoms are prominent in the morning (>1 hour), and patients can be symptomatic during the night. Buttock pain is common and correlates with sacroiliitis, which is typically bilateral. This patient has symptoms/signs consistent with ankylosing spondylitis, including more than 3 months of inflammatory back pain of primarily axial involvement, age of onset younger than 45 years, a positive HLA-B27, and a good response to an NSAID. The lack of sacroiliitis or other inflammatory changes on his radiographs does not rule out this diagnosis; these changes may not be evident early in the disease course and may not be seen on plain radiographs if there are no bone erosions. He fulfills the Assessment of SpondyloArthritis international Society (ASAS) classification criteria for axial spondyloarthritis because he has a positive HLA-B27 plus at least two other features of spondyloarthritis, including inflammatory back pain and a good response to NSAIDs. The ASAS classification criteria use a nomenclature that defines spondyloarthritis as axial or peripheral, and ankylosing spondylitis would be the prototype disease in the spectrum of axial spondyloarthritis. These criteria allow patients who have not yet developed radiographic sacroiliitis to be classified as having "non-radiographic" axial spondyloarthritis.

Distinguishing between inflammatory and noninflammatory joint pain is critical in evaluating patients with musculoskeletal conditions. Inflammation may be the only symptom that distinguishes ankylosing spondylitis from lumbar degenerative disk disease. Subjective manifestations of joint inflammation include morning stiffness for more than 1 hour. Lumbar degenerative disk disease is not likely in this patient because his radiographs are normal and he has inflammatory back pain.

Characteristic features of psoriatic arthritis include enthesitis, dactylitis, tenosynovitis, arthritis of the distal interphalangeal joints, asymmetric oligoarthritis, and spondylitis. The HLA-B27 antigen may be positive in patients with axial involvement. Psoriatic arthritis involving only the axial skeleton is possible in this patient but less likely because he has no evidence of psoriasis.

Reactive arthritis (formerly known as Reiter syndrome) is a postinfectious arthritis that occurs in both men and women. Infections may include urethritis or diarrhea, although patients may be asymptomatic. Arthritis, usually oligoarticular, develops several days to weeks after the infection. The HLA-B27 antigen may be positive in these patients. Reactive arthritis is also less likely as this patient has no history of a gastrointestinal or genitourinary infection preceding the onset of arthritis.

KEY POINT

- Ankylosing spondylitis is characterized by inflammatory back pain that manifests as pain and stiffness in the spine that is worse after immobility and better with use.

Bibliography

Rudwaleit M, van der Heijde D, Landewé R, et al. The Assessment of SpondyloArthritis International Society classification criteria for peripheral spondyloarthritis and for spondyloarthritis in general. Ann Rheum Dis. 2011 Jan;70(1):25-31. [PMID: 21109520]

Item 20   Answer: A

Educational Objective: **Recognize lymphoma in a patient with Sjögren syndrome.**

The most appropriate next step in the management of this patient is to obtain a lymph node biopsy. This patient has Sjögren syndrome, an immune-mediated disease manifesting primarily as inflammation of exocrine glands, including the major and minor salivary glands, lacrimal glands, and, less commonly, other exocrine glands such as the pancreas. Patients with Sjögren syndrome are at significant risk of developing lymphoma, the most common being diffuse B-cell and mucosa-associated lymphoid tissue (MALT) lymphomas; this risk is up to 44-fold higher than in the general population. It is thought that chronic B-cell activation may lead to the development of a clone of malignant B cells. Hypocomplementemia, splenomegaly, lymphadenopathy, gammopathy, skin vasculitis, and cryoglobulinemia predict the development of, and accompany, lymphoma. With this patient's clinical history and findings, lymphoma must be in the differential and should be evaluated with a lymph node biopsy.

Biopsy of the rash will demonstrate leukocytoclastic vasculitis, which frequently accompanies lymphoma, but will not be able to diagnose the underlying lymphoma.

Heterophile antibody testing is not indicated because the complete blood count results do not demonstrate lymphocytosis, and the patient's symptoms and findings are much more concerning for lymphoma.

Prednisone and cyclophosphamide therapy may be helpful for some of this patient's symptoms, including vasculitis, but are premature at this time until lymphoma has been either identified or excluded. If there is no lymphoma and Sjögren syndrome is believed to be active and causing vasculitis, then these therapies could be considered.

KEY POINT

- Patients with Sjögren syndrome have up to a 44-fold higher risk of developing lymphoma, the most common being diffuse B-cell and mucosa-associated lymphoid tissue (MALT) lymphomas.

Bibliography

Jonsson MV, Theander E, Jonsson R. Predictors for the development of non-Hodgkin lymphoma in primary Sjögren's syndrome. Presse Med. 2012 Sep;41(9 Pt 2):e511-6. [PMID: 22867948]

Item 21   Answer: D

Educational Objective: Utilize HLA-B27 testing to aid in the diagnosis of spondyloarthritis.

The most appropriate diagnostic test to perform next is HLA-B27 testing. The patient has uveitis and enthesitis at the Achilles tendon, which are suggestive of peripheral spondyloarthritis. The Assessment of SpondyloArthritis international Society classification criteria for peripheral and axial spondyloarthritis are primarily used for research purposes, although they include many of the common symptoms, signs, and tests that are useful in diagnosing these disorders. Classification criteria include several other manifestations, including psoriasis, inflammatory bowel disease, preceding infection, and sacroiliitis, which are absent in this patient. HLA-B27 is included in the criteria and, in the absence of other sufficient manifestations, can be helpful in supporting the diagnosis of peripheral or axial spondyloarthritis. HLA-B27 testing has limitations because of its approximately 5% prevalence in the general population, which can lead to false positives in diagnosis. Therefore, HLA-B27 is not a useful test in a patient in whom clinical suspicion for spondyloarthritis is low (for example, a 65-year-old patient with noninflammatory or mechanical back pain). Furthermore, it does not add anything in the setting of a high suspicion for spondyloarthritis when there are sufficient other findings to establish a diagnosis (for example, a 35-year-old man with a 12-month history

of anterior uveitis, chronic inflammatory back pain, and radiographic evidence of sacroiliitis).

Testing for anti–cyclic citrullinated peptide antibodies can be useful in patients with suspected rheumatoid arthritis, which is characterized by an inflammatory polyarthritis of small joints. Rheumatoid arthritis is unlikely in this patient because he only has enthesitis, an uncommon presentation of rheumatoid arthritis.

The ANCA-associated vasculitides include granulomatosis with polyangiitis (formerly known as Wegener granulomatosis), microscopic polyangiitis, and eosinophilic granulomatosis with polyangiitis (formerly known as Churg-Strauss syndrome). Granulomatosis with polyangiitis is a systemic necrotizing vasculitis that predominantly affects the upper and lower respiratory tract and kidneys. More than 70% of patients have upper airway manifestations such as sinusitis or nasal, inner ear, or laryngotracheal inflammation. Microscopic polyangiitis is a necrotizing vasculitis that predominantly affects the lungs and kidneys. Eosinophilic granulomatosis with polyangiitis is an eosinophil-rich necrotizing vasculitis predominantly affecting the respiratory tract and other major organs. This patient does not have clinical evidence of ANCA-associated vasculitis; therefore, testing for ANCA is not indicated.

Antinuclear antibody testing is useful for patients with suspected systemic lupus erythematosus (SLE); however, SLE does not usually cause enthesitis or uveitis as seen in this patient.

KEY POINT

- HLA-B27 testing can be helpful in supporting the diagnosis of spondyloarthritis in the absence of other sufficient manifestations.

Bibliography

Rudwaleit M, van der Heijde D, Landewé R, et al. The Assessment of SpondyloArthritis International Society classification criteria for peripheral spondyloarthritis and for spondyloarthritis in general. Ann Rheum Dis. 2011 Jan;70(1):25-31. [PMID: 21109520]

Item 22   Answer: B

Educational Objective: Treat a patient who has familial Mediterranean fever with colchicine.

Colchicine is appropriate for this patient who has familial Mediterranean fever (FMF), an autosomal recessive disease characterized by episodes of fever, polyserositis, arthritis, erysipeloid rash around the ankles, and elevated acute phase reactants. Attacks last 1 to 3 days and are self-limited but can be dramatic. FMF is associated with mutation of the $MEFV_1$ gene; testing for $MEFV$ mutations is available and should be considered as an aid to diagnosis, although not all mutations have been identified. AA amyloidosis is a potential long-term consequence of FMF due to the production and accumulation of serum amyloid A. Colchicine affects the function of various inflammatory cells that are thought to play a role in the cytokine overproduction seen in FMF. A response to colchicine is useful in the clinical diagnosis of FMF because it can prevent attacks as well as AA amyloidosis. Treatment with colchicine is therefore indicated for this patient who most likely has FMF, as manifested by her history of febrile attacks of abdominal serositis, erysipelas-like skin lesions that mimic cellulitis, and inflammatory arthritis occurring independently of the febrile episodes.

FMF genetic mutations affect the function of pyrin that results in overactivation of the inflammasome. The inflammasome is an important constituent of the innate immune system that is responsible for production of interleukin (IL)-1; dysregulation of the inflammasome, as in FMF, results in overproduction of IL-1. The IL-1 inhibitor anakinra can be used in patients with FMF who are unresponsive to colchicine; however, this agent is not first-line therapy.

NSAIDs and prednisone have not been shown to have a significant impact on the disease progression or symptoms associated with FMF.

KEY POINT

- Familial Mediterranean fever is characterized by episodes of fever, polyserositis, arthritis, erysipeloid rash around the ankles, and elevated acute phase reactants; a response to colchicine is useful in the clinical diagnosis.

Bibliography

Ben-Chetrit E, Touitou I. Familial Mediterranean fever in the world. Arthritis Rheum. 2009 Oct 15;61(10):1447-53. [PMID: 19790133]

Item 23   Answer: B

Educational Objective: Treat osteoarthritis with duloxetine.

The serotonin-norepinephrine reuptake inhibitor duloxetine is appropriate for this patient with osteoarthritis. The pharmacologic management of osteoarthritis pain can be difficult because therapy for symptom relief does not halt or reverse the disease process. Furthermore, all potential agents have side effects, some severe, and elderly patients can be at particularly high risk for developing them. The optimal choice of therapy relies on the risks and benefits of each agent in the context of the patient's comorbidities. This patient has already tried an NSAID (ibuprofen) as well as glucocorticoid and hyaluronic injections without symptomatic relief and has recently experienced an episode of gastrointestinal bleeding. Duloxetine is a reasonable choice given the patient's comorbidities and recent history of gastrointestinal bleeding. Compared with placebo, duloxetine significantly reduces pain and improves physical functioning in patients with knee osteoarthritis. In short-term studies, duloxetine was not associated with an increase in the adverse event rate compared with placebo. Unlike NSAIDs, duloxetine does not increase the risk for a recurrence of peptic ulcer disease. There are no medication interactions that contraindicate its use in this patient.

In an elderly patient who has had a recent bleeding peptic ulcer, the use of any NSAID, including the cyclooxy-

genase-2 inhibitor celecoxib, is inadvisable because the risk of recurrence with repeated exposure is high.

Narcotic use in the elderly, although not associated with ulcer risk or gastrointestinal bleeding, should also be approached cautiously. Short-acting narcotics should be tried first, and long-acting agents such as fentanyl may be used when other agents have failed. However, in this elderly patient at risk for falling due to her recent hospitalization, debilitation, quadriceps weakness, and a history of osteoporosis, fentanyl is not the optimal choice.

Although intra-articular glucocorticoids can be of benefit in the management of individual joints in osteoarthritis, there is no evidence that oral glucocorticoids would be of benefit. Furthermore, the likelihood of adverse effects with extended use is high in this patient.

KEY POINT

- Compared with placebo, duloxetine significantly reduces pain and improves physical functioning in patients with knee osteoarthritis.

Bibliography

Hochberg MC, Altman RD, Toupin AK, et al. American College of Rheumatology 2012 recommendations for the use of nonpharmacologic and pharmacologic therapies in osteoarthritis of the hand, hip, and knee. Arthritis Care Res (Hoboken). 2012 Apr;64(4):465-74. [PMID: 22563589]

Item 24   Answer: A

Educational Objective: Treat a patient who has interstitial lung disease associated with diffuse cutaneous systemic sclerosis.

Cyclophosphamide is appropriate for this patient who has interstitial lung disease (ILD) associated with diffuse cutaneous systemic sclerosis (DcSSc). This patient with DcSSc presents with dyspnea, decreased exercise tolerance, and characteristic Velcro-like crackles. These clinical findings are strongly suggestive of ILD and are supported by the imaging studies and confirmed by open lung biopsy. Patients with systemic sclerosis who have active inflammatory lung disease may be treated with immunosuppressive agents. Cyclophosphamide is the only treatment shown to have some benefit in patients with ILD associated with DcSSc. Cyclophosphamide given orally or intravenously for 1 year provides modest benefit. Although it has shown limited clinical improvement, it is the only evidence-based therapy and is therefore appropriate. High-dose glucocorticoids are frequently used in these patients but are of unclear benefit and may precipitate scleroderma renal crisis; therefore, if used, low doses are typically recommended by experts. Azathioprine may have a role as maintenance therapy.

Agents such as D-penicillamine or methotrexate have not been shown to be beneficial in these patients and should not be used to treat ILD.

Biologic agents, including tumor necrosis factor α inhibitors such as infliximab, have not been shown to have therapeutic benefit in ILD or systemic sclerosis and should not be used in this patient.

Answers and Critiques

Bibliography

Neogi T. Clinical practice. Gout. N Engl J Med. 2011 Feb 3;364(5):443-52. [PMID: 21288096]

KEY POINT

- Cyclophosphamide has been shown to have some benefit in patients who have interstitial lung disease associated with diffuse cutaneous systemic sclerosis.

Bibliography

Tashkin DP, Elashoff R, Clements PJ, et al; Scleroderma Lung Study Research Group. Cyclophosphamide versus placebo in scleroderma lung disease. New Engl J Med. 2006 Jun 22;354(25):2655-66. [PMID: 16790698]

Item 25   Answer: C

Educational Objective: Perform joint aspiration to diagnose acute monoarticular arthritis.

Aspiration of the right knee is the most appropriate next step in management. This patient is likely to have gout based on his risk factors (older man, hypertension, diabetes mellitus, obesity), the description of the symptoms (sudden onset at night with severe pain), and the recent episode of great toe swelling consistent with podagra. The gold standard for diagnosing gout is identification of monosodium needle-shaped urate crystals within leukocytes via synovial fluid analysis. Furthermore, infectious arthritis must be excluded in a patient with monoarticular arthritis. This patient is at increased risk for joint infection given his age and presence of diabetes. Thus, joint aspiration should be performed and synovial fluid sent for Gram stain, cultures, leukocyte count, and crystal analysis. Although uncommon, it is important to note that gout and an infected joint can coexist.

MRI may be useful for a patient with a history of trauma or other reason to suspect a mechanical cause for knee pain. Although MRI may demonstrate inflammation, it does not typically distinguish between infectious and noninfectious causes. Therefore, MRI is not currently indicated in this patient with warmth over the joint as well as fever, which suggests an inflammatory process.

Obtaining a serum urate level may assist in the diagnosis of this patient because an elevated level (>6.8 mg/dL [0.40 mmol/L]) would help support a diagnosis of gout. However, this test is not definitive for the diagnosis. An elevated level does not prove that the patient has gout because asymptomatic hyperuricemia is common in the general population. A relatively low serum urate level also does not exclude gout because serum urate levels can be paradoxically low during acute gout attacks.

Starting colchicine would be an option for the treatment of acute gout in this patient, and resolution of inflammation with colchicine may in fact support a diagnosis of crystal-induced arthritis. However, the diagnosis must first be established and infectious arthritis excluded.

KEY POINT

- Analysis of synovial fluid from joint aspiration is the gold standard to diagnose gout and exclude infection.

Item 26   Answer: C

Educational Objective: Diagnose psoriatic arthritis.

The most likely diagnosis is psoriatic arthritis. Although estimates of the prevalence of psoriatic arthritis in patients with psoriasis vary, more recent studies using standardized diagnostic criteria indicate that psoriatic arthritis is present in approximately 15% to 20% of those with psoriasis. Patients who have features consistent with psoriatic arthritis should be examined closely for psoriasiform skin lesions on the umbilicus, gluteal cleft, extensor surfaces, posterior auricular region, and scalp. Nails should be examined for pitting or onycholysis. Characteristic features of psoriatic arthritis include enthesitis, dactylitis, tenosynovitis, arthritis of the distal interphalangeal joints, asymmetric oligoarthritis, and spondylitis. The recently developed Classification Criteria for Psoriatic Arthritis (CASPAR) have a sensitivity and specificity of more than 90%, especially for the diagnosis of early psoriatic arthritis. This patient fulfills the CASPAR criteria because she has inflammatory articular disease with psoriasis, psoriatic nail dystrophy, dactylitis, and a negative rheumatoid factor.

This patient does not have symptoms or findings of inflammatory back pain associated with ankylosing spondylitis; her back pain is related to use and improves with rest, which is noninflammatory. HLA-B27 positivity alone is insufficient to diagnose this disease, and peripheral articular disease is not typical for ankylosing spondylitis.

Nearly 50% of patients with inflammatory bowel disease (IBD) develop musculoskeletal symptoms. Peripheral arthritis may be acute and remitting with a pauciarticular distribution commonly involving the knee. Peripheral arthritis can also be chronic or relapsing, with prominent involvement of the metacarpophalangeal joints and less correlation with intestinal inflammation. IBD-associated arthritis is also unlikely because this patient has no symptoms of bowel disease.

Reactive arthritis (formerly known as Reiter syndrome) is a postinfectious arthritis triggered by infections causing urethritis or diarrhea, although patients may be asymptomatic. Arthritis, usually oligoarticular, develops several days to weeks after the infection. Reactive arthritis can cause dactylitis; however, this patient has no history of a preceding infection, making this an unlikely diagnosis.

KEY POINT

- Psoriatic arthritis is associated with psoriasis, enthesitis, dactylitis, tenosynovitis, arthritis of the distal interphalangeal joints, asymmetric oligoarthritis, and spondylitis.

Bibliography

Coates LC, Conaghan PG, Emery P, et al. Sensitivity and specificity of the classification of psoriatic arthritis criteria in early psoriatic arthritis, Arthritis Rheum. 2012 Oct;64 (10):3150-5. [PMID: 22576997]

Item 27   Answer: B

Educational Objective: Diagnose eosinophilic granulomatosis with polyangiitis.

This patient most likely has eosinophilic granulomatosis with polyangiitis (EGPA; formerly known as Churg-Strauss syndrome). EGPA is characterized by eosinophilia, migratory pulmonary infiltrates, purpuric skin rash, and mononeuritis multiplex in the setting of antecedent atopy. Although EGPA is considered an ANCA-associated vasculitis (specifically, antimyeloperoxidase/p-ANCA), 40% of patients with EGPA are negative for ANCA. This patient has involvement of the lungs (likely capillaritis with hemoptysis), nerves (mononeuritis multiplex), and skin. In the presence of systemic eosinophilia, elevated serum IgE levels, and a history of asthma, this patient's most likely diagnosis is EGPA. Other systemic multiorgan system diseases are less likely. For example, granulomatosis with polyangiitis (GPA; formerly known as Wegener granulomatosis) and microscopic polyangiitis would be unusual in the absence of ANCA and the presence of eosinophilia (and, in the case of GPA, lack of sinus involvement). Diagnosis of EGPA can be made most definitively by tissue biopsy. Sural nerve biopsy is most likely to yield pathology specific for EGPA, specifically, the presence of necrotizing vasculitis with eosinophilic granulomas. In addition, confirmation that the patient's neurologic findings are due to EGPA is important for characterizing the extent of disease and the level of immunosuppression needed. Such a biopsy would also allow the exclusion of other eosinophilic diseases, such as hypereosinophilic syndrome.

Although cryoglobulinemia commonly affects the nerves and skin (along with the kidneys, which are not involved in this patient), it uncommonly affects the lungs. Furthermore, the high level of eosinophilia is inconsistent with cryoglobulinemia.

KEY POINT

- Eosinophilic granulomatosis with polyangiitis is characterized by eosinophilia, migratory pulmonary infiltrates, purpuric skin rash, and mononeuritis multiplex in the setting of antecedent atopy.

Bibliography

Mahr A, Moosig F, Neumann T, et al. Eosinophilic granulomatosis with polyangiitis (Churg-Strauss): evolutions in classification, etiopathogenesis, assessment and management. Curr Opin Rheumatol. 2014 Jan;26(1):16-23. [PMID: 24257370]

Item 28   Answer: D

Educational Objective: Treat polymyositis using prednisone.

Treatment with prednisone is indicated. This patient's findings of weakness, elevated muscle enzymes, electromyogram and MRI abnormalities, and no skin involvement suggest polymyositis. A definitive diagnosis can only be made by muscle biopsy, and every effort should be done to obtain it quickly.

Nonetheless, treatment should be started as soon as possible to prevent complications of active disease, improve symptoms, and have a better long-term prognosis. Treatment should not be withheld if the biopsy is delayed or cannot be obtained. The initial treatment of polymyositis or dermatomyositis with muscle involvement is systemic glucocorticoids, most commonly prednisone given at 1 mg/kg/d. Some patients with severe disease require treatment with intravenous methylprednisolone, and many physicians use methotrexate or azathioprine at onset for their glucocorticoid-sparing benefits. If refractory or recurrent disease is noted, additional agents such as mycophenolate mofetil, intravenous immune globulin, rituximab, cyclophosphamide, or tumor necrosis factor (TNF)-α inhibitors can also be considered.

The TNF-α inhibitor adalimumab is not recommended as initial therapy prior to a trial of prednisone with or without a glucocorticoid-sparing agent in patients with polymyositis or dermatomyositis. TNF-α inhibitors have been reported to be effective in some patients with refractory disease.

Cyclosporine is an immunosuppressant agent that preferentially targets T cells and demonstrates efficacy in several rheumatologic and autoimmune diseases, including rheumatoid arthritis, systemic lupus erythematosus, inflammatory myositis, psoriasis, pyoderma gangrenosum, and inflammatory bowel disease. Toxicity is relatively common (hypertension, nephrotoxicity, tremor, hirsutism); therefore, cyclosporine is mainly used as a third-line agent in rheumatologic diseases.

Leflunomide is approximately as effective as methotrexate for rheumatoid arthritis; its use in other diseases is less explored. Toxicities include liver and hematopoietic abnormalities, infection, and interstitial lung disease. This agent has an extremely long half-life (months) and undergoes enterohepatic circulation.

KEY POINT

- The initial treatment of polymyositis or dermatomyositis with muscle involvement is glucocorticoids, most commonly prednisone.

Bibliography

Amato AA, Griggs RC. Treatment of idiopathic inflammatory myopathies. Curr Opin Neurol. 2003 Oct;16(5):569-75. [PMID: 14501840]

Item 29   Answer: C

Educational Objective: Diagnose diffuse idiopathic skeletal hyperostosis.

The most likely diagnosis is diffuse idiopathic skeletal hyperostosis (DISH), which is defined by the presence of flowing osteophytes involving the anterolateral aspect of the thoracic spine at four or more contiguous vertebrae with preservation of the intervertebral disk space and the absence of apophyseal joint or sacroiliac inflammatory changes such as erosions. DISH may occur with or without osteoarthritis or inflammatory arthritis and represents a separate finding of calcification

Answers and Critiques

and ossification of spinal ligaments and the regions where tendons and ligaments attach to bone (entheses). DISH is a noninflammatory condition of unknown cause that is common in the elderly population. Patients may be asymptomatic or may describe stiffness and reduced range of motion, particularly at the thoracic spine.

Ankylosing spondylitis is an inflammatory disorder that usually becomes symptomatic in adolescence and early adulthood. It is characterized by progressive morning stiffness and low back pain and typically becomes symptomatic in the lumbar spine rather than the thoracic spine early in the course. Radiographs of DISH and ankylosing spondylitis have similarities; however, ankylosing spondylitis demonstrates vertical bridging syndesmophytes rather than the flowing osteophytes that occur in DISH. Plain radiographs of ankylosing spondylitis also characteristically show changes of the sacroiliac joints that can include erosions, evidence of sclerosis, and widening, narrowing, or partial ankylosis.

Degenerative disk disease is thought to arise from age-related changes in proteoglycan content in the nucleus pulposus of the disk. Disks shrink as they become desiccated and more friable. Age-related changes also occur in the annulus fibrosus, which becomes more fibrotic, less elastic, and can shift its position. Vertebral body endplates adjacent to the disk develop sclerosis, and osteophyte formation occurs at the vertebral margins.

Psoriatic arthritis is an inflammatory disorder that can affect the spine as well as peripheral joints. When axial involvement is prominent, sacroiliitis and spondylitis can both be present; however, axial disease rarely presents in the absence of frank inflammatory arthritis of peripheral joints.

KEY POINT

- Diffuse idiopathic skeletal hyperostosis is a noninflammatory condition defined by the presence of flowing osteophytes involving the anterolateral aspect of the thoracic spine at four or more contiguous vertebrae with preservation of the intervertebral disk space and the absence of apophyseal joint or sacroiliac inflammatory changes such as erosions.

Bibliography

Mader R, Verlaan JJ, Buskila D. Diffuse idiopathic skeletal hyperostosis: clinical features and pathogenic mechanisms. Nat Rev Rheumatol. 2013 Dec;9(12):741-50. [PMID: 24189840]

Item 30   Answer: C

Educational Objective: Diagnose the acute prodromal arthritis of hepatitis B virus infection.

The most likely diagnosis is hepatitis B virus (HBV)–associated arthritis. The patient has rapid-onset symmetric polyarthritis, rash, and elevated aminotransferase levels, which are consistent with the prodromal phase of HBV infection. The differential diagnosis of this symmetric pattern encompasses numerous arthritides; however, the presence of ele-

vated aminotransferase levels, a history of possible exposure risk (works as a home health aide), and the presence of a rash point toward the acute prodromal arthritis of HBV infection, which often presents before frank jaundice. Testing to document acute HBV infection, specifically assessment of hepatitis B core IgM and hepatitis B surface antigen, is indicated in this patient.

Hemochromatosis is characterized by excessive body stores of iron and can cause joint symptoms and liver dysfunction; unlike HBV-associated arthritis, it tends to occur gradually rather than abruptly, and the arthritis tends to resemble osteoarthritis without frank synovitis. Hemochromatosis is also uncommon in women, who are protected from iron accumulation due to menstruation.

Primary biliary cirrhosis and autoimmune hepatitis can cause acute liver enzyme elevation but do not cause acute arthritis or rash.

KEY POINT

- The prodromal stage of hepatitis B virus infection is characterized by rapid-onset symmetric polyarthritis, which is often present before frank jaundice.

Bibliography

Vassilopoulos D, Calabrese LH. Viral hepatitis: review of arthritis complications and therapy for arthritis in the presence of active HBV/HCV. Curr Rheumatol Rep. 2013 Apr;15(4):319. [PMID: 23436024]

Item 31   Answer: C

Educational Objective: Diagnose vasculitis as a cause of scleritis.

The most likely diagnosis associated with this patient's scleritis is granulomatosis with polyangiitis (formerly known as Wegener granulomatosis). Scleritis is inflammation of the fibrous layer of the eye underlying the conjunctiva and episclera. Scleritis can be caused by autoimmune diseases such as rheumatoid arthritis, relapsing polychondritis, inflammatory bowel disease, or vasculitis. This patient has evidence of systemic inflammation on laboratory testing, hypertension, and an abnormal urinalysis that could represent glomerulonephritis but no clinical evidence of rheumatoid arthritis, chondritis, or inflammatory bowel disease. Vasculitis, especially ANCA-associated vasculitis, should always be considered in the differential diagnosis of scleritis because delay in diagnosis can result in permanent loss of vision. In this case, the sinus symptoms, abnormal urinalysis suggestive of glomerulonephritis, and scleritis are suggestive of granulomatosis with polyangiitis.

Ankylosing spondylitis is characterized by inflammatory back pain that usually presents during the second to third decade of life. The type of ocular inflammation most commonly associated with this entity is anterior uveitis, not scleritis. Uveitis (inflammation of the uvea) commonly presents as a red eye with pain, photophobia, and blurred vision. Anterior uveitis is characterized by circumferential redness (ciliary flush) at the corneal limbus (junction of the cornea and sclera). Furthermore, the duration of this patient's back pain (which began after age 45 years) and evidence of osteoarthritis in her fingers suggest degenerative, rather than inflammatory, disease of the spine.

Behçet syndrome is characterized by recurrent oral and/or genital ulcers, eye and skin involvement, and pathergy. This patient has no clinical symptoms to suggest this diagnosis, and it is more commonly associated with uveitis rather than scleritis.

Sarcoidosis is a multisystem disease characterized by granulomas that form in tissues and most commonly affects the lungs. Sarcoidosis is more likely to cause uveitis than scleritis, and this patient has no other clinical symptoms such as respiratory complaints or an abnormal chest radiograph to suggest this diagnosis.

KEY POINT

- Scleritis can be caused by autoimmune diseases such as rheumatoid arthritis, relapsing polychondritis, inflammatory bowel disease, or vasculitis.

Bibliography

Sims J. Scleritis: presentations, disease associations and management. Postgrad Med J. 2012 Dec;88(1046):713-18. [PMID: 22977282]

Item 32   Answer: D

Educational Objective: Treat a suspected infected joint in the setting of gout.

Antibiotics are appropriate for this patient who has an acute inflammatory monoarthritis, possibly infectious arthritis. Acute crystalline attack can also cause fever and an inflammatory monoarthritis, but a negative Gram stain and/or the presence of crystals do not rule out infection. If infection is suspected, even if not yet confirmed on cultures, empiric therapy with antibiotics should be started without delay. The crystals seen in this patient's synovial fluid are extracellular, which is consistent with a diagnosis or history of gout but not diagnostic of an acute gouty attack; only intracellular crystals are diagnostic of an acute crystalline attack. In the absence of positive findings on Gram stain, initial empiric therapy usually includes coverage for gram-positive organisms (including methicillin-resistant *Staphylococcus aureus* [MRSA], which is increasing in prevalence in many communities) as well as coverage for gram-negative organisms if immunocompromised, at risk for gonococcal infection, or with trauma to the joint. Therapy can be adjusted once results from stains and cultures are available.

Probenecid is sometimes added to allopurinol to control gout when allopurinol alone is insufficient. If the patient were to experience persistent gout, increasing allopurinol to lower the serum urate below 6.0 mg/dL (0.35 mmol/L) would be more appropriate than combination therapy with two agents.

Allopurinol is considered a first-line agent for serum urate reduction in patients with gout. Increasing this patient's allopurinol will not be helpful in treating an acute

gouty attack, and it will not treat an infected joint. It may be indicated long term if the patient has persistently elevated serum urate with recurrent attacks of gout.

An intra-articular glucocorticoid injection can be used to treat an acute crystalline attack; however, if an infected joint were suspected, it would not be appropriate because it may worsen infection. It is therefore inappropriate at this time because the cause of this patient's acute inflammatory monoarthritis has not been determined.

Similarly, prednisone should not be started because it may cause worsening of infection. Prednisone is sometimes used short term to treat acute attacks of gout, but if a single large joint is involved, a local injection would avoid the systemic side effects of prednisone therapy.

KEY POINT

- Empiric therapy with antibiotics should be started immediately in the setting of an acute inflammatory monoarthritis if infection is suspected, even if not yet confirmed on cultures.

Bibliography

Yu KH, Luo SF, Liou LB, et al. Concomitant septic and gouty arthritis–an analysis of 30 cases. Rheumatology (Oxford). 2003 Sep;42(9):1062-6. [PMID: 12730521]

Item 33   Answer: E

Educational Objective: Monitor ankylosing spondylitis disease activity with physical examination.

No new imaging is required for this patient with ankylosing spondylitis. She is currently feeling well, continues to respond well to treatment, and has normal inflammatory markers, making new imaging unnecessary. As with any test, imaging to follow disease activity should be performed only if clearly indicated by the clinical situation (for example, if the result is likely to change management). According to the 2010 Assessment of SpondyloArthritis international Society/European League Against Rheumatism (ASAS/EULAR) guidelines, serial imaging of patients with ankylosing spondylitis can be part of a comprehensive monitoring plan that also includes patient history (such as questionnaires like the Bath Ankylosing Spondylitis Functional Index [BASFI] or Bath Ankylosing Spondylitis Disease Activity Index [BASDAI]), clinical parameters (such as physical examination findings like the Schober test), and laboratory tests (such as erythrocyte sedimentation rate and C-reactive protein). The ASAS/EULAR recommendations state that spinal radiography should not be repeated more frequently than every 2 years unless absolutely necessary in specific cases. The Schober test measures range of motion of the lumbar spine and is an inexpensive and noninvasive physical examination tool for assessing spine involvement and progression; greater than 4 cm is normal.

Bone scan, CT, MRI, and plain radiography may demonstrate evidence of inflammation and/or progression of disease, but without a clear indication may unnecessarily expose the patient to radiation and to expense. This patient is feeling well, has intact activities of daily living, and had radiographs less than 2 years ago; therefore, no additional imaging is necessary at this time.

KEY POINT

- Patients with ankylosing spondylitis who are responding well to treatment should be monitored clinically and do not require periodic imaging studies less than every 2 years unless absolutely necessary.

Bibliography

Braun J, van den Berg R, Baraliakos X, et al. 2010 update of the ASAS/EULAR recommendations for the management of ankylosing spondylitis. Ann Rheum Dis. 2011 Jan;70(6):896-904. [PMID: 21540199]

Item 34   Answer: B

Educational Objective: Diagnose Lyme arthritis.

Serologic testing for Lyme disease is appropriate for this patient with arthritis characterized by prominent swelling with stiffness without significant joint pain. He has a risk factor for Lyme arthritis, given his frequent hiking in an endemic area. Patients may not recall a tick bite; therefore, Lyme disease should be suspected even without this history. The knee is most commonly affected, although other large joints can also be involved, usually in a monoarticular or oligoarticular pattern. Serologic testing for *Borrelia burgdorferi* is the diagnostic test of choice for this disease and is typically done with an enzyme-linked immunosorbent assay (ELISA) screening test, followed by confirmation by Western blot.

Blood cultures should always be obtained when there is a suspicion for bacterial infectious arthritis. This patient does not have risk factors for infectious arthritis, with Lyme being the most compelling diagnosis. Arthrocentesis is recommended for routine synovial fluid analysis and symptomatic relief, but blood cultures will not provide the correct diagnosis.

An MRI of the knee is unlikely to have diagnostic benefit in new-onset Lyme arthritis (and even in recurrent cases, it tends to be a nonerosive arthritis). MRI can be helpful in cases in which mechanical damage needs to be excluded or if there is concern for osteomyelitis or other bone pathology.

Synovial fluid cultures tend to be negative in Lyme arthritis. Synovial fluid will show inflammatory fluid with a neutrophil predominance. *B. burgdorferi* can be detected by polymerase chain reaction in synovial fluid.

KEY POINT

- In patients with risk factors for Lyme arthritis (even without a history of a tick bite), serologic tests showing an immunologic response to *Borrelia burgdorferi* are indicated to establish the diagnosis.

Bibliography

Hu LT. In the clinic. Lyme disease. Ann Intern Med. 2012 Aug 7;157(3):ITC2-2-16. [PMID: 22868858]

Item 35   Answer: D

Educational Objective: Treat a patient with drug-induced lupus erythematosus caused by minocycline.

Discontinuation of minocycline is indicated for this patient. Minocycline is one of the known causes of drug-induced lupus erythematosus (DILE). Criteria for DILE include a positive antinuclear antibody (ANA) test, exposure to a drug associated with DILE, and at least one clinical feature of lupus in a patient without a known history of lupus. Common symptoms include malaise, fever, arthritis, and rash. Diagnosis is typically confirmed when symptoms resolve several weeks to months after discontinuation of the offending agent. The agents classically associated with DILE, such as procainamide and methyldopa, are not commonly used at present. However, the spectrum of DILE includes other medications that are more commonly used, including hydralazine, diltiazem, isoniazid, minocycline, and certain tumor necrosis factor α inhibitors (such as infliximab and etanercept). Other agents that possibly cause DILE include specific anticonvulsants, antithyroid agents, and certain antibiotics.

The diagnostic laboratory evaluation for DILE is similar to that for patients with suspected idiopathic systemic lupus erythematosus. Antinuclear antibodies are typically positive, whereas anti–double-stranded DNA antibodies are usually negative in DILE, as are most other lupus-associated extractable nuclear autoantibodies. Antihistone antibodies have traditionally been associated with DILE caused by older medications, but their presence may be more variable with DILE induced by newer agents. In addition to causing DILE, certain medications, such as minocycline and hydralazine, may be associated with a p-ANCA syndrome that may also cause a small- to medium-vessel vasculitis with organ involvement. Treatment of DILE, regardless of offending agent, requires discontinuation of the drug. The patient can also be treated symptomatically until manifestations resolve. An NSAID such as naproxen may be helpful, as can low-dose prednisone. Rarely, more substantial therapy may be needed if there is internal organ involvement.

Neither azathioprine nor high-dose prednisone is indicated in this patient because she does not have evidence of internal organ involvement.

Famotidine has not been associated with DILE.

KEY POINT

- The diagnosis of drug-induced lupus erythematosus is typically confirmed when symptoms resolve several weeks to months after discontinuation of the offending agent.

Bibliography

Chang C, Gershwin ME. Drug-induced lupus erythematosus: incidence, management and prevention. Drug Saf. 2011 May 1;34(5):357-74. [PMID: 21513360]

Item 36   Answer: B

Educational Objective: Diagnose inclusion body myositis.

The most likely diagnosis is inclusion body myositis (IBM), an insidious and slowly progressive inflammatory myopathy that occurs more commonly in men and in those over the age of 50 years. Muscle weakness may be diffuse and involve both the distal and proximal muscles. Although typically symmetric, IBM muscle involvement may be asymmetric in up to 15% of patients. Skin is generally spared. IBM is rarely associated with extramuscular manifestations such as rash, fever, or pulmonary involvement. Patients with IBM typically have only mildly elevated (typically <1000 U/L), or even normal, levels of muscle enzymes. The characteristic triad of electromyographic findings for myopathy includes short-duration, small, low-amplitude polyphasic potentials; fibrillation potentials at rest; and bizarre, high-frequency, repetitive discharges. This older male patient has developed slowly progressive weakness affecting both the proximal and distal muscles without any significant pain or stiffness. This presentation suggests a myopathy with weakness based on his history and physical examination, mild elevation of muscle enzymes, and abnormal electromyogram (EMG) results, all of which are most consistent with IBM.

Amyotrophic lateral sclerosis is characterized by progressive dysfunction of both upper motoneuron and lower motoneuron pathways in one or more areas of the body. Common upper motoneuron features are spasticity, hyperreflexia, and pathologic reflexes, including extensor plantar responses. Typical lower motoneuron features are muscle weakness, atrophy, fasciculations, and cramps. These findings are not present in the patient.

Myasthenia gravis is characterized by fluctuating, fatigable muscle weakness that worsens with activity and improves with rest. Neurologic examination may reveal bilateral asymmetric ptosis worsened by prolonged upward gaze, an expressionless or sagging appearance of facial muscles, a "snarling" smile, nasal speech worsened by prolonged speaking, and limb weakness that increases with exercise. None of these findings are present in this patient.

Statin-induced myopathy most commonly presents with muscle pain, tenderness, and cramping typically within the first 6 months of therapy, and EMG results are normal. This patient has no muscle pain, has an abnormal EMG, and has been taking a stable dose of a stain for years, making statin-induced myopathy unlikely.

KEY POINT

- Inclusion body myositis has an insidious onset, with muscle weakness that may be diffuse and involve both the distal and proximal muscles.

Bibliography

Engel WK, Askanas V. Inclusion body myositis: clinical, diagnostic, and pathologic aspects. Neurology. 2006 Jan 24;66(2 Suppl 1):S20. [PMID: 16432141]

Item 37   Answer: C

Educational Objective: Diagnose knee osteoarthritis with standing plain radiography.

Standing plain radiography is appropriate for this patient who most likely has osteoarthritis. Osteoarthritis is often clinically identifiable by the presence of bony hypertrophy in a characteristic pattern of joint involvement and the absence of overt inflammatory synovitis. The history generally consists of long-standing and gradually worsening symptoms in middle-aged or older patients. Confirmatory plain radiographs are appropriate to solidify the diagnosis and rule out less common findings such as osteonecrosis, fractures, or malignancies. They are also noninvasive, widely available, and the least expensive radiographic modality. Standing views of the knees can demonstrate a more accurate picture of the joint-space narrowing that is present during functioning, including standing and walking, than radiographs that are obtained supine.

Bone scintigraphy can visualize areas of bone turnover change due to osteophyte formation, subchondral sclerosis, subchondral cyst formation, and bone marrow lesions. However, its limited anatomic resolution and the use of ionizing radiation make it less useful for the diagnosis of osteoarthritis.

MRI is capable of demonstrating numerous findings in soft tissue and cartilage that provide information about the joint as a whole organ. As such, MRI is a critical tool in osteoarthritis research, but its high cost argues against its routine use, particularly because there are no end points apart from joint-space narrowing (easily assessed on plain radiographs as well) visualized on MRI that confer prognostic information.

Although ultrasonography is noninvasive and is appealing because it provides real-time information, its primary use in the management of osteoarthritis is for needle placement in difficult arthrocenteses. Limitations of ultrasonography include that it is an operator-dependent technique and that the physical properties of sound limit its ability to assess deep articular structures and the subchondral bone.

KEY POINT

- In patients with suspected osteoarthritis, confirmatory plain radiographs with standing views are appropriate to solidify the diagnosis and rule out less common findings such as avascular necrosis, fractures, and malignancies.

Bibliography

Guermazi A, Hayashi D, Roemer FW, DT Felson. Osteoarthritis: a review of strengths and weaknesses of different imaging options. Rheum Dis Clin N Am. 2013 Aug;39(3):567-91. [PMID: 23719076]

Item 38   Answer: B

Educational Objective: Treat dry eyes in a patient with Sjögren syndrome.

Cyclosporine drops are appropriate for this patient. She has primary Sjögren syndrome with dry eyes (keratoconjunctivitis sicca), which has not responded to topical lubrication or punctal plugs. Sjögren syndrome is an immune-mediated disease of unknown cause manifesting primarily as inflammation of exocrine glands, including the major and minor salivary glands, lacrimal glands, and, less commonly, other exocrine glands such as the pancreas. The most prominent clinical feature is dryness (sicca), particularly of the eyes and mouth. Dry eyes can lead to corneal damage and visual impairment. Sicca symptoms are primarily treated with hydration and lubrication, although other local measures and medications may be helpful. Topical cyclosporine has been demonstrated in trials to improve the symptoms of dry eyes in patients with primary Sjögren syndrome. An alternative therapy is punctal occlusion (placement of plugs in the tear drainage duct openings of the lower eyelids to increase eye moisture). There is controversy as to the timing and type of plug to use when performing this procedure.

Certolizumab pegol is a tumor necrosis factor (TNF)-α inhibitor used to treat diseases such as rheumatoid arthritis, psoriatic arthritis, and ankylosing spondylitis. This agent is not appropriate for this patient because trials of other TNF-α inhibitors (etanercept and infliximab) did not demonstrate benefit for sicca symptoms.

Hydroxychloroquine is used to treat diseases such as systemic lupus erythematosus and rheumatoid arthritis. This agent has not been demonstrated to improve sicca symptoms, although it could be useful for treating arthritic and other systemic symptoms associated with Sjögren syndrome.

Olopatadine drops reduce histamine release from mast cells and are used to treat allergic conjunctivitis; they would therefore not be helpful for Sjögren-related sicca symptoms.

Prednisone is a potent anti-inflammatory agent that is very effective in many rheumatologic diseases. It has not been demonstrated to improve sicca symptoms, although it could be useful for treating systemic manifestations of Sjögren syndrome.

KEY POINT

- Topical cyclosporine improves the symptoms of dry eyes in patients with primary Sjögren syndrome.

Bibliography

Ramos-Casals M, Tzioufas AG, Stone JH, Sisó A, Bosch X. Treatment of primary Sjögren syndrome: a systematic review. JAMA. 2010 Jul 28;304(4): 452-60. [PMID: 20664046]

Item 39   Answer: C

Educational Objective: Monitor a patient with Marfan syndrome using echocardiography.

Echocardiography to evaluate for aortic root dilatation is the most appropriate routine monitoring test for this patient with Marfan syndrome. This autosomal dominant condition is characterized by a mutation in the gene *FBN1* responsible for producing fibrillin 1, a structural protein in tissues that contain elastic fibers, such as the arterial wall. Clinical features include tall stature, arachnodactyly, anterior thoracic deformity, spinal curvature, and skin hyperextensibility. The most common cause of morbidity and mortality is aortic root dilatation with possible dissection, rupture, or aortic valve insufficiency. Current guidelines recommend that echocardiography should be performed at the time of diagnosis to determine aortic root and ascending aortic diameters and 6 months later to determine their rate of enlargement. Annual imaging is recommended if stability of the aortic diameter is documented. If the maximal aortic diameter is 4.5 cm or greater, more frequent imaging should be considered.

Patients with Marfan syndrome may develop abdominal aortic aneurysm, but thoracic involvement or thoracic and abdominal aneurysms are much more common. There currently are no recommendations from any organization to routinely screen these patients with abdominal ultrasonography.

Apical lung bullae can form and lead to pneumothorax in patients with Marfan syndrome; however, there are no data to suggest that monitoring with annual chest radiography has any impact on morbidity or mortality.

Likewise, routine monitoring for progressive skeletal abnormalities, including annual spine radiography to monitor this patient's scoliosis, is not indicated because it has no impact on outcome and should be evaluated only when symptomatic. However, counseling regarding joint protection to prevent osteoarthritis is useful.

KEY POINT

- In patients with Marfan syndrome, echocardiography should be performed at the time of diagnosis to determine aortic root and ascending aortic diameters and 6 months later to determine their rate of enlargement.

Bibliography

Dean JCS. Marfan's syndrome: clinical diagnosis and management 2007 Jul;15(7):727-33. [PMID: 17487218]

Item 40   Answer: A

Educational Objective: Treat a patient who has hypersensitivity vasculitis.

Discontinuation of trimethoprim-sulfamethoxazole is indicated for this patient who developed palpable purpura within days of starting trimethoprim-sulfamethoxazole for a urinary tract infection. The most likely diagnosis is hypersensitivity vasculitis, which is caused by a hypersensitivity reaction to antigens such as medication or infection. Hypersensitivity vasculitis typically resolves when the offending agent is removed. Similar to other forms of small-vessel vasculitis, hypersensitivity vasculitis results from antibodies directed toward the antigens that result in immune complex formation. Complement is activated, and neutrophils are attracted to accumulate in capillaries, arterioles, and post-capillary venules. Although a similar reaction associated with the infection itself may occur, this is less likely given the time course of onset and the high degree of association of trimethoprim-sulfamethoxazole with this reaction. Because her reaction is mild and limited to the skin, the most important aspect of treatment is to remove the likely offending agent, after which the condition will resolve.

Prednisone has shown efficacy in hypersensitivity vasculitis and can be used if the vasculitis is severe, is causing discomfort of the skin or other organ damage, or if it is imperative that the agent be continued despite the reactions. Because this is not the case, discontinuing the offending agent remains the highest priority.

Antihistone antibodies occur frequently in patients with either systemic or drug-induced lupus erythematosus. This patient's disease is more consistent with hypersensitivity vasculitis without specific features of drug-induced lupus (for example, malar rash); however, even if drug-induced lupus were the likely diagnosis, discontinuing the offending agent would still be the highest priority.

Palpable purpura is a clinical diagnosis for which a skin biopsy is not generally needed. A skin biopsy could be useful in cases where the mechanism of the rash needs to be understood to facilitate diagnosis or treatment, or when the rash fails to resolve despite management. In this case, the cause of the rash is known, and management should consist of removal of the offending agent before any further work-up is considered.

KEY POINT

- Hypersensitivity vasculitis is caused by a hypersensitivity reaction to antigens such as medication or infection and typically resolves when the offending agent is removed.

Bibliography
Chen KR, Carlson JA. Clinical approach to cutaneous vasculitis. Am J Clin Dermatol. 2008;9(2):71-92. [PMID: 18284262]

Item 41   Answer: B

Educational Objective: Treat mild systemic lupus erythematosus.

Hydroxychloroquine is an appropriate agent to address milder systemic manifestations of systemic lupus erythematosus (SLE) such as arthritis and pericarditis, and it can act as a glucocorticoid-sparing agent. All patients with SLE who can tolerate it should be taking hydroxychloroquine. Antimalarial therapy such as hydroxychloroquine in SLE has documented benefit for reducing disease activity, improving survival, and reducing the risk of SLE-related thrombosis and myocardial infarction.

Azathioprine is generally reserved for more severe manifestations of SLE not responsive to low-dose prednisone and hydroxychloroquine but can be associated with serious

toxicity. Azathioprine has generally been supplanted by the use of mycophenolate mofetil in SLE.

Mycophenolate mofetil may be appropriate for this patient if she had more serious disease activity such as nephritis or if her arthritis or pericarditis recurred while taking hydroxychloroquine.

NSAIDs, often with colchicine, are first-line therapy for most patients with pericarditis, although glucocorticoids may be indicated in patients with pericarditis associated with a systemic inflammatory disease such as in this patient. However, there is no indication to start an NSAID now given resolution of her symptoms, and doing so would increase her risk of gastrointestinal complications if used along with her daily glucocorticoid.

KEY POINT

- Antimalarial therapy such as hydroxychloroquine in systemic lupus erythematosus (SLE) has documented benefit for reducing disease activity, improving survival, and reducing the risk of SLE-related thrombosis and myocardial infarction.

Bibliography
Lee SJ, Silverman E, Bargman JM. The role of antimalarial agents in the treatment of SLE and lupus nephritis. Nat Rev Nephrol. 2011 Oct 18;7(12):718-29. [PMID: 22009248]

Item 42   Answer: C

Educational Objective: Treat gout with urate-lowering therapy.

Initiation of allopurinol is appropriate for this patient with gout who has had two attacks of podagra within the past year. The American College of Rheumatology (ACR) guidelines currently recommend that urate-lowering therapy should be initiated in patients with gout who have had two or more attacks within a 1-year period, one attack in the setting of chronic kidney disease of stage 2 or worse, one attack with the presence of tophi visible on examination or imaging, or one attack with a history of urolithiasis. Allopurinol, a xanthine oxidase inhibitor, is an appropriate first-line agent for urate reduction. Flare prophylaxis should be maintained when urate-lowering therapy is undertaken.

Low-dose aspirin can increase serum urate due to effects on renal uric acid transport; however, the ACR does not currently recommend aspirin discontinuation in patients for whom it is indicated, such as this patient with coronary artery disease.

This patient needs to begin urate-lowering therapy, and his flare prophylaxis (colchicine) should be maintained during this period given the paradoxical increased risk of flare during acute serum urate reduction. In the absence of active disease, the ACR currently recommends that prophylaxis should be continued for the greater of the following: 6 months; 3 months after achieving the target serum urate level for a patient without tophi; or 6 months after achieving the target serum urate level where there has been resolution of tophi.

Probenecid is a uricosuric agent (promotes kidney uric acid excretion) and is a viable alternative first-line urate-lowering agent in patients who cannot tolerate or have a contraindication to xanthine oxidase inhibitor therapy. However, allopurinol is generally more appropriate in patients such as in this case who have no contraindication to urate-lowering therapy. Moreover, the patient's history of urolithiasis makes probenecid relatively contraindicated because this medication increases the risk of kidney stones.

KEY POINT

- Urate-lowering therapy should be initiated in patients with gout who have had two or more attacks within a 1-year period, one attack in the setting of chronic kidney disease of stage 2 or worse, one attack with the presence of tophi visible on examination or imaging, or one attack with a history of urolithiasis.

Bibliography

Khanna D, Fitzgerald JD, Khanna PP, et al; American College of Rheumatology. 2012 American College of Rheumatology guidelines for management of gout. Part 1: systematic nonpharmacologic and pharmacologic therapeutic approaches to hyperuricemia. Arthritis Care Res (Hoboken). 2012 Oct;64(10):1431-46. [PMID: 23024028]

Item 43   Answer: E

Educational Objective: Clinically diagnose osteoarthritis of the hands.

No further testing is necessary for this patient who clinically appears to have hand osteoarthritis. Osteoarthritis is a clinical diagnosis, and the cardinal symptom is pain with activity that is relieved with rest. Affected patients also typically experience morning stiffness that lasts for less than 30 minutes daily. Bony hypertrophy is commonly detected in the fingers, and Heberden and Bouchard nodes may be easily palpated. Osteoarthritis also may cause squaring or boxing of the carpometacarpal joint at the base of the thumb.

This patient has no clinical signs or symptoms suggestive of a systemic inflammatory disease and therefore does not require diagnostic testing with antinuclear antibodies (ANA) or anti–double-stranded DNA antibodies. A positive ANA test result has low predictive value when the pretest probability of systemic lupus erythematosus or a related disease is low. Therefore, this test should not be used to screen indiscriminately for the presence of rheumatologic disease. The American College of Rheumatology recommends not testing ANA subserologies such as anti–double-stranded DNA without the combination of a positive ANA and elevated clinical suspicion of autoimmune disease, which is not present in this patient.

Radiography is not needed to confirm the diagnosis of osteoarthritis in patients with a history and physical examination compatible with this condition. Clinical examination is more sensitive and specific for the diagnosis of hand osteoarthritis compared with radiography.

The key features of rheumatoid arthritis (RA) are swelling and tenderness in and around the joints. Prominent morning stiffness that usually lasts more than 1 hour characterizes early RA. Rheumatoid factor positivity is characteristic of RA, although rheumatoid factor has a low specificity for diagnosis of RA. Rheumatoid factor may be present in healthy persons, especially at older ages. Because this patient has no clinical evidence of RA, testing for rheumatoid factor is unnecessary.

KEY POINT

- Additional testing such as autoantibody measurements or radiography is unnecessary in patients with clinically diagnosed hand osteoarthritis.

Bibliography

Hunter DJ. In the clinic. Osteoarthritis. Ann Intern Med. 2007 Aug 7;147(3):ITC8-1-16. [PMID: 17679702]

Item 44   Answer: D

Educational Objective: Treat polymyalgia rheumatica with low-dose prednisone.

Treatment with prednisone, 15 mg/d, is appropriate. This 74-year-old man presents with shoulder and hip girdle pain and limitation accompanied by signs of systemic inflammation, including low-grade fever, weight loss, malaise, and a markedly elevated erythrocyte sedimentation rate (ESR). This constellation of findings is classic for polymyalgia rheumatica (PMR), especially in this age group. Treatment of PMR, typically prednisone initiated at a dose of 10 to 20 mg/d, is warranted and should result in rapid resolution of symptoms. Prednisone can be tapered over a 6-month period in some patients, but others experience flares with tapering and require more prolonged therapy, for as long as 1 to 3 years. Methotrexate can be tried as a glucocorticoid-sparing agent, but studies suggest limited efficacy.

Low-dose aspirin (81 mg/d) may be useful to reduce ocular complications in patients with giant cell arteritis (GCA), which can co-occur with PMR; however, this patient has no signs or symptoms consistent with GCA such as jaw claudication, temporal headache, or visual loss.

Aspirin, 650 mg three times daily, functions in a manner similar to other traditional NSAIDs, with analgesic, anti-inflammatory, and antipyretic effects. However, like other NSAIDs, it is not a treatment for PMR and is not effective for this condition.

Duloxetine is a dual serotonin-norepinephrine reuptake inhibitor that is used as an antidepressant, to modulate pain due to fibromyalgia and other chronic central pain syndromes, and for chronic musculoskeletal pain. Although the patient has pain and a depressed affect–a common constellation in fibromyalgia–his pain is in a classic distribution for PMR and his depressed affect is common in patients with PMR pain. Since low-dose prednisone will likely be curative, duloxetine therapy should not be needed.

High-dose prednisone is indicated for GCA and severe or life-threatening forms of autoimmunity but carries a high rate of toxicity. This patient has no signs or symptoms of GCA or any other disease except PMR; therefore, high-dose prednisone is not warranted.

Answers and Critiques

KEY POINT

- Treatment of polymyalgia rheumatica typically consists of low-dose prednisone, initially at 10 to 20 mg/d, which should result in rapid resolution of symptoms.

Bibliography

Kermani TA, Warrington KJ. Polymyalgia rheumatica. Lancet. 2013 Jan 5;381(9860):63-72. [PMID: 23051717]

Item 45   Answer: C

Educational Objective: Diagnose chlamydia infection associated with reactive arthritis.

The most appropriate diagnostic test to perform next is a DNA amplification urine test for *Chlamydia trachomatis*. This patient has a presentation consistent with reactive arthritis (oligoarticular lower extremity dactylitis, keratoderma blennorrhagicum). Up to 30% of patients with reactive arthritis develop keratoderma blenorrhagicum, a hyperkeratotic rash found on the soles and palms that may be indistinguishable from pustular psoriasis. Chlamydia infection is a common cause of reactive arthritis and is often asymptomatic. Patients with reactive arthritis, even if asymptomatic, should be tested for chlamydia because they may have persistent infection or carriage of this organism. If chlamydia is identified, these patients, as well as their partners, should receive treatment to prevent recurrence or transmission of infection. More studies are needed to determine whether antibiotics are helpful in treating arthritic symptoms. Antibiotics are not indicated for non–chlamydia-related reactive arthritis unless there is documentation of persistent infection because they have not been shown to alter the course of arthritis.

Anti-cyclic citrullinated peptide antibodies are associated with rheumatoid arthritis, which is characterized by a symmetric small joint polyarthritis typically without dactylitis. This patient does not have this typical presentation; therefore, testing for these antibodies is not indicated.

Antinuclear antibodies are associated with systemic lupus erythematosus (SLE); with the exception of arthritis, this patient has no clinical evidence of SLE, including alopecia, aphthous ulcers, pericardial and pleural serositis, kidney disease, rash, and cytopenias, and does not need to be tested for these antibodies.

Although many patients with reactive arthritis are positive for HLA-B27, it will not add any further value to the diagnosis or management. This patient has several typical features to establish a diagnosis of reactive arthritis, and management with anti-inflammatory medication for arthritis will be effective in the presence or absence of HLA-B27.

KEY POINT

- Patients with reactive arthritis, even if asymptomatic, should be tested for chlamydia infection using a DNA amplification urine test.

Bibliography

Carter JD, Inman RD. Chlamydia-induced reactive arthritis: hidden in plain sight? Best Pract Res Clin Rheumatol. 2011 Jun;25(3):359-74. [PMID: 22100286]

Item 46   Answer: A

Educational Objective: Treat inadequately controlled rheumatoid arthritis.

Addition of a tumor necrosis factor (TNF)-α inhibitor such as etanercept is indicated for this patient with inadequately controlled rheumatoid arthritis (RA). He has been appropriately started on the recommended initial agent, methotrexate, with the dose appropriately titrated up because of continued disease activity. Symptomatic relief has been sought with the use of prednisone and naproxen, but he continues to have active synovitis. Because he has been given an appropriate dose of methotrexate for an adequate period of time, the most appropriate next step is to add a TNF-α inhibitor such as etanercept. TNF-α inhibitors remain the most widely used biologics for RA and are highly effective in the treatment of RA, leading to a 20% improvement in signs and symptoms of disease within weeks for over half of patients.

Rituximab is indicated for use in patients with moderate to severe RA who are also taking methotrexate but have not responded to TNF-α inhibitors. Having never been treated with a TNF-α inhibitor, it is most appropriate to add a TNF-α inhibitor to this patient's regimen rather than rituximab. Other biologics are available, and a number have different mechanisms of action and can be used in combination with methotrexate.

The patient has been on methotrexate since diagnosis and is taking a dose that would be expected to improve his symptoms; however, he continues to have significant disease activity. It is unlikely that continuing to increase the dose will adequately control his disease; this will also increase the risk of toxicity.

Increasing prednisone may offer short-term relief of flares in patients with RA. However, this patient has been on chronic glucocorticoids and high-dose methotrexate, yet continues to have a considerable amount of synovitis. Given the chronic nature of RA and need for long-term treatment, exposing patients to the numerous side effects associated with higher doses of glucocorticoids is not optimal. Furthermore, in this patient with known seropositive erosive disease, therapy with disease-modifying agents is required, and prednisone does not halt bony destruction.

KEY POINT

- In patients with inadequately controlled rheumatoid arthritis who are taking methotrexate, the addition of a tumor necrosis factor α inhibitor is appropriate to improve signs and symptoms of disease.

Bibliography

Singh JA, Furst DE, Bharat A, et al. 2012 Update of the 2008 American College Of Rheumatology recommendations for the use of disease-modifying antirheumatic drugs and biologic agents in the treatment of rheumatoid arthritis. Arthritis Care Res (Hoboken). 2012 May;64(5):625-39. [PMID: 22473917]

Item 47   Answer: E

Educational Objective: Diagnose cryoglobulinemic vasculitis.

Measurement of serum cryoglobulin levels is most likely to establish the diagnosis of cryoglobulinemic vasculitis. This patient presents with palpable purpura, glomerulonephritis (elevated serum creatinine, active urine sediment with cellular casts), mononeuritis, and skin infarctions of the fingers and ears. Although several vasculitic diseases may present with this picture, the presence of ear infarctions is most consistent with a diagnosis of cryoglobulinemia. Moreover, low C4 with a normal (or relatively unaffected) C3, in the presence of rheumatoid factor and a monoclonal paraprotein (the rheumatoid factor itself), is the classic pattern for cryoglobulinemic vasculitis. Thus, the test most likely to establish the diagnosis is a serum cryoglobulin level. Because more than 90% of patients with essential mixed cryoglobulinemia are infected with hepatitis C virus, this patient should be screened and treated for this infection.

Anti–cyclic citrullinated peptide antibodies are found in patients with rheumatoid arthritis (RA). Because this patient lacks arthritis, this diagnosis can be excluded, with the rheumatoid factor (also associated with RA) explained by the patient's cryoglobulinemia.

Anti–glomerular basement membrane antibodies can produce glomerulonephritis but would be less likely to cause the skin findings that are seen in this patient and would be inconsistent with the other serologies presented.

Antinuclear antibodies are present in nearly all patients with systemic lupus erythematosus, a disease of protean manifestations that could indeed present in this manner. However, the presence of a normal C3 with a low C4 is atypical in lupus.

p-ANCA is found in several forms of vasculitis, all of which may involve the kidneys and the skin. However, external auricular involvement is not classic, and the C4 is not reduced.

KEY POINT

- Patients presenting with a multisystem vasculitic disease should be considered for cryoglobulinemia, particularly if the C4 is low, the C3 is relatively preserved, and rheumatoid factor is present.

Bibliography

Saadoun D, Landau DA, Calabrese LJ, Cacoub PP. Hepatitis C–associated mixed cryoglobulinaemia: a crossroad between autoimmunity and lymphoproliferation. Rheumatology. 2007 Aug;46(8):1234-42. [PMID: 17566058]

Item 48   Answer: C

Educational Objective: Diagnose basic calcium phosphate deposition.

This patient has Milwaukee shoulder syndrome, caused by basic calcium phosphate deposition. Milwaukee shoulder syndrome is characterized by symptoms of pain, stiffness, and swelling that tend to occur gradually over time, often with a preceding trauma or history of overuse on the affected side; this entity is classically described in women over the age of 70 years. This patient has typical features of the syndrome, including a large effusion on examination and synovial fluid that is blood tinged with a low leukocyte count. The crystals are often not visible by routine light microscopy due to their small size, and they are not birefringent (hence, not appreciated with a polarizing microscope); however, they may be revealed with alizarin red staining (with crystals visualized as red, globular clumps). This patient's shoulder radiograph reveals narrowing of the glenohumeral joint, calcification of the periarticular cartilage, and erosive changes of the humeral head, all typical findings in this syndrome. Upward subluxation of the humeral head due to rotator cuff destruction and bony cysts are also common.

Acute calcium pyrophosphate crystal arthritis (also known as pseudogout) can lead to significant joint swelling; however, the absence of inflammatory synovial fluid makes this diagnosis unlikely.

This patient has a history of gout; however, her current symptoms are atypical for a gout attack, particularly the gradual onset of these symptoms. The synovial fluid is also very uncharacteristic for gout, which typically causes an inflammatory effusion. The absence of crystals in the synovial fluid further speaks against gout, although monosodium urate crystals are sometimes missed on synovial fluid analysis.

Monoarticular joint swelling must always raise suspicion for an infected joint; however, in this case, the slow onset of symptoms, lack of fever, and normal serum leukocyte count go against this diagnosis. Synovial fluid with low leukocyte count and negative Gram stain also point away from a diagnosis of an infected joint.

KEY POINT

- Milwaukee shoulder syndrome, caused by basic calcium phosphate deposition, is characterized by pain, stiffness, and swelling that tend to occur gradually over time, often with a preceding trauma or history of overuse on the affected side, with a predilection for women older than the age of 70 years.

Bibliography

Halverson PB. Crystal deposition disease of the shoulder (including calcific tendonitis and Milwaukee shoulder syndrome). Curr Rheumatol Rep. 2003 Jun;5(3):244-77. [PMID: 12744818]

Item 49   Answer: A

Educational Objective: Diagnose disseminated gonococcal infection.

Cervical culture is the most appropriate diagnostic test to perform in this patient who most likely has disseminated gonococcal infection (DGI). DGI occurs in up to 3% of patients with *Neisseria gonorrhoeae* and can cause two distinct clinical presentations. In the setting of bacteremia from DGI, patients present with vesiculopustular or hemorrhagic macular skin lesions, fever, polyarthralgia, and tenosynovitis. Arthritis typically is nonpurulent, and synovial fluid cultures tend to be negative. Blood cultures or cultures of the genitourinary tract or pharynx are often positive. Therefore, a cervical culture is appropriate for this patient; cultures of the throat, skin, and rectum should also be ordered to maximize the chance of organism identification.

The second presentation of DGI is purulent arthritis without the rash or other features of gonococcal bacteremia. Synovial fluid cultures are often positive for *N. gonorrhoeae* in these patients. This patient does not exhibit these symptoms; therefore, synovial fluid analysis is unnecessary.

Hepatitis B virus infection can also present with arthralgia, fever, and rash; however, this patient's rash is not typical for hepatitis B, and her liver chemistry studies are normal. Hepatitis B serologies therefore will not be diagnostic.

A positive rapid streptococcal antigen test is helpful to diagnose acute rheumatic fever; however, this patient lacks the sore throat, characteristic rash, and other findings such as cardiac or neurologic involvement that are associated with acute rheumatic fever.

KEY POINT

- Blood cultures or cultures of the genitourinary tract or pharynx are useful diagnostic tests in the setting of bacteremia from disseminated gonococcal infection.

Bibliography
Rice PA. Gonococcal arthritis (disseminated gonococcal infection). Infect Dis Clin North Am. 2005 Dec;19(4):853-61. [PMID: 16297736]

Item 50   Answer: B

Educational Objective: Manage rheumatoid arthritis medications in a patient of childbearing age.

Discontinuation of methotrexate is indicated for this patient with rheumatoid arthritis (RA) who is interested in becoming pregnant. This nonbiologic disease-modifying antirheumatic drug is both highly teratogenic and abortifacient and must be discontinued 3 months prior to attempting to conceive. Although this patient is taking folic acid to help reduce her incidence of methotrexate side effects, taking folic acid supplements during pregnancy can reduce the risk of certain neural tube birth defects. Therefore, she should not discontinue folic acid even if she discontinues methotrexate.

Considerable epidemiologic evidence in patients with systemic lupus erythematosus as well as RA supports the use of hydroxychloroquine during pregnancy. The risks to mothers and their fetuses appear low, particularly when balanced against the consequences of discontinuing treatment in anticipation of pregnancy. Greater disease activity during pregnancy is associated with small gestational age and preterm delivery. In addition, patients in whom all medications are stopped, including hydroxychloroquine, run the risk of flare, which can impair their physical functioning and make coping with pregnancy more difficult. No increases in adverse maternal or fetal outcomes have been observed in a number of studies in which hydroxychloroquine has been continued throughout pregnancy.

Low-dose glucocorticoids are frequently used but should be avoided if possible before 14 weeks of gestation because of the risk of cleft palate. Glucocorticoid use can contribute to gestational diabetes and hypertension. However, they can be useful in the management of RA in pregnancy if the benefit of treatment is thought to exceed risk.

KEY POINT

- Women taking methotrexate must discontinue this medication 3 months prior to attempting to conceive.

Bibliography
Barbhaiya M, Bermas BL. Evaluation and management of systemic lupus erythematosus and rheumatoid arthritis during pregnancy. Clin Immunol. 2013 Nov;149(2):225-35. [PMID: 23773975]

Item 51   Answer: B

Educational Objective: Diagnose IgG4-related disease.

The most likely diagnosis is IgG4-related disease, a recently described condition characterized by lymphoplasmacytic infiltration and enlargement of various structures, including the pancreas, lymph nodes, salivary glands, periaortic region leading to retroperitoneal fibrosis, kidneys, and skin. Most patients are men (60%-80%) over the age of 50 years. Typical presentation is the subacute development of a mass in the affected organ (for example, an orbital pseudotumor) or diffuse organ enlargement. Up to 90% of patients have multiple organ involvement. Lymphadenopathy is common, as is lacrimal and salivary gland involvement. Most patients lack constitutional symptoms at the time of diagnosis and generally feel well. Staining for IgG4-producing plasma cells reveals large numbers in the tissue.

Hodgkin lymphoma usually presents with palpable lymphadenopathy or a mediastinal mass that requires tissue biopsy for diagnosis. Biopsy is likely to show mainly clonal malignant Hodgkin/Reed-Sternberg cells in a background of granulocytes, plasma cells, and lymphocytes. Reed-Sternberg cells appear as large cells with large, pale nuclei containing large purple nucleoli, and their appearance is indicative of Hodgkin disease. The patient's biopsy findings are not consistent with Hodgkin lymphoma.

Sarcoidosis is a multisystem disease characterized by noncaseating granulomas that form in tissues and most commonly affects the lungs. The absence of granulomas on biopsy is helpful to distinguish IgG4-related disease from sarcoidosis.

Sjögren syndrome can present with enlargement of the salivary glands. However, it is associated with focal, centrilobular collections of lymphocytes on biopsy without the histology characteristic for IgG4-related disease present in this patient. Patients with Sjögren syndrome also usually have positive anti-Ro/SSA and anti-La/SSB antibodies, which are not present in this patient.

Answers and Critiques

KEY POINT

- IgG4-related disease is characterized by the lympho-plasmacytic infiltration and enlargement of various structures, including the pancreas, lymph nodes, salivary glands, periaortic region leading to retroperitoneal fibrosis, kidneys, and skin.

Bibliography

Mahajan VS, Matto H, Deshpande V, Pillai SS, Stone JS. IgG4-Related disease. Ann Rev Pathol. 2014;24(9):315-47. [PMID: 24111912]

Item 52   Answer: A

Educational Objective: **Diagnose erosive osteoarthritis.**

The most likely diagnosis is erosive osteoarthritis (OA). Distinguishing erosive OA from rheumatoid arthritis (RA) can be difficult because both diseases disproportionately affect women, are polyarticular, and preferentially affect the hand joints. Signs of inflammation (warmth, erythema, swelling, tenderness, reduced function) are present in both entities, although generally involving more joints for longer periods of time in RA. In contrast to RA, erosive OA is common in the distal interphalangeal and carpometacarpal joints, does not typically affect the wrists or elbows, and is not associated with rheumatoid factor, anti-cyclic citrullinated peptide antibodies, or an elevated erythrocyte sedimentation rate or C-reactive protein level. Both types of arthritis can lead to erosions seen on plain radiographs. In erosive OA, these erosions are centrally located in the joint and are accompanied by proliferative changes. In RA, erosions are located at the joint margins, and periarticular osteopenia is likely to be present.

Reactive arthritis is a noninfectious inflammatory arthritis that can occur after a gastrointestinal or genitourinary infection. It is not commonly associated with erosive changes on radiographs.

Tophaceous gout can occur in either gender and is more frequent in women after menopause. It can occasionally have a polyarticular presentation in the hands, but extensive disease is typically accompanied by the obvious presence of multiple tophi in the skin. When inflammation is evident, an acute gout flare is occurring in the presence of tophaceous gout. Tophi can occur in many locations and can create the appearance of erosions with overhanging edges in affected bones, which are sometimes found adjacent to joints. Highly destructive changes can occur that can lead to loss of joint space with long-standing tophaceous gout.

KEY POINT

- In contrast to rheumatoid arthritis, erosive osteoarthritis is common in the distal interphalangeal and carpometacarpal joints, is associated with erosions that are centrally located in the joint and accompanied by proliferative changes, does not typically affect the wrists or elbows, and is not associated with inflammatory markers.

Bibliography

Kwok WY, Kloppenburg M, Rosendaal FR, et al. Erosive hand osteoarthritis: its prevalence and clinical impact in the general population and symptomatic hand osteoarthritis. Ann Rheum Dis. 2011 Jul;70(7):1238-42. [PMID: 21474485]

Item 53   Answer: B

Educational Objective: **Diagnose limited cutaneous systemic sclerosis.**

The most likely diagnosis is limited cutaneous systemic sclerosis (LcSSc), a form of systemic sclerosis that is characterized by distal (face, neck, and hands) but not proximal skin thickening and is typically not accompanied by internal organ fibrosis. Patients with LcSSc may display features of the CREST (calcinosis cutis, Raynaud phenomenon, esophageal dysmotility, sclerodactyly, and telangiectasia) syndrome and are more likely to develop Raynaud phenomenon early in the disease course. Pulmonary arterial hypertension is more common in patients with LcSSc compared with diffuse cutaneous systemic sclerosis. This patient presents with skin thickening involving the distal extremities and face as well as Raynaud phenomenon; he also has nodules on the extremities, which are suggestive of calcinosis cutis. A number of patients may present with only one or two clinical features, and negative serologies (including antinuclear antibodies) are seen in up to 10% to 25% of patients with LcSSc. He does not have CREST syndrome, which is a variant of LcSSc characterized by the presence of telangiectasias and esophageal dysmotility as well as positive antinuclear and anticentromere antibodies.

Eosinophilia myalgia syndrome is characterized by fasciitis and dermal induration linked to consuming contaminated L-tryptophan, a nutritional supplement. Patients also develop neuropathy and myopathy but not Raynaud phenomenon or scleroderma-specific autoantibodies. New cases are rare since the identification of the toxin several years ago. This patient consumes no nutritional supplements and has Raynaud phenomenon, making eosinophilia myalgia syndrome unlikely.

Morphea is characterized by a localized area of skin thickening, usually on the torso; systemic manifestations or Raynaud phenomenon is extremely rare in patients with this condition.

Primary biliary cirrhosis (PBC) is a chronic cholestatic liver disease of unknown cause affecting middle-aged women. Fatigue, dry eyes, dry mouth, and pruritus are the most common symptoms. Jaundice, cutaneous hyperpigmentation, hepatosplenomegaly, and xanthelasmas are rarely observed at diagnosis. Raynaud phenomenon and skin thickening are not consistent with PBC.

KEY POINT

- Limited cutaneous systemic sclerosis is characterized by distal skin thickening (face, neck, and hands) and is typically not accompanied by internal organ fibrosis; patients may display features of the CREST (calcinosis cutis, Raynaud phenomenon, esophageal dysmotility, sclerodactyly, and telangiectasia) syndrome.

Bibliography

Van den Hoogen F, Khanna D, Fransen J, et al. 2013 classification criteria for systemic sclerosis: an American College of Rheumatology/European League against Rheumatism collaborative initiative. Arthritis Rheum. 2013 Nov;65(11):2737-47. [PMID: 24122180]

Item 54   Answer: B

Educational Objective: Treat rheumatoid arthritis with methotrexate.

Treatment with methotrexate is indicated for this patient with rheumatoid arthritis (RA). She has a polyarticular inflammatory arthritis involving the small joints of the hands as well as a wrist and an ankle, with radiographically demonstrated marginal erosions and periarticular osteopenia and positive anti–cyclic citrullinated peptide antibodies and rheumatoid factor, all of which support a diagnosis of RA. Methotrexate with or without the addition of another disease-modifying antirheumatic drug (DMARD) should be instituted immediately in patients with erosive disease documented at disease onset. Methotrexate is the gold standard therapy because it is usually better tolerated than other DMARDs and has good efficacy, long-term compliance rates, and relatively low cost.

Hydroxychloroquine is indicated to treat early, mild, and nonerosive disease. Hydroxychloroquine therapy alone has not been shown to retard radiographic progression of RA and therefore should be used only in patients whose disease has remained nonerosive for several years. This patient has erosive disease, and hydroxychloroquine as a single agent is not appropriate.

Rituximab, the anti–CD20 B-cell depleting monoclonal antibody, is FDA approved for the treatment of moderately to severely active RA in combination with methotrexate in patients who have had an inadequate response to tumor necrosis factor α inhibitor therapy. Rituximab may also be considered for patients with high disease activity and poor prognostic features despite sequential nonbiologic DMARDs or methotrexate in combination with other DMARDs. It is not appropriate initial treatment for RA in a patient who has not been given a trial of methotrexate.

Tofacitinib is also indicated for use in the management of RA but only in patients who have already not responded to methotrexate alone. This relatively recent addition to the treatment armamentarium for RA is the first oral agent to be introduced in decades but is indicated for use in patients who are intolerant to or have had an inadequate response to methotrexate.

KEY POINT

- Methotrexate is the initial treatment of choice for patients with new-onset, rapidly progressive, or erosive rheumatoid arthritis.

Bibliography

Singh JA, Furst DE, Bharat A, et al. 2012 Update of the 2008 American College Of Rheumatology recommendations for the use of disease-modifying antirheumatic drugs and biologic agents in the treatment of rheumatoid arthritis. Arthritis Care Res (Hoboken). 2012 May;64(5):625-39. [PMID: 22473917]

Item 55   Answer: A

Educational Objective: Diagnose mixed connective tissue disease.

The most likely diagnosis is mixed connective tissue disease (MCTD), an overlap syndrome that includes features of systemic lupus erythematosus (SLE), systemic sclerosis, and/or polymyositis in the setting of positive anti–U1-ribonucleoprotein (RNP) antibodies. Patients with MCTD must have positive anti–U1-RNP antibodies and at least three of the following five features: Raynaud phenomenon, edema of the hands, sclerodactyly, synovitis, and myositis. Patients with MCTD usually have positive antinuclear antibodies (ANA), negative anti–double-stranded DNA antibodies, normal complement levels, and a low incidence of kidney disease. These criteria have a sensitivity of 63% and specificity of 86% in the diagnosis of MCTD. These patients are more likely to have myositis and pulmonary hypertension, an important cause of mortality, than patients with SLE.

Polymyositis is a form of inflammatory myopathy characterized by symmetric proximal muscle weakness with little or no pain, and muscle enzymes such as creatine kinase are usually elevated 10- to 50-fold the upper limit of normal. However, polymyositis is not associated with anti–U1-RNP antibodies and does not result in puffy hands or sicca symptoms.

Although the patient has a positive ANA, the diagnosis of SLE is less likely in the context of the negative anti–Smith and anti–double-stranded DNA antibodies as well as the normal complement levels, serum creatinine, and urinalysis.

The absence of sclerodactyly, sclerodermatous skin changes, and esophageal involvement makes systemic sclerosis an unlikely diagnosis.

Undifferentiated connective tissue disease (UCTD) is not an overlap syndrome but instead refers to nonspecific clinical features (such as Raynaud phenomenon and arthralgia), no disease-specific findings, and nonspecific positive autoantibodies (such as ANA). UCTD may exist for some time prior to a clear emergence of symptoms characteristic enough to define a single rheumatologic disease.

KEY POINT

- Mixed connective tissue disease is an overlap syndrome that includes features of systemic lupus erythematosus, systemic sclerosis, and/or polymyositis in the setting of positive anti–U1-ribonucleoprotein antibodies.

Bibliography

Hajas A, Szodoray P, Nakken B, et al. Clinical course, prognosis, and causes of death in mixed connective tissue disease. J Rheumatol. 2013 Jul;40(7):1134-42. [PMID: 23637328]

Item 56   Answer: A

Educational Objective: Diagnose diffuse alveolar hemorrhage in a patient with systemic lupus erythematosus.

Bronchoscopy with bronchoalveolar lavage (BAL) and biopsy is the most appropriate diagnostic test to perform next in this

Answers and Critiques

CONT.

patient with suspected diffuse alveolar hemorrhage (DAH), a rare but severe manifestation of systemic lupus erythematosus (SLE). The triad of hypoxemia, new infiltrates found on chest radiograph, and decreasing hematocrit is highly predictive of underlying DAH; only about 50% of patients have hemoptysis. DAH occurs in the setting of active SLE, and up to 90% of patients have evidence of nephritis. Chest radiograph demonstrates bilateral infiltrates often sparing the lung apices. Diagnosis is by BAL during bronchoscopy to demonstrate bleeding and rule out infection. Lung biopsy is the definitive diagnostic test, which typically shows a capillaritis with immune complex deposition. Mechanical ventilation and aggressive immunosuppression are generally required, but mortality rates still are as high as 70%.

Although DAH can be suggested by the presence of ground-glass opacities on chest CT, the diagnosis is established only with bronchoalveolar lavage and biopsy.

MRI of the chest can be used to determine if the infiltrates are blood and could be used in rare cases in which bronchoalveolar lavage and biopsy are unable to be done.

Because DAH is typically a pulmonary capillaritis, angiography will not image vessels of this size and will not be useful in establishing the diagnosis.

KEY POINT

- The triad of hypoxemia, new pulmonary infiltrates on chest radiograph, and decreasing hematocrit is highly predictive of underlying diffuse alveolar hemorrhage associated with systemic lupus erythematosus.

Bibliography
Martinez-Martinez MU, Abud-Mendoza C. Predictors of mortality in diffuse alveolar haemorrhage associated with systemic lupus erythematosus. Lupus. 2011 May;20(6):568-74. [PMID: 21558137]

Item 57   Answer: D

Educational Objective: Treat a patient who has Löfgren syndrome.

An NSAID such as naproxen is appropriate for this patient who has Löfgren syndrome, a self-limiting form of sarcoidosis characterized by a triad of acute arthritis in combination with bilateral hilar lymphadenopathy and erythema nodosum. The "arthritis" associated with Löfgren syndrome is actually a nondestructive periarthritis of the soft tissue, entheses, and tenosynovium around the joints. Symmetric involvement of the ankles is classic, but knees, wrists, and elbows can also be involved. Ninety percent of patients remit within 12 months. When the triad of features occurs, it has a 95% specificity for diagnosis, and further diagnostic tests (such as radiography or serologic testing) are unnecessary. This patient presents with the classic triad of hilar lymphadenopathy, erythema nodosum, and acute arthritis involving the ankles and therefore has Löfgren syndrome. Erythema nodosum may occur in association with a wide array of causes, including infections, medications, and systemic disease, or it may be idiopathic. Sarcoidosis

and inflammatory bowel disease are the most frequently associated systemic diseases. The lesions of erythema nodosum are tender, subcutaneous nodules presenting as barely appreciable convexities on the skin surface, with a reddish hue in the acute phase. As the lesions resolve, a dull brown circular patch is often left behind. Erythema nodosum is frequently bilateral and symmetric, and it usually occurs on the distal lower extremities. Löfgren is more common among Europeans. Initial treatment is generally with NSAIDs (such as naproxen), colchicine, or low-dose prednisone.

Methotrexate, high-dose prednisone, or a tumor necrosis factor α inhibitor such as adalimumab are reserved for patients with chronic, organ-damaging forms of sarcoidosis.

KEY POINT

- Löfgren syndrome is a self-limiting form of sarcoidosis characterized by acute arthritis, bilateral hilar lymphadenopathy, and erythema nodosum.

Bibliography
O'Regan A, Berman JS. Sarcoidosis. Ann Intern Med. 2012 May 1;156(9): ITC5:1-16. [PMID: 22547486]

Item 58   Answer: C

Educational Objective: Diagnose reactive arthritis.

The most likely diagnosis is reactive arthritis (formerly known as Reiter syndrome), a noninfectious inflammatory arthritis that can occur approximately 3 to 6 weeks after a gastrointestinal or genitourinary infection. It is common for infection to have resolved and stool culture to become negative by the time arthritis begins. Asymmetric monoarthritis or oligoarthritis in the lower extremities is the most common presentation, but up to 20% of patients have polyarthritis. Enthesopathy (inflammation at the site where ligaments, tendons, joint capsule or fascia attaches to bone), dactylitis, and sacroiliitis may occur. Erosive disease is uncommon. Ophthalmologic inflammation is a feature of this disease in up to 30% of patients and can manifest as uveitis or conjunctivitis. This patient's manifestations, including a diarrheal illness that preceded the onset of arthritis by 2 to 3 weeks, inflammatory oligoarticular involvement of lower extremities, inflammation of the insertion of the Achilles tendon, and anterior uveitis, are typical of reactive arthritis.

In bacterial infections, synovial fluid analysis typically reveals a neutrophilic leukocytosis (typically >50,000/μL [50 × 10^9/L]), but synovial fluid leukocyte counts ≤50,000/μL (50 × 10^9/L) do not definitively rule out infection. In this patient, infectious arthritis is less likely because this patient has no fever or leukocytosis on complete blood count.

Although psoriatic arthritis can present as an oligoarthritis, it is also less likely because the patient has no evidence of psoriasis on physical examination.

Rheumatoid arthritis is unlikely because it usually is a symmetric small joint polyarthritis rather than large joint oligoarthritis, and enthesopathy is not common.

KEY POINT

- Reactive arthritis can occur after a gastrointestinal or genitourinary infection and is characterized by an asymmetric monoarthritis or oligoarthritis in the lower extremities as well as enthesopathy, dactylitis, and sacroiliitis.

Bibliography

Morris D, Inman RD. Reactive arthritis: developments and challenges in diagnosis and treatment. Curr Rheumatol Rep. 2012 Oct;14(5):390-4. [PMID: 22821199]

Item 59   Answer: C

Educational Objective: **Treat tophaceous gout.**

Continuation of colchicine for flare prophylaxis and allopurinol for urate lowering is indicated for this patient with tophaceous gout. He is having a good response to colchicine and allopurinol, with a serum urate level currently at the target goal of less than 6.0 mg/dL (0.35 mmol/L), resolution of flares, and reduction in size of tophi (reservoirs of monosodium urate). The American College of Rheumatology currently recommends continuation of flare prophylaxis if there is any evidence of active disease, including flares or tophi as seen in this patient. Hence, both agents should be continued at this time. The guidelines further suggest that in the absence of active disease and once target serum urate is reached, colchicine should be continued for the longer of the following: 6 months; 3 months after reaching target serum urate in a patient without baseline tophi; or 6 months after reaching target serum urate in a patient with baseline tophi that have resolved.

Changing this patient's urate-lowering regimen by adding probenecid or changing allopurinol to febuxostat is unnecessary in this patient who has reached the target serum urate level by taking allopurinol. His gout symptoms have improved, and the tophi have begun to shrink in size. If he was not at goal or was having ongoing flares or resistance of tophi to dissolve on his current regimen, options would be to further increase allopurinol, switch to febuxostat (a newer, more expensive xanthine oxidase inhibitor), or add probenecid.

Colchicine should be maintained at daily dosing because the patient still needs ongoing protection against flares, given the presence of tophi.

KEY POINT

- In patients with gout, continuation of flare prophylaxis and urate-lowering therapy is currently indicated if there is any evidence of active disease, including flares or tophi.

Bibliography

Khanna D, Khanna PP, Fitzgerald JD, et al; American College of Rheumatology. 2012 American College of Rheumatology guidelines for management of gout. Part 2: therapy and antiinflammatory prophylaxis of acute gouty arthritis. Arthritis Care Res (Hoboken). 2012 Oct;64(10):1447-61. [PMID: 23024029]

Item 60   Answer: A

Educational Objective: **Treat ankylosing spondylitis with a tumor necrosis factor α inhibitor.**

Treatment with adalimumab is appropriate for this patient with ankylosing spondylitis, a form of spondyloarthritis that predominantly affects the axial skeleton. Inflammatory back pain is a hallmark feature, manifesting as pain and stiffness in the spine that is worse after immobility and better with use. Symptoms are prominent in the morning and can be symptomatic during the night. Buttock pain is common and correlates with sacroiliitis. Fusion of the spine may occur over time, leading to rigidity and kyphosis. Exercise to preserve range of motion and strengthen the spine extensor muscles to prevent kyphosis is essential. Physical therapy may be indicated to assist patients in developing a home exercise routine. NSAIDs are considered first-line therapy for symptomatic patients. If the patient does not adequately respond to a minimum of two different trials of NSAIDs used at least 4 weeks total, the Assessment of SpondyloArthritis international Society/European League Against Rheumatism (ASAS/EULAR) guidelines recommend treatment with a tumor necrosis factor (TNF)-α inhibitor. This patient has not adequately responded to either naproxen or indomethacin; therefore, a TNF-α inhibitor such as adalimumab is appropriate. The currently available TNF-α inhibitors appear to be equally effective when compared with placebo. Response is rapid, often within the first 6 weeks of therapy. Patients who do not respond to one agent may respond to an alternative. Because long-term safety is unknown, TNF-α inhibitors remain second-line therapy to NSAIDs.

Nonbiologic disease-modifying antirheumatic drugs (DMARDs) such as methotrexate and sulfasalazine have not been demonstrated to be efficacious for axial disease but may be considered for peripheral arthritis.

Rituximab is a biologic DMARD used to treat moderate to severe rheumatoid arthritis in combination with methotrexate in patients who have had an inadequate response to TNF-α inhibitor therapy and is also used in ANCA-associated vasculitis. There is no evidence showing benefit of this agent in ankylosing spondylitis.

KEY POINT

- In patients with ankylosing spondylitis, treatment with a tumor necrosis factor α inhibitor is currently recommended if first-line therapy with NSAIDs is inadequate.

Bibliography

van der Heijde D, Sieper J, Maksymowych WP, et al; Assessment of SpondyloArthritis international Society. 2010 Update of the international ASAS recommendations for the use of anti-TNF agents in patients with axial spondyloarthritis. Ann Rheum Dis. 2011 Jun;70(6):905-8. [PMID: 21540200]

Item 61   Answer: B

Educational Objective: **Diagnose acute osteonecrosis in a patient with systemic lupus erythematosus.**

MRI of the left hip is the most appropriate diagnostic test to perform next in this patient with systemic lupus erythematosus (SLE) who has symptoms associated with osteonecrosis. Patients with SLE who have pain or limitation of motion of the large joints, especially the hips, should be evaluated for osteonecrosis. MRI is the best method for detecting early bone edema caused by osteonecrosis when plain radiographs are normal. MRI can also be prognostic: If more than 20% of the femoral volume demonstrates necrosis and edema on MRI, progressive disease (subchondral fracture and femoral head collapse) is the rule, whereas smaller infarcts rarely progress. Up to 37% of patients with SLE may have osteonecrosis by serial MRI monitoring, although less than 10% become symptomatic. Cushingoid features indicate a risk for osteonecrosis because enlargement of fat cells in the face is a marker for enlargement of fat cells in the ends of long bones. Increased adipose volume causes compression of small sinusoidal vessels that leads to interosseous hypertension and impairment of arterial inflow. Use of daily oral prednisone more than 20 mg/d for 4 to 6 weeks is also a risk factor, whereas use of intravenous glucocorticoids may not have the same risk. This patient has hip pain, cushingoid features, and recent use of high-dose prednisone, all indicators that she should be evaluated for osteonecrosis despite the normal hip radiograph.

MRI remains the gold standard to diagnose osteonecrosis. CT is less sensitive than MRI and exposes the patient to unnecessary radiation.

Plain radiography may not detect changes of osteonecrosis for several months following the onset of symptoms. Early radiographic findings include bone density changes, sclerosis, and, eventually, cyst formation. Subchondral radiolucency producing the "crescent sign" indicates subchondral collapse. End-stage disease is characterized by collapse of the femoral head, joint-space narrowing, and degenerative changes.

Ultrasonography can be used to evaluate for trochanteric bursitis as the cause of lateral hip pain but would not be useful to check for osteonecrosis. Trochanteric bursitis can be confirmed in patients in whom hip adduction intensifies the pain or in those in whom the examination reveals pain and tenderness over the bursa. Pain at night is present when the patient sleeps on the affected side.

KEY POINT

- Patients with systemic lupus erythematosus who have pain or limitation of motion of the large joints, especially the hips, should be evaluated for osteonecrosis using MRI when plain radiographs are normal.

Bibliography

Shigemura T, Nakamura J, Kishida S, et al. Incidence of osteonecrosis associated with corticosteroid therapy among different underlying diseases: prospective MRI study. Rheumatology (Oxford). 2011 Nov;50(11):2023-8. [PMID: 21865285]

Item 62   Answer: E

Educational Objective: Diagnose ovarian cancer in a patient with dermatomyositis.

Transvaginal pelvic ultrasonography is indicated for this patient with dermatomyositis, which may be associated with an underlying malignancy, especially in the first 2 years after diagnosis. Malignancy risk may also be higher in the presence of vasculitis (as seen in this patient) or cutaneous necrosis as well as in patients who are of older age at onset. Patients with dermatomyositis have an increased standardized incidence ratio of solid malignancies such as adenocarcinomas of the lung, cervix, ovaries, pancreas, colorectal, stomach, and bladder as well as non-Hodgkin lymphoma. Risk of ovarian cancer may be especially increased. In a population-based study, the standardized incidence ratio was 10.5 for ovarian cancer, highest among all cancers diagnosed. Therefore, obtaining a transvaginal pelvic ultrasonography to look for ovarian pathology, especially ovarian cancer, is recommended for this patient who has worsening dermatomyositis and new-onset ascites on examination.

Chest CT is helpful in diagnosing interstitial lung disease in patients with myositis and in evaluating malignancy; however, this patient has no evidence of respiratory symptoms but does have new-onset ascites, making ovarian cancer a more likely diagnosis.

Although this patient has elevated aspartate aminotransferase, it is likely of muscle origin and abnormal due to active myositis. Liver biopsy is not needed prior to obtaining other noninvasive studies for her abnormal liver chemistry tests and evaluation for ovarian cancer.

The diagnosis of advanced ovarian cancer is usually made by CT- or ultrasound-guided biopsy of a suspicious mass or cytologic examination of ascitic fluid. PET scan is likely to show abnormalities in her abdomen but will not lead to the correct diagnosis and is not cost-effective.

Thigh muscle MRI with specialized (STIR protocol) images may show evidence of actively involved muscle with myositis and support the diagnosis of dermatomyositis. However, this study is not needed in this patient who already has been diagnosed with dermatomyositis and has evidence of the classic rash, weakness, and elevated muscle enzymes.

KEY POINT

- The risk of ovarian cancer may be especially increased in women with dermatomyositis.

Bibliography

Hill CL, Zhang Y, Felson DT, et al. Frequency of specific cancer types in dermatomyositis and polymyositis: a population-based study. Lancet. 2001 Jan 13;357(9250):96. [PMID: 11197446]

Item 63   Answer: D

Educational Objective: Diagnose polyarteritis nodosa.

The most likely diagnosis is polyarteritis nodosa (PAN), the most common medium-sized vasculitis that affects the mesenteric and renal arteries. Patients usually present with nonspecific inflammatory symptoms as well as abdominal symptoms (chronic or intermittent ischemic pain), neurologic involvement (mononeuritis multiplex), and skin findings (livedo reticularis, purpura, and painful subcutaneous nodules). Kidney disease is based on decreased renal artery blood flow rather than glomerulonephritis. The presence of hepatitis B virus (HBV) infection is a strong risk factor for the development of PAN, although in areas where HBV vaccination is common, the incidence of HBV-associated PAN has diminished greatly. This patient with HBV infection (positive hepatitis B surface antigen) presents with involvement of the abdomen, kidneys, nerves, joints, and skin, accompanied by hypertension but sparing the upper and lower respiratory tracts. He also has mononeuropathy, arthralgia, fever, and livedo reticularis (shown in the figure) but lacks the active urine sediment characteristic of glomerulonephritis. Together these findings suggest a systemic vasculitis of which PAN is the most likely. Testicular involvement is also common, as in this case. Diagnosis of PAN is best established by demonstrating necrotizing arteritis in biopsy specimens, or characteristic medium-sized artery aneurysms and stenoses on imaging studies of the mesenteric or renal arteries using either angiography or CT angiography.

Goodpasture syndrome affects the kidneys and often the lungs. The lack of active urine sediment and the presence of medium arterial involvement are inconsistent with Goodpasture syndrome, as are the abdominal symptoms.

Granulomatosis with polyangiitis (GPA; formerly known as Wegener granulomatosis) can involve the kidneys, and neuropathy and purpura can occur; however, this disease is associated with glomerulonephritis, which is absent in this patient. Furthermore, medium-sized artery involvement does not occur in GPA, and the absence of ANCA makes GPA much less likely.

Henoch-Schönlein purpura (HSP) can affect the kidneys, nerves, and skin as well as cause abdominal pain. However, HSP is an immune complex disease affecting small vessels; active urine sediment is common, complements (particularly C4) are typically low, and IgA levels may be elevated, none of which is the case in this patient.

KEY POINT

- Patients with polyarteritis nodosa typically present with fever, arthralgia, myalgia, skin findings, abdominal pain, weight loss, and peripheral nerve manifestations, most commonly mononeuropathy or mononeuritis multiplex.

Bibliography

Ebert EC, Hagspiel KD, Nagar M, Schlesinger N. Gastrointestinal involvement in polyarteritis nodosa. Clin Gastroenterol Hepatol. 2008 Sep;6(9):960-6. [PMID: 18585977]

Item 64   Answer: C

Educational Objective: Recognize the risk of early-onset knee osteoarthritis following meniscectomy.

The most likely cause of this patient's left knee osteoarthritis is meniscectomy. The history of prior injury followed by meniscectomy puts this patient at substantial risk for the development of osteoarthritis at an earlier age than would otherwise be predicted. A recent prospective study with a

40-year follow-up concluded that meniscectomy leads to osteoarthritis of the knee with a resultant 132-fold increase in the rate of total knee replacement in comparison to their matched controls. The risk of osteoarthritis of the knee following meniscus injury and removal is also well documented for adolescent athletes and, as recognition of this link has become more widespread, the incidence of meniscus repair rather than meniscectomy has risen.

Other factors for osteoarthritis are advancing age, obesity, female gender, and genetic factors. For example, obesity is the most important modifiable risk factor for osteoarthritis of the knee, but this patient is not obese. The incidence of knee osteoarthritis is also increased by occupations with repetitive bending, which this patient does not experience. The prevalence of osteoarthritis of the hip and knee is nearly two times higher in women than in men. Osteoarthritis of the hand has strong female and genetic predilections; it is also associated with obesity. His mother's hand osteoarthritis is probably not relevant for this patient who developed knee osteoarthritis at an early age following meniscectomy.

KEY POINT

- There is an increased risk of early-onset knee osteoarthritis in patients with a history of prior injury followed by meniscectomy.

Bibliography

Pengas IP, Assiotis A, Nash W, et al. Total meniscectomy in adolescents: a 40-year follow-up. J Bone Joint Surg Br. 2012 Dec;94(12):1649-54. [PMID: 23188906]

Item 65   Answer: B

Educational Objective: Manage a prosthetic joint infection.

Obtaining blood and synovial fluid cultures is the most appropriate next step in management for this patient with suspected prosthetic joint infection. Infections may occur early (within 3 months of surgery), have delayed onset (3-12 months), or have late onset (>12 months after surgery). Early-onset infections typically present with joint swelling, erythema, wound drainage, and/or fever. Delayed-onset infections present more insidiously with prolonged joint pain, often without fever. Late-onset infections present as acute pain and swelling, often in the setting of a nidus for hematogenous seeding such as a vascular catheter or other site of infection remote from the affected joint. This patient has acute onset of pain and swelling of the right knee, along with fevers, an elevated leukocyte count with a left shift, and elevated inflammatory markers, occurring 2 months after knee replacement. Urgent surgical consultation is warranted, and blood and synovial fluid cultures should be obtained before administration of antibiotics, whenever possible, to allow for more accurate culture data. Blood cultures are essential (even when fever is absent); although the infection likely arose locally at the surgical site in this patient, most cases of infectious arthritis arise from hematogenous spread. Blood cultures are also important

CONT.

because, even in cases in which the infection arises directly at the joint, the organism may occasionally be identified in the blood cultures. Before initiating antibiotics, synovial fluid cultures should be obtained via arthrocentesis or in the operating room if surgical intervention is imminent and the patient is stable enough to withhold antibiotics until surgery.

This patient will need antibiotics shortly, but she is stable enough to await surgical evaluation and collection of blood and synovial fluid cultures.

More advanced imaging such as a CT, bone scan, or MRI is generally not indicated in the preliminary evaluation and treatment of a suspected prosthetic joint infection because these studies delay the more urgent management of the patient and do not change the initial management.

KEY POINT

- In patients with suspected prosthetic joint infection, blood and synovial fluid cultures should be obtained before initiation of antibiotics to allow for more accurate culture data.

Bibliography

Osmon DR, Berbari EF, Berendt AR, et al; Infectious Diseases Society of America. Diagnosis and management of prosthetic joint infection: clinical practice guidelines by the Infectious Diseases Society of America. Clin Infect Dis. 2013 Jan;56(1):e1-e25. [PMID: 23223583]

Item 66   Answer: B

Educational Objective: Manage gout with dietary modifications.

The addition of low-fat dairy products is appropriate for this patient with gout. Low-fat dairy products have been shown to decrease the risk of gout flares both through uricosuric and anti-inflammatory properties. He should also be advised to reduce intake of high-fructose beverages such as soft drinks because they are associated with gout flares due to metabolic pathways utilized in the metabolism of fructose, which lead to increased uric acid generation. Obesity is also a risk factor for gout and should be addressed as needed.

Some leafy green vegetables are high in purines, the nucleic acid component that is metabolized to uric acid. Thus, a recommendation to increase leafy greens as a dietary approach to gout treatment would be incorrect. However, intake of leafy green vegetables has not been shown to increase the risk of flares in population-based studies.

Alcohol is a well-established trigger for gout, probably due to several mechanisms, including uric acid production and kidney urate handling. Although wine has been found less likely to trigger gout flares than beer, alcohol consumption of any sort will increase the risk of flares overall.

Shellfish have long been established as a food that is likely to trigger a gout flare due to the high purine load and should therefore be restricted in this patient's diet.

KEY POINT

- In patients with gout, lifestyle and dietary modifications, including weight loss if appropriate, reduction of high-fructose and high-purine foods, alcohol restriction, and increased low-fat dairy intake, may help decrease the risk of gout flares.

Bibliography

Choi HK, Atkinson K, Karlson EW, Willett W, Curhan G. Purine-rich foods, dairy and protein intake, and the risk of gout in men. N Engl J Med. 2004 Mar 11;350(11):1093-1103. [PMID: 15014182]

Item 67   Answer: D

Educational Objective: Treat a patient who has fibromyalgia.

An aerobic exercise program is appropriate for this patient with fibromyalgia, which is characterized by chronic widespread pain, tenderness of skin and muscles to pressure, fatigue, sleep disturbance, and exercise intolerance. Nonpharmacologic therapy is the cornerstone of treatment and should be initiated in all affected patients. Regular aerobic exercise has been shown to be effective in this setting. Exercise regimens should be individualized and titrated up to 30 minutes most days of the week. Physical therapy may also be helpful initially to develop a stretching and progressive aerobic program. Cognitive behavioral therapy has been shown to be beneficial but is not always covered by insurance plans.

NSAIDs such as ibuprofen have not been shown to be particularly useful in fibromyalgia, and most patients have tried them before seeking medical care for their symptoms. Although possibly helpful when taken on an as-needed basis for other musculoskeletal pain, NSAIDs as a primary therapy for fibromyalgia would not be appropriate.

This patient also has hypothyroidism but has a normal thyroid-stimulating hormone level, indicating that she is being treated properly and does not need an increase of her levothyroxine dose.

Fibromyalgia may co-occur in patients with inflammatory diseases such as rheumatoid arthritis, systemic lupus erythematosus, and Sjögren syndrome, but this patient does not have any clinical signs or laboratory features that would suggest an inflammatory disease. Thus, an antinuclear antibody (ANA) panel would not be helpful, and a clinically insignificant low-level positive ANA may actually lead to further unnecessary testing and specialist referral.

KEY POINT

- Nonpharmacologic therapy, including regular aerobic exercise, is the cornerstone of fibromyalgia treatment and should be initiated in all affected patients.

Bibliography

Fitzcharles MA, Ste-Marie PA, Pereira JX; Canadian Fibromyalgia Guidelines Committee. Fibromyalgia: evolving concepts over the past 2 decades. CMAJ. 2013 Sep 17;185(13):E645-51. [PMID: 23649418]

Answers and Critiques

Item 68   Answer: C

Educational Objective: Manage NSAID gastrointestinal risk in an older patient by using topical NSAID therapy.

Discontinuation of oral naproxen and initiation of a topical NSAID is the most appropriate therapy for this 75-year-old patient with knee osteoarthritis. The major risks of NSAIDs include gastrointestinal toxicity, cardiovascular disease, hypertension, and kidney disease. Among these, NSAID gastrointestinal risk is higher among older patients and needs to be managed. The American College of Rheumatology currently recommends topical NSAIDs rather than oral NSAIDs for patients aged 75 years or older. A 2012 Cochrane review of topical NSAIDs for chronic musculoskeletal pain included 34 studies with 7688 participants. Topical NSAIDs were superior to placebo for pain relief, with the most data available for topical diclofenac. Topical and oral NSAIDs did not differ with regard to pain relief. Topical NSAIDs led to more skin reactions than placebo or oral NSAIDs and fewer gastrointestinal events than oral NSAIDs.

Discontinuing naproxen and adding celecoxib would reduce the risk of gastrointestinal toxicity to an extent similar to that of adding a proton pump inhibitor (PPI) to naproxen but would be unwarranted in the setting of a good response to topical naproxen. In patients with particularly high risk who require therapy with oral NSAIDs, simultaneously switching to celecoxib and adding a PPI could be considered.

Joint replacement should be considered in patients who have knee osteoarthritis with function and/or pain that cannot be managed using nonsurgical interventions. Because this patient has neither pain nor limitation on his current therapy, consideration of joint replacement would be premature.

KEY POINT

- Older patients with osteoarthritis who require NSAID therapy to control pain should be considered for topical NSAID therapy to manage gastrointestinal toxicity.

Bibliography
Hochberg MC, Altman RD, April KT, et al; American College of Rheumatology. American College of Rheumatology 2012 recommendations for the use of nonpharmacologic and pharmacologic therapies in osteoarthritis of the hand, hip, and knee. Arthritis Care Res (Hoboken). 2012 Apr;64(4):465-74. [PMID: 22563589]

Item 69   Answer: B

Educational Objective: Diagnose seronegative rheumatoid arthritis.

The most likely diagnosis is rheumatoid arthritis (RA), which is characterized by a symmetric inflammatory polyarthritis of the small joints. Autoantibodies such as rheumatoid factor or anti–cyclic citrullinated peptide (CCP) antibodies may be present, although autoantibodies are neither necessary nor sufficient for diagnosis. Anti-CCP antibodies occur less frequently than rheumatoid factor, but their presence has more diagnostic specificity for RA. Some patients with RA also lack rheumatoid factor. Seronegative RA has an identical clinical appearance as seropositive RA but is more likely to occur in men. Despite a negative rheumatoid factor and anti-CCP antibodies, this patient's clinical presentation of polyarticular inflammatory arthritis involving multiple and bilateral interphalangeal joints of the fingers, metacarpophalangeal joints, a wrist, and an ankle as well as prolonged morning stiffness and radiographic findings of marginal erosion and periarticular osteopenia, is characteristic of RA. Over time, some patients who are initially seronegative develop a positive rheumatoid factor.

This patient does not have monoarticular or oligoarticular disease or radiographs showing bony sclerosis or osteophyte formation, all of which are typical of osteoarthritis. This patient's symmetric polyarticular inflammatory arthritis associated with prolonged morning stiffness is not consistent with osteoarthritis, in which joint swelling is not found and morning stiffness lasts less than 30 minutes.

Although sarcoidosis can occasionally cause joint involvement, it is unlikely to present with joint symptoms alone. Chronic sarcoid arthropathy most commonly involves the ankles, knees, hands, wrists, and metacarpophalangeal and proximal interphalangeal joints and is usually accompanied by parenchymal pulmonary disease. It is unlikely to be the cause of inflammatory polyarthritis in a previously healthy middle-aged man.

Although systemic lupus erythematosus (SLE) can cause seronegative polyarticular inflammatory arthritis, the initial presentation in a middle-aged man as an explanation for polyarticular inflammatory arthritis would be exceedingly unlikely, and erosions are not seen as a result of arthritis in SLE. The patient has no signs or symptoms otherwise suggestive of SLE such as brain, kidney, lung, heart, or skin manifestations.

KEY POINT

- Seronegative rheumatoid arthritis has an identical clinical appearance as seropositive rheumatoid arthritis but is more likely to occur in men.

Bibliography
Aletaha D, Neogi T, Silman AJ, et al. 2010 rheumatoid arthritis classification criteria: an American College of Rheumatology/European League Against Rheumatism collaborative initiative. Arthritis Rheum. 2010 Sep;62(9)2569-81. [PMID: 20872595]

Item 70   Answer: B

Educational Objective: Diagnose adult-onset Still disease.

The most likely diagnosis is adult-onset Still disease (AOSD), a multisystem inflammatory disease characterized by high spiking fevers, arthritis, rash, high neutrophil counts, and markedly elevated serum ferritin. The rash is a nonpruritic salmon-colored macular/maculopapular rash on the trunk or extremities. Serum ferritin is elevated in many patients, often to extremely high levels, and is a marker of macrophage activation. Erythrocyte sedimentation rate and C-reactive protein can also be impressively elevated. Diagnosis is clinical, based on exclusion of infection, malignancy, or other rheumatologic diseases. Clinical criteria have been developed to assist in the diagnosis of AOSD. The most sensitive of these are the Yamaguchi classification criteria. Diagnosis requires fulfilling at least five criteria, two of which must be major. This patient fulfills three major criteria (fever, rash, joint involvement) and three minor criteria (splenomegaly, lymphadenopathy, elevated liver chemistries). Very few other diseases elevate ferritin to this level, although this is not currently one of the criteria.

Acute myeloid leukemia (AML) is a malignancy of myeloid progenitor cells. Clinical manifestations of bone marrow failure develop over days to months and include fatigue, dyspnea, and easy bleeding. Fever is commonly caused by infection. The leukocyte count can be low, normal, or high, but circulating myeloblasts are present in most cases. This patient has a significant leukocytosis but no circulating blasts, thus excluding the diagnosis of AML.

Granulomatosis with polyangiitis (formerly known as Wegener granulomatosis) is also a multisystem disorder characterized by upper respiratory, lower respiratory, and kidney involvement. More than 70% of patients have upper airway manifestations such as sinusitis or nasal, inner ear, or laryngotracheal inflammation. This patient has none of these manifestations.

Systemic lupus erythematosus (SLE) is also a multisystem disease with early nonspecific constitutional symptoms, including fever, fatigue, and weight loss. Common presentations include a photosensitive rash and symmetric polyarthritis. Cytopenia is common, whereas leukocytosis and extremely elevated serum ferritin levels are not characteristic of SLE.

KEY POINT

- Adult-onset Still disease is characterized by high spiking fevers, arthritis, rash, high neutrophil counts, and markedly elevated serum ferritin.

Bibliography

Iliou C, Papagoras C, Tsifetaki N, Voulgari PV, Drosos AA. Adult-onset Still's disease: clinical, serological and therapeutic considerations. Clin Exp Rheumatol. 2013 Jan-Feb;31(1):47-52. [PMID: 23010097]

Item 71   Answer: A

Educational Objective: Diagnose Behçet syndrome.

The most likely diagnosis is Behçet syndrome, a form of vasculitis that can affect small to large arterial vessels and is one of the few forms of vasculitis that also can affect veins. Behçet syndrome has an increased prevalence in a belt from East Asia to Turkey and therefore conveys an ethnic/genetic risk in those with a Mediterranean/Asian background. Behçet syndrome is characterized by recurrent painful oral ulcers plus at least two of the following: recurrent painful genital ulcers, eye involvement, skin involvement (typically acneiform lesions),

and pathergy (development of a pustule following a needle stick). Oral ulcers typically resolve spontaneously after 1 to 3 weeks. Eye involvement can be severe, especially when there is a posterior uveitis/retinal vasculitis, and can lead to blindness. Hypopyon (suppurative fluid seen in the anterior chamber) is also a distinctive feature. The combination of recurrent painful oral ulcerations, genital ulcerations, and uveitis make Behçet syndrome the most likely diagnosis in this patient. Other clinical findings include gastrointestinal ulceration that may make it challenging to differentiate Behçet syndrome from Crohn disease with extraintestinal manifestations. Arthritis affecting medium and large joints is common, and the vasculitic process may cause neurologic, cardiopulmonary, kidney, and vascular complications.

Clinical manifestations of cytomegalovirus infection (CMV) include a mononucleosis-like illness with findings ranging from fever and lymphadenopathy to colitis, hepatitis, and even retinitis. Oral ulcers, genital ulcers, and hypopyon are not features of acute CMV infection.

Herpes simplex virus type 1 (HSV-1) infection has been classically associated with causing recurrent painful oral ulcerations. Although HSV-1 is being increasingly recognized as a cause of genital ulceration, it is much less common than with HSV type 2 infection. Systemic symptoms, such as fever, may be associated with primary herpes virus infection but are less common with recurrent episodes of viral activation. Additionally, HSV-1 may also be associated with ocular disease, although keratitis is the most common manifestation seen with HSV-1 infection and not hypopyon, as seen in this patient.

Reactive arthritis (formerly known as Reiter syndrome) is a postinfectious, noninfectious arthritis that occurs in both men and women. Arthritis, usually oligoarticular, develops several days to weeks after a genitourinary or gastrointestinal infection and can be associated with oral and genital lesions as well as uveitis. Unlike Behçet, the oral ulcers are painless, the genital lesions are hyperkeratotic rather than ulcerative, and hypopyon is not typical.

KEY POINT

- Behçet syndrome is characterized by recurrent painful oral ulcers plus at least two of the following: recurrent painful genital ulcers, eye involvement, skin involvement, and pathergy.

Bibliography

Dalvi SR, Yildirim R, Yazici Y. Behçet's Syndrome. Drugs. 2012 Dec 3;72(17):2223-41. [PMID: 23153327]

Item 72   Answer: A

Educational Objective: Select acetaminophen as a first-line pharmacologic agent in the treatment of knee osteoarthritis.

Treatment with acetaminophen is appropriate for this patient with knee osteoarthritis (OA). The presence of progressive knee pain in this older individual that is worse with walking

Answers and Critiques

and is accompanied by unicompartmental joint-space narrowing and osteophytosis in the absence of extensive inflammation is pathognomonic for OA. Although OA includes a component of low-level inflammation, the goal of treatment is relief of pain and restoration of function. Most treatment guidelines suggest the initial use of acetaminophen for pain control in patients with knee OA. Acetaminophen is usually at least moderately effective in OA management; at doses of up to 3 to 4 g/d, it is considered safe and well tolerated. Additionally, it causes little or no gastrointestinal intolerance in most patients, does not affect blood pressure, and has significantly less nephrotoxicity than NSAIDs.

Both selective cyclooxygenase (COX)-2 inhibitors and traditional nonselective NSAIDs (such as ibuprofen) are of proven benefit in patients with OA and may be incrementally more effective than acetaminophen; selective COX-2 inhibitors have improved gastrointestinal tolerance and might be a better choice than a traditional NSAID in this patient given his gastric symptoms. However, both selective COX-2 inhibitors and traditional NSAIDs promote hypertension and can cause or exacerbate kidney disease; this patient's chronic kidney disease therefore makes them even less desirable as first-line therapy compared with acetaminophen. Other options for pharmacotherapy include local and topical therapy, intra-articular management, tramadol, and, if absolutely necessary, opiates.

Colchicine is an anti-inflammatory agent commonly used in gout and is not recommended for OA therapy.

KEY POINT

- In patients with osteoarthritis, initial treatment with acetaminophen for pain control is generally recommended.

Bibliography

Hochberg MC, Altman RD, April KT, et al; American College of Rheumatology. American College of Rheumatology 2012 recommendations for the use of nonpharmacologic and pharmacologic therapies in osteoarthritis of the hand, hip and knee. Arthritis Care Res (Hoboken). 2012 Apr;64(4):465-74. [PMID: 22563589]

Item 73   Answer: D

Educational Objective: Evaluate a patient with primary Raynaud phenomenon.

Clinical observation is the most appropriate next step in management. This patient's presentation is suggestive of primary Raynaud phenomenon, a common occurrence in young women that may be seen in up to 30% of women who are white. Raynaud phenomenon may also be the initial symptom of an underlying fibrosing connective tissue disease (CTD) such as mixed connective tissue disease or systemic sclerosis; the predictors/features include severe and prolonged episodes of vasospasm, asymmetric involvement of the digits, and abnormal nailfold capillary examination and/or digital pitting. This patient has none of these features, has a negative family history for CTD, and has undergone nailfold capillary examination, which is normal. She is at a

low risk for progressing to a CTD, should be reassured, and can be followed periodically. In these patients, most episodes of Raynaud phenomenon are self-limiting and do not require treatment. Persistently symptomatic patients can be treated with a peripherally acting calcium channel blocker such as nifedipine or amlodipine. Sildenafil and endothelin-1 blockers can be used in refractory cases.

This patient's likelihood of developing a CTD is low, and measuring antinuclear and anti-U1-ribonucleoprotein antibodies would be of extremely low yield and would not be cost-effective.

Similarly, obtaining an antiphospholipid antibody panel and cryoglobulins in a patient who has no history or evidence of thrombosis, pregnancy loss, or vasculitis is unnecessary and not cost-effective.

Digital arteriography is an invasive test and is usually normal in patients with Raynaud phenomenon. Obtaining this study would be appropriate if thromboangiitis obliterans ("Buerger disease") were suspected, which is a nonatherosclerotic vascular inflammatory disease affecting the medium and small vessels of the extremities and digits that has a strong association with smoking and male gender.

KEY POINT

- Raynaud phenomenon may be the initial symptom of an underlying connective tissue disease; the predictors/features include severe and prolonged vasospastic episodes, asymmetric involvement of the digits, and abnormal nailfold capillary examination and/or digital pitting.

Bibliography

Lambova SN, Müller-Ladner U. The role of capillaroscopy in differentiation of primary and secondary Raynaud's phenomenon in rheumatic diseases: a review of the literature and two case reports. Rheumatology Int. 2009 Sep;29(11):1263-71. [PMID: 19547979]

Item 74   Answer: D

Educational Objective: Evaluate a patient for primary angiitis of the central nervous system.

The most appropriate next step in management is to obtain an intracerebral angiography and brain biopsy. This patient, presenting with recurrent headaches and rapidly progressive encephalopathy but no clear evidence of stroke or infection, requires consideration for primary angiitis of the central nervous system (PACNS). PACNS is a rare and challenging, but treatable, diagnosis because it is isolated to the CNS with no evidence of systemic involvement. His change in mental status could alternatively represent Alzheimer disease, or dementia on a vascular basis given his history of hypertension and smoking; however, the time course would be unusual, headaches are somewhat atypical for dementia, and the presence of an abnormal cerebrospinal fluid suggests an inflammatory process. Other diagnoses to consider include reversible vasoconstriction syndrome, infection, and intravascular malignancy. MR angiography (MRA) is insufficiently sensitive for a

H
CONT.

Answers and Critiques

negative result, as in this patient's case, to suggest an absence of vasculitis, and insufficiently specific for a positive finding to abrogate further work-up. Because treatment of PACNS is aggressive and not without hazard, it is important to definitively establish a diagnosis whenever possible. Angiography is generally used to define the extent of vasculitic disease. Although it is more sensitive than MRA, it is still insufficiently sensitive and specific to establish a PACNS diagnosis alone. Brain biopsy is the gold standard, although it also has sensitivity limitations. The combination of intracerebral angiography and brain biopsy is therefore the preferred approach.

If PACNS were confirmed, treatment would generally require initiation of cyclophosphamide and high-dose glucocorticoids; however, such treatment should only be initiated after the brain biopsy or empirically if a brain biopsy cannot be carried out.

Azathioprine is a somewhat safer immunosuppressant than cyclophosphamide but has not been shown to be a treatment of first choice in PACNS; however, azathioprine may be utilized to reduce relapse rates among patients already treated and in remission.

Functional MRI (fMRI) could provide information about this patient's overall brain functioning; however, to date there are no specific signatures on fMRI that would permit specific diagnosis of PACNS.

KEY POINT

- Intracerebral angiography with brain biopsy can provide a definitive diagnosis in patients with suspected primary angiitis of the central nervous system.

Bibliography

Birnbaum J, Hellmann DB. Primary angiitis of the central nervous system. Arch Neurol. 2009 Jun;66(6):704-9. [PMID: 19506130]

Item 75   Answer: B

Educational Objective: Manage liver toxicity in a patient taking leflunomide.

Discontinuation of the nonbiologic disease-modifying antirheumatic drug leflunomide is appropriate for this patient with rheumatoid arthritis who has developed abdominal pain and tenderness with acute hepatitis. The most likely diagnosis is leflunomide-induced hepatitis. Leflunomide-induced elevation of liver chemistries can occur in up to 20% of patients taking the medication, and a threefold elevation of serum aminotransferase levels has been noted in up to 13% of patients treated with leflunomide. She is at a slight increased risk for it due to concomitant NSAID use. Mild elevations less than three times the upper limit of normal are usually reversible with dose reduction or drug discontinuation. Hence, temporary or permanent discontinuation of leflunomide is indicated in this patient. In patients with more severe elevations (> three times), additional therapy with cholestyramine to quickly decrease the drug levels would also be indicated because leflunomide undergoes significant enterohepatic circulation. The current American College of Rheumatology

treatment guidelines recommend periodic monitoring of liver chemistry tests (every 8-12 weeks) in patients being treated with leflunomide.

Etanercept is a receptor fusion protein, which blocks tumor factor necrosis α. Etanercept-induced liver disease is extremely rare and should not be considered the likely diagnosis.

The usual presentation of biliary colic is episodic, with severe abdominal pain typically in the epigastrium and/or right upper quadrant. The pain rapidly intensifies over a 15-minute interval to a steady plateau that lasts as long as 3 hours and resolves slowly. The pain is often associated with nausea or vomiting, and there is no jaundice. This patient's symptoms are not suggestive of biliary colic; therefore, cholecystectomy is not indicated.

Liver biopsy may be needed to evaluate the cause of liver disease, but it is an invasive process and is only recommended if repeat testing and discontinuation of a known offending agent do not lead to resolution, if the cause of liver disease is uncertain, or if there is evidence of chronic liver disease.

KEY POINT

- Leflunomide can induce elevation of liver chemistries, which is usually reversible with dose reduction or drug discontinuation.

Bibliography

Singh JA, Furst DE, Bharat A, et al. 2012 update of the 2008 American College of Rheumatology recommendations for the use of disease-modifying antirheumatic drugs and biologic agents in the treatment of rheumatoid arthritis. Arthritis Care Res (Hoboken). 2012 May;64(5):625-39. [PMID: 22473917]

Item 76   Answer: A

Educational Objective: Identify azathioprine as a contraindication to the use of febuxostat.

Azathioprine is a contraindication to the use of febuxostat in this patient with gout. Febuxostat is a purine analogue that blocks urate synthesis by inhibiting xanthine oxidase, the final enzyme in the pathway of urate synthesis from purine precursors. It can be utilized when a patient has intolerance to or failure of allopurinol. Azathioprine, a purine analogue used in the treatment of inflammatory bowel disease, undergoes metabolism via xanthine oxidase. Thus, concomitant use of febuxostat (a xanthine oxidase inhibitor) can lead to dangerously high levels of azathioprine. Of note, use of allopurinol (also a xanthine oxidase inhibitor) concomitantly with azathioprine also poses a risk and is relatively contraindicated; however, some practitioners have used allopurinol in this setting with dose reduction and careful monitoring.

Use of diltiazem is a relative contraindication to colchicine, not febuxostat. Diltiazem is a moderate CYP34A inhibitor, and coadministration of this agent with colchicine can cause elevated colchicine levels.

Moderate chronic kidney disease (estimated glomerular filtration rate, 30-59 mL/min/1.73 m^2) is not a contraindication to the use of febuxostat; no dose adjustment to this medication is needed in the setting of mild to moderate kidney impairment.

Nonalcoholic fatty liver disease is not a contraindication to febuxostat use, although monitoring of hepatic function with administration of the drug is indicated.

KEY POINT

- The xanthine oxidase inhibitor febuxostat is contraindicated in patients taking azathioprine, which undergoes metabolism via xanthine oxidase; concomitant use of these agents can lead to dangerously high levels of azathioprine.

Bibliography
Khanna D, Fitzgerald JD, Khanna PP, et al; American College of Rheumatology. 2012 American College of Rheumatology guidelines for management of gout. Part 1: systematic nonpharmacologic and pharmacologic therapeutic approaches to hyperuricemia. Arthritis Care Res (Hoboken). 2012 Oct;64(10):1431–46. [PMID: 23024028]

Item 77   Answer: C

Educational Objective: Diagnose Takayasu arteritis.

The most appropriate diagnostic test to perform next is aortic arteriography in this patient who most likely has Takayasu arteritis. She presents with arterial compromise in the setting of a systemic febrile illness. Asymmetric blood pressure in the arms suggests arm involvement, and a midabdominal bruit, leg symptoms, and hypertension suggest aortic and renal artery obstruction. The differential diagnosis includes other forms of vasculitis and/or thrombosis. Given her age, sex, and high erythrocyte sedimentation rate, a diagnosis of Takayasu arteritis is likely. Because there are no specific laboratory tests used to diagnose or define Takayasu arteritis, arteriography of the aorta and its branches is used to confirm the diagnosis and define the extent of the problem. Alternative imaging modalities such as CT angiography or MR angiography might also be used for the same purpose.

An antimyeloperoxidase antibody assay would be useful if microscopic polyangiitis (MPA) were a diagnostic consideration; however, the kidney disease seen in this patient is due to renal artery obstruction and occurs in the absence of active urine sediment such as would be expected in MPA glomerulonephritis. Moreover, peripheral artery involvement would not be expected in MPA, a small-vessel disease.

The presence of antiphospholipid antibodies would be consistent with the antiphospholipid antibody syndrome and with the presence of thrombotic disease potentially occluding the arm, aorta, and renal arteries. However, her normal prothrombin and partial thromboplastin times indicate the absence of a lupus anticoagulant (one criterion for antiphospholipid antibody syndrome), and the lack of elevation in fibrin degradation products (D-dimer) argues against a thrombotic disease.

Although Takayasu arteritis and giant cell arteritis (GCA) share remarkably similar pathology, GCA occurs in older patients and is characterized by temporal arteritis, whereas Takayasu arteritis is a disease of the young that rarely, if ever, involves temporal arteries. Thus, a temporal artery biopsy is not indicated.

KEY POINT

- Arteriography of the aorta and its branches can be used to confirm the diagnosis of Takayasu arteritis.

Bibliography
Wen D, Ma CS. Takayasu arteritis: diagnosis, treatment and prognosis. Int Rev Immunol. 2012 Dec;31(6):462–73. [PMID: 23215768].

Item 78   Answer: B

Educational Objective: Manage pregnancy planning in a patient with systemic lupus erythematosus who is taking mycophenolate mofetil.

Discontinuation of mycophenolate mofetil is indicated for this patient with systemic lupus erythematosus (SLE) who plans to become pregnant. Pregnancy outcomes in patients with SLE are better if their disease has been well controlled for 6 months prior to becoming pregnant. SLE can worsen during pregnancy in up to one third of patients, and hydroxychloroquine can reduce this risk. In addition, most rheumatologists continue stable low-dose prednisone during the pregnancy. Many medications used in SLE are contraindicated in pregnancy; permitted medications include prednisone, hydroxychloroquine, and azathioprine. Mycophenolate mofetil was developed to prevent transplant rejection but in recent years has been used as a treatment for SLE. Mycophenolate works by inhibiting the purine pathway in nucleotide synthesis and may be at least as effective as cyclophosphamide for SLE (including lupus nephritis) but with fewer and milder side effects. This agent is teratogenic and must be stopped for 3 months prior to becoming pregnant. Mycophenolate mofetil use may also be associated with difficulty in conception in some cases. This patient with SLE plans to become pregnant and has stable disease, and her laboratory parameters show no significant activity. Stopping mycophenolate is the only necessary intervention, and both hydroxychloroquine and prednisone should be continued unchanged.

Stopping all three medications would put this patient at unnecessary increased risk of a flare-up during pregnancy.

KEY POINT

- Mycophenolate mofetil is teratogenic and must be stopped for 3 months prior to becoming pregnant.

Bibliography
Østensen M, Förger F. How safe are anti-rheumatic drugs during pregnancy? Curr Opin Pharmacol. 2013 Jun;13(3):470–5. [PMID: 23522967]

Item 79   Answer: B

Educational Objective: Diagnose *Mycobacterium tuberculosis* infection.

The most likely diagnosis is *Mycobacterium tuberculosis* infection of the hip. Joint infections with *M. tuberculosis* present as an indolent process, often in the hip, knee, or spine (Pott disease). Constitutional symptoms are frequently absent, and imaging may reveal nonspecific erosions that may be interpreted as osteoarthritis. Moderate elevation of the erythrocyte sedimentation rate is common. The diagnosis is made by joint aspiration with fluid sent for mycobacterial cultures. This patient is at increased risk due to origination from and travel to an endemic area (India) and the recent initiation of the tumor necrosis factor (TNF)–α inhibitor etanercept for treatment of rheumatoid arthritis. TNF–α inhibitors increase the risk of tuberculosis reactivation. Patients should be screened for latent infection prior to start of therapy and monitored for signs of infection during therapy. In this case, the patient had appropriate treatment for latent tuberculosis infection in the past but may have had an incomplete response or contracted another latent infection.

Gout rarely occurs in premenopausal women and typically presents in peripheral joints, with the great toe (podagra) the classic site of the first attack.

This patient is not sexually active and thus is not at risk for *Neisseria gonorrhoeae* infection. Furthermore, gonococcal arthritis typically spares the axial skeleton.

Rheumatoid arthritis (RA) is always a consideration in a patient with RA and joint pain. However, it is unusual for a single joint to be involved in an RA flare, and her arthritis appears well controlled overall. Isolated inflammation of a single joint out of proportion to other joints is a clue to infection.

KEY POINT

- Patients should be screened for latent tuberculosis prior to start of tumor necrosis factor α inhibitor therapy and monitored for signs of infection during therapy.

Bibliography

Mariconda M, Cozzolino A, Attingenti P, Cozzolino F, Milano C. Osteoarticular tuberculosis in a developed country. J Infect. 2007 Apr;54(4):375-80. [PMID: 16860392]

Item 80 Answer: B

Educational Objective: Evaluate a patient with systemic lupus erythematosus who has developed mononeuritis multiplex.

Electromyography (EMG) and nerve conduction studies (NCS) are appropriate for this patient with systemic lupus erythematosus (SLE) who most likely has mononeuritis multiplex. Mononeuritis multiplex is characterized by abnormal findings in the territory of two or more nerves in separate parts of the body. She has a foot drop with normal reflexes that suggests an injury to the peroneal nerve and wrist drop that suggests injury to the radial nerve. EMG/NCS would most likely document a peripheral neuropathy. Mononeuritis multiplex is highly specific for vasculitic disorders that affect the vasa vasorum or nerve vascular supply but can also occur in systemic inflammatory disorders such as SLE.

The peroneal nerve is the most commonly affected nerve. Approximately 14% of patients with SLE have a peripheral neuropathy with the majority (60%) due to SLE. Risk factors for the development of SLE–associated peripheral neuropathy include moderate to severe disease and the presence of other neuropsychiatric SLE manifestations. Approximately two thirds of patients improve with more aggressive immunosuppression. EMG/NCS can identify a nerve (usually the sural nerve) that might be amenable to biopsy to document the vasculitis prior to aggressive immunosuppression.

Hydroxychloroquine can cause a neuromyopathy manifested by proximal muscle weakness and areflexia. Biopsy demonstrates vacuoles in the muscle cells. However, hydroxychloroquine has not been associated with mononeuritis multiplex.

SLE may rarely cause transverse myelitis, which is characterized by a rapidly progressing paraparesis associated with a sensory level. Autonomic symptoms, including increased urinary urgency, bladder and bowel incontinence, and sexual dysfunction, may be present. The patient has no symptoms suggesting transverse myelitis, and a spine MRI is not indicated.

A small–fiber neuropathy causes a burning pain in the extremities and has been associated with autoimmune diseases such as SLE but does not cause motor symptoms. Diagnosis is made by skin biopsy, which demonstrates a reduced density of small sensory nerve fibers in the skin.

KEY POINT

- Mononeuritis multiplex is characterized by abnormal findings in the territory of two or more nerves in separate parts of the body and is highly specific for vasculitis but can occur in systemic inflammatory disorders such as systemic lupus erythematosus.

Bibliography

Florica B, Aghdassi E, Su J, et al. Peripheral neuropathy in patients with systemic lupus erythematosus. Semin Arthritis Rheum. 2011 Oct;41(2):203-11. [PMID: 21641018]

Item 81 Answer: B

Educational Objective: Diagnose HIV infection as the cause of a severe flare of psoriatic arthritis.

HIV antibody testing is indicated for this patient with a severe flare of psoriatic arthritis. HIV infection can trigger the onset of or exacerbate preexisting psoriatic arthritis and psoriasis. Skin and joint symptoms tend to be severe. Explosive onset or severe flare-up of psoriatic arthritis should therefore raise suspicion for concomitant HIV infection. This patient had previously well-controlled psoriatic arthritis until a recent severe flare, as manifested by severe pain and swelling of multiple joints and psoriasis, and should therefore be tested for HIV infection.

Although viral infections other than HIV can trigger flares of psoriasis, infectious mononucleosis is characterized by sore throat, lymphadenopathy, and splenomegaly, none of which (except adenopathy) is seen in this patient. Therefore, heterophile antibody testing is not indicated.

HLA-B27 is associated with psoriatic arthritis but not with psoriasis; furthermore, it neither confirms the diagnosis nor explains the flare-up of psoriasis.

The initial clinical manifestation of early localized Lyme disease is erythema migrans, an erythematous skin lesion that is noted in 70% to 80% of patients with confirmed infection. Early disseminated Lyme disease develops several weeks after the initial infection. Patients frequently present with a febrile illness associated with myalgia, headache, fatigue, and lymphadenopathy. Although Lyme disease may trigger a flare of psoriasis, as most acute infections can, it cannot account for the patient's thrush.

Streptococcal pharyngitis is a common trigger of guttate psoriasis, especially in children. Guttate psoriasis can also be the first sign of a flare in previously stable chronic plaque psoriasis. Guttate psoriasis consists of many small raindrop-like papules and plaques on the trunk. This patient's psoriatic pattern does not suggest guttate psoriasis, and testing for streptococcal infection is not indicated.

KEY POINT

- The development of explosive onset or severe flare of psoriatic arthritis should raise suspicion for concomitant HIV infection.

Bibliography

Fernandes S, Pinto GM, Cardoso J. Particular clinical presentations of psoriasis in HIV patients. Int J STD AIDS. 2011 Nov;22(11):653-4. [PMID: 22096050]

Item 82   Answer: B

Educational Objective: Treat a patient who has parvovirus B19 infection.

This patient has parvovirus B19 infection, and an NSAID such as ibuprofen is the appropriate initial treatment. This infection most commonly occurs in children and is characterized by acute polyarthritis with symmetric swelling and stiffness, the classic "slapped cheek" rash, and flu-like symptoms. Adults tend to contract the virus from children, but the rash may be absent or atypical in adults. Therefore, diagnosis should be suspected in adults with other characteristic findings as well as exposure to sick children. This patient shows evidence of a symmetric, small joint arthritis of the hands, a pattern consistent with rheumatoid arthritis as well as several forms of viral arthritis, most characteristically the arthritis that accompanies parvovirus B19 infection. This patient is at risk for parvovirus B19 infection given her occupation as an elementary school teacher, and the presence of IgM antibodies for parvovirus is definitive and establishes the diagnosis. Parvovirus B19 infection and its associated arthritis are generally self-limited; therefore, management is symptomatic, and an NSAID such as ibuprofen should alleviate symptoms until the episode resolves.

Azithromycin therapy may be appropriate for treatment of *Chlamydia* infection associated with reactive arthritis, a form of spondyloarthritis associated with a specific group of urogenital and gastrointestinal pathogens. However, antibiotic therapy is not indicated for parvovirus B19 infection.

Interferon alfa is of value for treating some viruses, particularly hepatitis. However, this agent is not needed to treat parvovirus B19 infection, which is self-limited.

Glucocorticoid therapy is not indicated in uncomplicated parvovirus B19 infection due to the self-limited nature of the infection and associated arthritis.

KEY POINT

- Parvovirus B19 infection and its associated arthritis are generally self-limited; therefore, management is symptomatic, and an NSAID such as ibuprofen should alleviate symptoms until the episode resolves.

Bibliography

Young NS, Brown KE. Parvovirus B19. N Engl J Med. 2004 Feb 5;350(6):586-97. [PMID: 14762186]

Item 83   Answer: C

Educational Objective: Diagnose granulomatosis with polyangiitis.

The presence of antiproteinase 3 (PR3) antibodies will be diagnostic in this patient who most likely has granulomatosis with polyangiitis (formerly known as Wegener granulomatosis), a systemic necrotizing vasculitis that predominantly affects the upper and lower respiratory tract and kidneys. More than 70% of patients have upper airway manifestations such as sinusitis or nasal, inner ear, or laryngotracheal inflammation. Purpura and ulcers are common skin manifestations. Mononeuritis multiplex may also occur. Pulmonary manifestations can present as cough, hemoptysis, and pleurisy. Characteristic radiographic findings include multifocal infiltrates or nodules, some of which may cavitate; diffuse opacities are seen in patients with pulmonary hemorrhage. Pauci-immune glomerulonephritis occurs in up to 80% of patients. Diagnosis is best established by lung or kidney biopsy. However, the presence of anti-PR3 antibodies is sufficient to establish a diagnosis in patients with classic upper airway manifestations, pulmonary infiltrates/nodules, and urinary abnormalities consistent with glomerulonephritis.

Anti–double-stranded DNA antibodies are specific but relatively insensitive for systemic lupus erythematosus (SLE). SLE is an unlikely diagnosis in this patient because the involvement of the upper airways, particularly with erosion of the sinuses, is uncommon in SLE, the disease is much less common in men than women, and complement levels are typically reduced during active disease.

Antimyeloperoxidase antibodies reflect the presence of ANCA in a perinuclear rather than cytosolic pattern and are associated with microscopic polyangiitis, eosinophilic granulomatosis with polyangiitis (formerly known as Churg-Strauss syndrome), and rapidly progressive glomerulonephritis. However, the presence of upper airway disease essentially rules out these conditions in this patient.

Answers and Critiques

Serum cryoglobulins can be elevated in cryoglobulinemia, which can characteristically affect the kidneys, skin, and nerves and can less commonly affect the lungs. However, upper airway involvement is uncommon, and the normal complement levels, especially a normal C4, also argue against cryoglobulinemia as a diagnosis.

KEY POINT

- The presence of antiproteinase 3 antibodies is sufficient to establish a diagnosis of granulomatosis with polyangiitis in patients with classic upper airway manifestations, pulmonary infiltrates/nodules, and urinary abnormalities consistent with glomerulonephritis.

Bibliography

Lutalo PMK, D'Cruz DP. Diagnosis and classification of granulomatosis with polyangiitis (aka Wegener's granulomatosis). J Autoimmun. 2014 Feb-Mar;48-49:94-8. [PMID: 24485158]

Item 84   Answer: C

Educational Objective: Evaluate a patient with suspected lupus nephritis using a kidney biopsy.

A kidney biopsy is appropriate for this patient with systemic lupus erythematosus (SLE). Kidney disease occurs in some form in up to 70% of patients with SLE, especially in those who express anti–double-stranded DNA antibodies, which typically rise and fall with disease activity. Diagnosis of lupus nephritis is suggested by proteinuria (>500 mg/24 h) or cellular casts (erythrocytes or leukocytes) in the urine sediment of patients fulfilling the formal criteria for the diagnosis of SLE. Most patients with active lupus nephritis have low serum complement levels. According to the 2012 American College of Rheumatology guidelines for evaluating and treating lupus nephritis, this patient meets the criteria for kidney biopsy. Unless contraindicated, biopsy should be done before initiating therapy. This patient will most likely have a proliferative form of lupus nephritis (class III/IV) and will require aggressive immunosuppressive therapy.

The usual therapeutic agents for proliferative forms of lupus nephritis are either cyclophosphamide or mycophenolate mofetil. There are no data to suggest that methotrexate is useful in this setting. Methotrexate is renally excreted, and toxicity increases in the setting of kidney disease.

Without adequate management, class III, class IV, or class V combined with class III or class IV generally are progressive, with a probability of end-stage kidney disease as high as 50% to 70% after 5 to 10 years of diagnosis. Therefore, there is no reason to wait another month to repeat laboratory testing in this patient given the present abnormalities.

Because the vascular lesion in lupus nephritis is at the level of the arteriole, a renal artery Doppler examination will not be useful for treatment decisions.

KEY POINT

- The diagnosis of lupus nephritis, suggested by proteinuria (>500 mg/24 h) or cellular casts (erythrocytes or leukocytes) in the urine sediment, must be confirmed and classified with a kidney biopsy.

Bibliography

Hahn BH, McMahon MA, Wilkinson A, et al. American College of Rheumatology guidelines for screening, treatment, and management of lupus nephritis. Arthritis Care Res. 2012 Jun;64(6):797-808. [PMID: 22556106]

Item 85   Answer: C

Educational Objective: Treat hypertension in a patient with hyperuricemia who is at increased risk for acute gout.

The angiotensin receptor blocker (ARB) losartan is the most appropriate antihypertensive drug for this patient with hyperuricemia who is at increased risk for acute gout. Hypertension is a common comorbidity of gout and is found in approximately 74% of patients with gout. Antihypertensive drugs have variable effects on serum urate levels and risk of acute gout. A population-based, nested-case control study compared nearly 25,000 patients with a new diagnosis of gout with 50,000 control patients. The risk of gout was assessed according to antihypertensive drug class. Losartan, but not other ARBs, and calcium channel blockers were associated with a reduced risk of gout (relative risk for losartan: 0.81 [95% CI, 0.7-0.84]; relative risk for calcium channel blockers: 0.87 [95% CI, 0.82-0.93]). Both losartan and calcium channel blockers lower serum urate. Losartan, like probenecid, interferes with the urate-reabsorbing transporter, thereby promoting kidney urate excretion. The mechanism by which calcium channel blockers lower urate levels is unclear but may be mediated through increased glomerular filtration rate and increased urate clearance. Based upon these data, losartan and calcium channel blockers are the preferred antihypertensive agents if reducing the risk of gout is clinically relevant.

In this same study, ACE inhibitors, non-losartan ARBs, β-blockers, and diuretics were all associated with an increased risk of gout. The absolute risk of gout was greatest with diuretics, with an estimated risk of six events per 1000 person-years.

KEY POINT

- The angiotensin receptor blocker losartan and calcium channel blockers lower serum urate and may be useful to treat patients in whom hypertension and gout are both clinical concerns.

Bibliography

Choi HK, Soriano LC, Zhang Y, Rodríguez LA. Antihypertensive drugs and risk of incident gout among patients with hypertension: population based case-control study. BMJ. 2012 Jan 12;344:d8190. [PMID: 22240117]

Item 86　　　Answer:　D

Educational Objective: Treat tophaceous gout with pegloticase in a patient who has not responded to oral urate-lowering therapy.

Switching febuxostat to pegloticase is appropriate for this patient. He has severe tophaceous gout and persistent hyperuricemia and has not responded to oral urate-lowering therapy, including the xanthine oxidase inhibitors allopurinol and febuxostat. He therefore warrants a trial of the synthetic uricase replacement pegloticase, an intravenous medication FDA approved for treatment-failure gout. Patients with bothersome persistent tophi or recurrent gout flares despite oral urate-lowering therapy (or with contraindications to available oral therapy) should be considered for pegloticase treatment, in consultation with a rheumatologist.

Xanthine oxidase inhibitors such as febuxostat should be discontinued when initiating pegloticase. Immunogenicity to pegloticase can result in infusion reactions; loss of response to the drug suggests the presence of neutralizing antibodies to the drug and indicates increased risk of infusion reactions. Therefore, drugs that might otherwise lower the serum urate level should be discontinued because they may mask a rising serum urate level that would signal the presence of pegloticase antibodies and its attendant loss of effectiveness and increased risk of a serious infusion reaction. Pegloticase is contraindicated in patients with glucose-6-phosphate dehydrogenase deficiency.

This patient's current gout flare is nearly resolved and therefore does not require prednisone. Moreover, prednisone is not effective in reducing serum urate levels, and it is not an appropriate drug to prevent recurrent attacks of acute gout due to its many long-term side effects.

Colchicine is generally working well in reducing gout flares in this patient. If this were ineffective or not tolerated, another agent would need to be considered for prophylaxis (or treatment of acute flares). Anakinra is an interleukin-1β inhibitor that may be considered for off-label use for gout prophylaxis and flare treatment in patients in whom other more conventional agents are ineffective or contraindicated, which is not the case for this patient.

KEY POINT

- Pegloticase may be considered for patients with resistant gout who have not responded to oral urate-lowering therapy.

Bibliography

Khanna D, Fitzgerald JD, Khanna PP, et al; American College of Rheumatology. 2012 American College of Rheumatology guidelines for management of gout. Part 1: systematic nonpharmacologic and pharmacologic therapeutic approaches to hyperuricemia. Arthritis Care Res (Hoboken). 2012 Oct;64(10):1431-46. [PMID: 23024028]

Item 87　　　Answer:　A

Educational Objective: Confirm a flare of systemic lupus erythematosus with an anti–double-stranded DNA antibody measurement.

Measurement of anti–double-stranded DNA antibodies is appropriate for this patient who is having a flare of systemic lupus erythematosus (SLE). She has symptoms of fatigue, joint pain, rash, leukopenia, and lymphopenia. Urinalysis shows proteinuria and hematuria, indicating that she may have glomerulonephritis as well. Levels of anti–double-stranded DNA antibodies correlate with SLE disease activity; in particular, they correlate with active kidney disease or glomerulonephritis and might prompt further evaluation such as kidney biopsy. Thus, measuring anti–double-stranded DNA antibody titers may be useful in assessing this patient's recent symptoms. Following anti–double-stranded DNA antibody titers over time can be useful because it is a marker for risk of developing lupus nephritis.

Antinuclear antibody (ANA) testing is a useful screening tool for SLE because more than 95% of patients with SLE are positive for ANA; however, ANA does not correlate with disease activity.

Anti-Ro/SSA and anti-La/SSB antibodies can be present in patients with Sjögren syndrome as well as SLE. These antibodies correlate with SLE rashes and photosensitivity and are a risk factor for the development of neonatal lupus erythematosus; however, they do not correlate with disease activity.

Anti-Smith antibodies are highly specific for the diagnosis of SLE; however, these antibodies also do not correlate with disease activity.

Anti-U1-ribonucleoprotein antibodies are found in patients with SLE and with mixed connective tissue disease but do not correlate with disease activity.

KEY POINT

- Anti–double-stranded DNA antibodies correlate with systemic lupus erythematosus disease activity, particularly active kidney disease or glomerulonephritis.

Bibliography

Andrejevic S, Jeremic I, Sefik-Bukilica M, Nikolic M, Stojimirovic B, Bonaci-Nikolic B. Immunoserological parameters in SLE: high-avidity anti-dsDNA detected by ELISA are the most closely associated with the disease activity. Clin Rheumatol. 2013 Nov;32(11):1619-26. [PMID: 23857662]

Item 88　　　Answer:　A

Educational Objective: Treat a patient who has scleroderma renal crisis.

The ACE inhibitor captopril is the most appropriate treatment for this patient who most likely has scleroderma renal crisis (SRC) in the setting of diffuse cutaneous systemic sclerosis (DcSSc). SRC occurs in 10% to 15% of patients with systemic sclerosis and is more frequent in DcSSc compared with limited cutaneous systemic sclerosis. Vascular involvement of afferent arterioles leads to glomerular ischemia and hyperreninemia. The typical presentation is acute onset of oliguric kidney disease and severe hypertension, mild proteinuria, urinalysis with few cells or casts, microangiopathic hemolytic anemia, and thrombocytopenia.

H
CONT.

Some patients develop pulmonary edema and hypertensive encephalopathy. Normal blood pressure may be present in up to 10%. This patient presents acutely with a rapid rise in serum creatinine consistent with acute kidney injury, with a bland urinalysis and non–nephrotic-range proteinuria as well as neurologic symptoms suggestive of encephalopathy. Although her blood pressure is almost normal, these findings are highly suggestive of SRC. Treatment with an ACE inhibitor is essential to restore kidney function and manage hypertension associated with SRC. Captopril is the preferred ACE inhibitor because it has been the most extensively studied agent in this clinical setting, and its short half-life allows rapid titration.

Cyclophosphamide is a potent immunosuppressant used to treat severe or life-threatening manifestations of certain diseases such as systemic lupus erythematosus or systemic vasculitis. It is ineffective in treating SRC, which is vascular and noninflammatory.

This patient does not have inflammatory end-organ involvement; therefore, methylprednisolone is not needed. Glucocorticoids are not useful in SRC, and intravenous glucocorticoids may cause worsening symptoms.

Sildenafil can be used to treat pulmonary hypertension or finger ulcerations but is not appropriate for SRC, which is primarily mediated through the renin-angiotensin axis.

KEY POINT

- In patients with scleroderma renal crisis, treatment with an ACE inhibitor is essential to restore kidney function and manage hypertension.

Bibliography
Penn H, Howie AJ, Kingdon EJ, et al. Scleroderma renal crisis: patient characteristics and long-term outcomes. QJM. 2007 Aug;100(8):485-94. [PMID: 17601770]

Item 89   Answer: B

Educational Objective: Treat a patient who has inadequately controlled knee osteoarthritis.

An NSAID such as diclofenac is indicated for this patient with knee osteoarthritis. In addition to the implementation of nonpharmacologic measures such as an exercise regimen and/or assistive devices, the initial pharmacologic management of osteoarthritis recommended in guidelines issued by various societies is acetaminophen in doses ≤3 g/d. If this offers inadequate relief, NSAIDs can be used. NSAIDs are more efficacious than acetaminophen in the relief of osteoarthritis pain. Treatment guidelines suggest using the lowest possible effective dose for the shortest time period because side effects are common and occasionally severe. However, many patients require years of NSAID use given the prolonged timeframe over which the disease is symptomatic and the small number of alternative pharmacologic treatments. NSAIDs are associated with important toxicities, particularly with prolonged exposure. The risk of peptic ulcer disease and gastrointestinal bleeding can be reduced

with concomitant use of proton pump inhibitors. Cardiovascular risks can be mitigated by appropriate patient selection for chronic NSAID use.

Topical capsaicin can be used at any time to treat osteoarthritis as well; however, in the absence of an effect from acetaminophen, an NSAID is likely to give this patient more substantial relief of symptoms.

Duloxetine is a serotonin-norepinephrine reuptake inhibitor approved to treat osteoarthritis pain but is slower acting than NSAIDs and requires ongoing, rather than intermittent and as-needed, administration.

Hyaluronic acid injections have shown only a minimal degree of benefit in the treatment of knee osteoarthritis; they also require an invasive procedure for administration and are expensive. Therefore, they would not be preferred to treatment with an NSAID.

Narcotics such as hydrocodone should be reserved for patients who have not responded to nonpharmacologic measures in addition to NSAIDs. An alternative to hydrocodone is tramadol, a centrally acting synthetic opioid analgesic that binds to μ-opioid receptors and inhibits reuptake of norepinephrine and serotonin. It can be used for analgesia when NSAIDs are not tolerated or are contraindicated. Side effects include headaches and dizziness. Tolerance can occur with long-term use; withdrawal symptoms can occur with discontinuation.

KEY POINT

- An NSAID should be initiated in patients with osteoarthritis if first-line therapy with acetaminophen does not provide adequate relief.

Bibliography
Hochberg MC, Altman RD, Toupin AK, et al. American College of Rheumatology 2012 recommendations for the use of nonpharmacologic and pharmacologic therapies in osteoarthritis of the hand, hip, and knee. Arthritis Care Res (Hoboken). 2012 Apr;64(4):465-74. [PMID: 22563589]

Item 90   Answer: B

Educational Objective: Diagnose bladder cancer in a patient who has received cyclophosphamide.

Cystoscopy is the most appropriate diagnostic test to perform next in this patient. He has painless hematuria with a history of granulomatosis with polyangiitis (formerly known as Wegener granulomatosis), which was treated with the non-biologic disease-modifying antirheumatic alkylating agent cyclophosphamide. Both the underlying rheumatologic condition and the medication used for its treatment are associated with increased risk of malignancy, especially bladder cancer. Bladder cancer usually presents with painless frank (usually not microscopic) hematuria, and cystoscopy with biopsy is most likely to lead to the correct diagnosis. In contrast, kidney involvement due to the disease is associated with glomerulonephritis, and urinalysis shows erythrocyte casts or dysmorphic erythrocytes, which is not the case here. The risk of bladder cancer is higher if the patient has received oral cyclophosphamide because there is prolonged daily exposure to the metabolites associated with causing mucosal irritation and metaplasia. The incidence of cystitis and bladder cancer is lower with intermittent intravenous cyclophosphamide, especially when given with mesna, an adjuvant therapy given with cyclophosphamide to detoxify urotoxic metabolites. Importantly, bladder cancers associated with cyclophosphamide exposure may be more aggressive and should be urgently evaluated even when suspicion is low.

CT and ultrasonography may show large lesions affecting the kidneys and gastrointestinal tract but do not detect small and superficial lesions, which can only be detected on cystoscopy.

The patient had no new drug exposure, and urinalysis does not show significant findings of nephritis; therefore, there is no reason to suspect a drug reaction or interstitial nephritis and obtain urine eosinophils.

Urine protein-creatinine ratio to look for glomerular disease is not helpful in evaluating a patient with hematuria when suspicion for the underlying vasculitis is low, as seen in this patient with a negative p-ANCA.

KEY POINT

- The use of cyclophosphamide is associated with increased risk of malignancy, especially bladder cancer, and patients should be evaluated accordingly.

Bibliography

Talar-Williams C, Hijazi YM, Walther MM, et al. Cyclophosphamide-induced cystitis and bladder cancer in patients with Wegener granulomatosis. Ann Intern Med. 1996 Mar 1;124(5):477. [PMID: 8602705]

Item 91   Answer: A

Educational Objective: **Diagnose cardiomyopathy in a patient with systemic sclerosis.**

The most likely diagnosis is cardiomyopathy in this patient with systemic sclerosis. Cardiomyopathy due to systemic sclerosis–induced coronary vasospasm and microvascular disease leading to patchy myocardial fibrosis is the most common symptomatic manifestation of heart involvement in systemic sclerosis. Although accelerated macroscopic coronary atherosclerosis has been associated with other autoimmune inflammatory diseases, coronary vascular involvement in systemic sclerosis is most often microvascular, with ischemia due to structural changes and recurrent spasm of small vessels. This results in contraction band necrosis, a pathologic finding due to episodes of myocardial ischemia followed by reperfusion. This process may ultimately lead to patchy fibrosis resulting in cardiomyopathy and heart failure. Patients who have systemic sclerosis with symptomatic cardiac involvement have a poor prognosis and mortality rate of 75% at 5 years. This patient presents with evidence of fluid overload due to heart failure as seen on her physical examination and confirmed by an abnormal chest radiograph and an echocardiogram suggesting diffuse myocardial dysfunction, consistent with this cause. Infiltrative myocardial fibrosis and conduction abnor-

malities may also contribute to the cardiac dysfunction but are less common causes of systemic sclerosis heart disease.

Constrictive pericarditis is a chronic disorder resulting from inflammation and fibrosis of the pericardium with loss of elasticity and resulting noncompliance of the pericardium. Although it may be associated with connective tissue disease, this patient does not have specific clinical findings typically associated with constrictive pericarditis such as a pericardial knock or pulsus paradoxus; furthermore, her echocardiogram shows evidence of diffuse myocardial dysfunction and no evidence of impaired cardiac filling with normal ventricular function as would be expected with constrictive pericarditis.

Pulmonary arterial hypertension is a common complication of systemic sclerosis and may lead to cor pulmonale and primarily right-sided heart failure. This patient's clinical presentation is more consistent with generalized myocardial dysfunction due to cardiomyopathy.

The kidneys are frequently involved in systemic sclerosis, with scleroderma renal crisis (SRC) occurring in 10% to 15% of patients. SRC causes acute-onset oliguric kidney disease, severe hypertension, and often microangiopathic hemolysis and thrombocytopenia. Except for evidence of impaired kidney function likely due to heart failure, this patient's clinical presentation is not consistent with SRC.

KEY POINT

- Microvascular cardiomyopathy is the most common symptomatic manifestation of heart involvement in systemic sclerosis and presents with heart failure.

Bibliography

Tyndall AJ, Bannert B, Vonk M, et al. Causes and risk factors for death in systemic sclerosis: a study from the EULAR Scleroderma Trials and Research (EUSTAR) database. Ann Rheum Dis. 2010 Oct;69(10):1809-15. [PMID: 20551155]

Item 92   Answer: D

Educational Objective: **Diagnose bacterial overgrowth syndrome due to systemic sclerosis–associated intestinal disease.**

A glucose hydrogen breath test is indicated. This patient has an 8-year history of diffuse cutaneous systemic sclerosis (DcSSc) and now presents with weight loss, abdominal cramping, and loose stools. She is at high risk for developing malabsorption from bacterial overgrowth (also known as blind loop syndrome) due to altered peristalsis caused by fibrosis associated with her underlying disease. She has unexplained weight loss as well as loose stools without any increase in symptoms of dysphagia, nausea, or vomiting. The most appropriate study for her evaluation at this time is the glucose hydrogen breath test. The gold standard for the detection of bacterial overgrowth is small bowel aspiration, but this study is not frequently performed because it is invasive. By comparison, the glucose hydrogen breath test is noninvasive and has a high sensitivity and specificity. Barium study may also be done to confirm these findings, but obtaining a CT scan at this point is unnecessary and costly. MRI may also be useful in the future for assessment of disease and exclusion of other pathologies.

She does not have bloody bowel movements or colitis, and performing a colonoscopy is unlikely to lead to the correct diagnosis because the primary pathology is in the small bowel and not the colon.

Endoscopic retrograde cholangiopancreatography is the diagnostic test of choice for suspected pancreatic or extrahepatic biliary tract pathology. She has no evidence of biliary tract blockage or pancreatic disease.

> **KEY POINT**
> - In patients with systemic sclerosis, malabsorption due to bacterial overgrowth is evaluated by obtaining a glucose hydrogen breath test.

Bibliography

Forbes A, Marie I. Gastrointestinal complications: the most frequent internal complications of systemic sclerosis. Rheumatology. 2008 Jun;48(Suppl 3):iii36–39. [PMID: 19487222]

Item 93   Answer: B

Educational Objective: Diagnose osteoarthritis with calcium pyrophosphate deposition.

This patient most likely has pyrophosphate arthropathy, specifically osteoarthritis with calcium pyrophosphate deposition (CPPD). She has symptoms consistent with degenerative arthritis (pain worse with activity, brief morning stiffness) and signs of osteoarthritis of her hands. Her radiograph shows calcification (also known as chondrocalcinosis) of the triangular fibrocartilage, seen as calcific densities in the region of the distal ulna and ulnar styloid, consistent with CPPD; there is also some narrowing of the carpal metacarpal joints consistent with osteoarthritis. In osteoarthritis with CPPD, patients often have osteoarthritis in joints not typically involved with traditional osteoarthritis, including non–weight-bearing joints such as the shoulders and wrists.

This patient has risk factors for gout (postmenopausal woman, hypertension and taking a diuretic, diabetes mellitus, overweight). However, she lacks a history of episodic joint inflammation that typically precedes chronic gouty arthropathy.

The distribution of involved joints, including the distal interphalangeal (DIP) joints, is consistent with psoriatic arthritis; however, there is no evidence or symptoms of inflammatory arthritis. This patient also has no skin or nail findings to support the diagnosis of psoriasis. Although some patients develop skin involvement after the onset of arthritis, psoriatic arthritis cannot account for the finding of chondrocalcinosis seen in this patient.

The absence of synovial thickening and limited morning stiffness are not consistent with inflammatory arthritis such as rheumatoid arthritis. Rheumatoid factor is also negative, and inflammatory markers are within normal limits. Finally, examination and radiographic findings indicate involvement of the DIP joints, which tend to be spared in rheumatoid arthritis.

> **KEY POINT**
> - Osteoarthritis with calcium pyrophosphate deposition is a form of pyrophosphate arthropathy in which patients often have osteoarthritis in joints not typically involved with traditional osteoarthritis, including non–weight-bearing joints such as the shoulders and wrists.

Bibliography

Zhang W, Doherty M, Bardin T, et al. European League Against Rheumatism recommendations for calcium pyrophosphate deposition. Part I: terminology and diagnosis. Ann Rheum Dis. 2011 Apr;70(4):563-70. [PMID: 21216817]

Item 94   Answer: D

Educational Objective: Identify the cause of an elevated erythrocyte sedimentation rate.

Continuing this patient's current treatment is appropriate at this time. This patient has polymyalgia rheumatica (PMR); she feels well, and her laboratory studies have improved over time. Although her erythrocyte sedimentation rate (ESR) remains elevated, it likely does not represent ongoing disease activity. The most likely cause of this patient's persistently elevated ESR is her age; it may also be elevated because of uncontrolled diabetes mellitus (possibly exacerbated by prednisone). The degree of elevation is related to the serum globulin concentration, the albumin-globulin ratio, the serum fibrinogen concentration, and the percent of hemoglobin A_{1c} but not the fasting serum glucose concentrations. ESR is dictated by characteristics of the erythrocytes themselves and by the presence of specific plasma proteins that alter the normal repulsive forces between erythrocytes and influence their ability to aggregate, form rouleaux, and sediment more quickly. These plasma proteins include acute phase reactants (such as fibrinogen) produced by the liver in response to proinflammatory cytokines occurring in rheumatologic disease, infection, and malignancy that neutralize these negative surface charges and increase ESR. Noninflammatory conditions causing elevated fibrinogen, including kidney disease, diabetes, pregnancy, and obesity, can also result in an elevated ESR. Normal aging can also cause an elevated ESR; for this female patient, an equation to find the estimate of the maximal expected ESR is (age in years + 10)/2, resulting in 42 mm/h.

It is important to recognize underlying factors that influence laboratory studies such as ESR; misinterpreting an elevated ESR as indicative of persistent inflammation or other disease can lead to inappropriate treatment such as prolongation or increase of glucocorticoid therapy. Thus, increasing prednisone or adding methotrexate is not indicated at this time.

This patient reports no headache, jaw claudication, or visual changes, all of which are clinical signs of giant cell arteritis; therefore, temporal artery biopsy is not indicated.

KEY POINT

- Noninflammatory conditions (kidney disease, diabetes mellitus, pregnancy, obesity) as well as normal aging can cause an elevated erythrocyte sedimentation rate.

Bibliography

Colglazier C, Sutej P. Laboratory testing in the rheumatic disease: a practical review. South Med J. 2005 Feb;98(2):185–91. [PMID: 15759949]

Item 95   Answer: D

Educational Objective: Identify rheumatoid arthritis as the cause of pericarditis.

Rheumatoid arthritis (RA) is the most likely cause of this patient's pericarditis. RA is an independent risk factor for both coronary artery disease and heart failure; patients with severe extra-articular disease are at particularly increased risk of cardiovascular death. Pericarditis is the most common cardiac manifestation of RA and is often asymptomatic. Approximately one third of patients with RA can be found to have an asymptomatic pericardial effusion, and 10% of patients with RA will have symptomatic pericarditis at some point during the course of their disease. Most of those with symptomatic disease have a positive rheumatoid factor and active synovitis; however, when symptomatic, the manifestations are likely to be similar to those of any other cause of pericarditis. Diagnosis is most often made by confirming two of three classic findings: chest pain, often with a pleuritic component; friction rub; and diffuse ST-segment elevation on electrocardiogram.

Ankylosing spondylitis is a form of spondyloarthritis that manifests primarily by axial inflammation and bony ankylosis (fusion across joints). Inflammatory arthritis involvement of the hands tends to present as "sausage digits" rather than the symmetric polyarthritis seen in RA. Although conduction defects and aortitis with dilatation of the aortic valve ring and aortic regurgitation occur, pericarditis is not seen in patients with ankylosing spondylitis.

Polymyalgia rheumatica occurs in patients over the age of 50 years and causes diffuse achiness at the neck, shoulder girdle, and pelvic girdle. It is rarely associated with synovitis and is not associated with pericarditis.

Psoriatic arthritis is associated with an increased risk of coronary artery disease, as is RA. It can also cause a symmetric polyarticular inflammatory arthritis involving the small joints of the hands. However, psoriatic arthritis is not a common cause of pericarditis.

KEY POINT

- Pericarditis is the most common cardiac manifestation of rheumatoid arthritis and is often asymptomatic.

Bibliography

Kitas G, Banks MJ, Bacon PA. Cardiac involvement in rheumatoid disease. Clin Med. 2001 Jan–Feb;1(1):18–21. [PMID: 11358070]

Item 96   Answer: C

Educational Objective: Evaluate synovial fluid for infection and crystal-related disease.

Gram stain, culture, and crystal analysis are the most helpful and appropriate diagnostic tests to perform next on this patient's synovial fluid. Synovial fluid aspiration is essential when evaluating for infection and crystal-related disease and is useful in distinguishing between inflammatory and noninflammatory disease. On physical examination, this febrile patient has evidence of a monoarthritis with inflammation in her knee, which is confirmed by the cloudy appearance of the synovial fluid at the bedside and her elevated synovial fluid leukocyte count (15,000/μL [15 × 10^9/L]). Synovial fluid leukocyte counts greater than 2000/μL (2.0 × 10^9/L) are consistent with inflammatory fluid; the higher the count is, the more inflammatory the fluid and the greater the suspicion for crystal-related or infectious disease. An acute hospitalization or illness can precipitate an attack of crystal-related arthritis (either gout or pseudogout) and/or infection, and these entities can be evaluated for by synovial fluid analysis. It is important to note that the presence of crystals does not rule out concomitant infection. The most useful tests to obtain when analyzing synovial fluid are leukocyte count, stains, cultures, and crystal analysis. Sometimes the amount of synovial fluid available for analysis may be small; therefore, it is important to order only the most useful tests.

Antinuclear antibodies, glucose levels, and protein levels do not add any useful information and do not distinguish between infectious and noninfectious synovial fluid.

KEY POINT

- The most useful tests to obtain from synovial fluid are leukocyte count, Gram stains, cultures, and crystal analysis to evaluate for infection and crystal-related disease and to distinguish between inflammatory and noninflammatory disease.

Bibliography

Courtney P, Doherty M. Joint aspiration and injection and synovial fluid analysis. Best Pract Res Clin Rheumatol. 2013 Apr;27(2):137–69. [PMID: 23731929]

Index

ACP®

American College of Physicians
Leading Internal Medicine, Improving Lives

Medical Knowledge Self-Assessment Program® 17

A NAME AND ADDRESS (Please complete.)

Last Name   First Name   Middle Initial

Address

Address cont.

City   State   ZIP Code

Country

Email address

B Order Number

(Use the Order Number on your MKSAP materials packing slip.)

C ACP ID Number

(Refer to packing slip in your MKSAP materials for your ACP ID Number.)

TO EARN *AMA PRA CATEGORY 1 CREDITS*™ YOU MUST:

1. Answer all questions.
2. Score a minimum of 50% correct.

==

TO EARN *FREE* INSTANTANEOUS *AMA PRA CATEGORY 1 CREDITS*™ ONLINE:

1. Answer all of your questions.
2. Go to **mksap.acponline.org** and enter your ACP Online username and password to access an online answer sheet.
3. Enter your answers.
4. You can also enter your answers directly at **mksap.acponline.org** without first using this answer sheet.

To Submit Your Answer Sheet by Mail or FAX for a $15 Administrative Fee per Answer Sheet:

1. Answer all of your questions and calculate your score.
2. Complete boxes A–F.
3. Complete payment information.
4. Send the answer sheet and payment information to ACP, using the FAX number/address listed below.

COMPLETE FORM BELOW ONLY IF YOU SUBMIT BY MAIL OR FAX

Last Name   First Name   MI

Payment Information. Must remit in US funds, drawn on a US bank.

The processing fee for each paper answer sheet is $15.

☐ Check, made payable to ACP, enclosed

Charge to ☐ **VISA** ☐ **MasterCard** ☐ **AMERICAN EXPRESS** ☐ **DISCOVER**

Card Number _____

Expiration Date _____/_____   Security code (3 or 4 digit #s) _____
                 MM   YY

Signature _____

Fax to: 215-351-2799

Mail to:
Member and Customer Service
American College of Physicians
190 N. Independence Mall West
Philadelphia, PA 19106–1572

D

TEST TYPE

		Maximum Number of CME Credits
○	Cardiovascular Medicine	21
○	Dermatology	12
○	Gastroenterology and Hepatology	16
○	Hematology and Oncology	22
○	Neurology	16
○	Rheumatology	16
○	Endocrinology and Metabolism	14
○	General Internal Medicine	26
○	Infectious Disease	19
○	Nephrology	19
○	Pulmonary and Critical Care Medicine	19

E

CREDITS CLAIMED ON SECTION
(1 hour = 1 credit)

Enter the number of credits earned on the test to the nearest quarter hour. Physicians should claim only the credit commensurate with the extent of their participation in the activity.

F

Enter your score here.

Instructions for calculating your own score are found in front of the self-assessment test in each book.

You must receive a minimum score of 50% correct.

_____ %

Credit Submission Date: _____

1 Ⓐ Ⓑ Ⓒ Ⓓ Ⓔ
2 Ⓐ Ⓑ Ⓒ Ⓓ Ⓔ
3 Ⓐ Ⓑ Ⓒ Ⓓ Ⓔ
4 Ⓐ Ⓑ Ⓒ Ⓓ Ⓔ
5 Ⓐ Ⓑ Ⓒ Ⓓ Ⓔ

6 Ⓐ Ⓑ Ⓒ Ⓓ Ⓔ
7 Ⓐ Ⓑ Ⓒ Ⓓ Ⓔ
8 Ⓐ Ⓑ Ⓒ Ⓓ Ⓔ
9 Ⓐ Ⓑ Ⓒ Ⓓ Ⓔ
10 Ⓐ Ⓑ Ⓒ Ⓓ Ⓔ

11 Ⓐ Ⓑ Ⓒ Ⓓ Ⓔ
12 Ⓐ Ⓑ Ⓒ Ⓓ Ⓔ
13 Ⓐ Ⓑ Ⓒ Ⓓ Ⓔ
14 Ⓐ Ⓑ Ⓒ Ⓓ Ⓔ
15 Ⓐ Ⓑ Ⓒ Ⓓ Ⓔ

16 Ⓐ Ⓑ Ⓒ Ⓓ Ⓔ
17 Ⓐ Ⓑ Ⓒ Ⓓ Ⓔ
18 Ⓐ Ⓑ Ⓒ Ⓓ Ⓔ
19 Ⓐ Ⓑ Ⓒ Ⓓ Ⓔ
20 Ⓐ Ⓑ Ⓒ Ⓓ Ⓔ

21 Ⓐ Ⓑ Ⓒ Ⓓ Ⓔ
22 Ⓐ Ⓑ Ⓒ Ⓓ Ⓔ
23 Ⓐ Ⓑ Ⓒ Ⓓ Ⓔ
24 Ⓐ Ⓑ Ⓒ Ⓓ Ⓔ
25 Ⓐ Ⓑ Ⓒ Ⓓ Ⓔ

26 Ⓐ Ⓑ Ⓒ Ⓓ Ⓔ
27 Ⓐ Ⓑ Ⓒ Ⓓ Ⓔ
28 Ⓐ Ⓑ Ⓒ Ⓓ Ⓔ
29 Ⓐ Ⓑ Ⓒ Ⓓ Ⓔ
30 Ⓐ Ⓑ Ⓒ Ⓓ Ⓔ

31 Ⓐ Ⓑ Ⓒ Ⓓ Ⓔ
32 Ⓐ Ⓑ Ⓒ Ⓓ Ⓔ
33 Ⓐ Ⓑ Ⓒ Ⓓ Ⓔ
34 Ⓐ Ⓑ Ⓒ Ⓓ Ⓔ
35 Ⓐ Ⓑ Ⓒ Ⓓ Ⓔ

36 Ⓐ Ⓑ Ⓒ Ⓓ Ⓔ
37 Ⓐ Ⓑ Ⓒ Ⓓ Ⓔ
38 Ⓐ Ⓑ Ⓒ Ⓓ Ⓔ
39 Ⓐ Ⓑ Ⓒ Ⓓ Ⓔ
40 Ⓐ Ⓑ Ⓒ Ⓓ Ⓔ

41 Ⓐ Ⓑ Ⓒ Ⓓ Ⓔ
42 Ⓐ Ⓑ Ⓒ Ⓓ Ⓔ
43 Ⓐ Ⓑ Ⓒ Ⓓ Ⓔ
44 Ⓐ Ⓑ Ⓒ Ⓓ Ⓔ
45 Ⓐ Ⓑ Ⓒ Ⓓ Ⓔ

46 Ⓐ Ⓑ Ⓒ Ⓓ Ⓔ
47 Ⓐ Ⓑ Ⓒ Ⓓ Ⓔ
48 Ⓐ Ⓑ Ⓒ Ⓓ Ⓔ
49 Ⓐ Ⓑ Ⓒ Ⓓ Ⓔ
50 Ⓐ Ⓑ Ⓒ Ⓓ Ⓔ

51 Ⓐ Ⓑ Ⓒ Ⓓ Ⓔ
52 Ⓐ Ⓑ Ⓒ Ⓓ Ⓔ
53 Ⓐ Ⓑ Ⓒ Ⓓ Ⓔ
54 Ⓐ Ⓑ Ⓒ Ⓓ Ⓔ
55 Ⓐ Ⓑ Ⓒ Ⓓ Ⓔ

56 Ⓐ Ⓑ Ⓒ Ⓓ Ⓔ
57 Ⓐ Ⓑ Ⓒ Ⓓ Ⓔ
58 Ⓐ Ⓑ Ⓒ Ⓓ Ⓔ
59 Ⓐ Ⓑ Ⓒ Ⓓ Ⓔ
60 Ⓐ Ⓑ Ⓒ Ⓓ Ⓔ

61 Ⓐ Ⓑ Ⓒ Ⓓ Ⓔ
62 Ⓐ Ⓑ Ⓒ Ⓓ Ⓔ
63 Ⓐ Ⓑ Ⓒ Ⓓ Ⓔ
64 Ⓐ Ⓑ Ⓒ Ⓓ Ⓔ
65 Ⓐ Ⓑ Ⓒ Ⓓ Ⓔ

66 Ⓐ Ⓑ Ⓒ Ⓓ Ⓔ
67 Ⓐ Ⓑ Ⓒ Ⓓ Ⓔ
68 Ⓐ Ⓑ Ⓒ Ⓓ Ⓔ
69 Ⓐ Ⓑ Ⓒ Ⓓ Ⓔ
70 Ⓐ Ⓑ Ⓒ Ⓓ Ⓔ

71 Ⓐ Ⓑ Ⓒ Ⓓ Ⓔ
72 Ⓐ Ⓑ Ⓒ Ⓓ Ⓔ
73 Ⓐ Ⓑ Ⓒ Ⓓ Ⓔ
74 Ⓐ Ⓑ Ⓒ Ⓓ Ⓔ
75 Ⓐ Ⓑ Ⓒ Ⓓ Ⓔ

76 Ⓐ Ⓑ Ⓒ Ⓓ Ⓔ
77 Ⓐ Ⓑ Ⓒ Ⓓ Ⓔ
78 Ⓐ Ⓑ Ⓒ Ⓓ Ⓔ
79 Ⓐ Ⓑ Ⓒ Ⓓ Ⓔ
80 Ⓐ Ⓑ Ⓒ Ⓓ Ⓔ

81 Ⓐ Ⓑ Ⓒ Ⓓ Ⓔ
82 Ⓐ Ⓑ Ⓒ Ⓓ Ⓔ
83 Ⓐ Ⓑ Ⓒ Ⓓ Ⓔ
84 Ⓐ Ⓑ Ⓒ Ⓓ Ⓔ
85 Ⓐ Ⓑ Ⓒ Ⓓ Ⓔ

86 Ⓐ Ⓑ Ⓒ Ⓓ Ⓔ
87 Ⓐ Ⓑ Ⓒ Ⓓ Ⓔ
88 Ⓐ Ⓑ Ⓒ Ⓓ Ⓔ
89 Ⓐ Ⓑ Ⓒ Ⓓ Ⓔ
90 Ⓐ Ⓑ Ⓒ Ⓓ Ⓔ

91 Ⓐ Ⓑ Ⓒ Ⓓ Ⓔ
92 Ⓐ Ⓑ Ⓒ Ⓓ Ⓔ
93 Ⓐ Ⓑ Ⓒ Ⓓ Ⓔ
94 Ⓐ Ⓑ Ⓒ Ⓓ Ⓔ
95 Ⓐ Ⓑ Ⓒ Ⓓ Ⓔ

96 Ⓐ Ⓑ Ⓒ Ⓓ Ⓔ
97 Ⓐ Ⓑ Ⓒ Ⓓ Ⓔ
98 Ⓐ Ⓑ Ⓒ Ⓓ Ⓔ
99 Ⓐ Ⓑ Ⓒ Ⓓ Ⓔ
100 Ⓐ Ⓑ Ⓒ Ⓓ Ⓔ

101 Ⓐ Ⓑ Ⓒ Ⓓ Ⓔ
102 Ⓐ Ⓑ Ⓒ Ⓓ Ⓔ
103 Ⓐ Ⓑ Ⓒ Ⓓ Ⓔ
104 Ⓐ Ⓑ Ⓒ Ⓓ Ⓔ
105 Ⓐ Ⓑ Ⓒ Ⓓ Ⓔ

106 Ⓐ Ⓑ Ⓒ Ⓓ Ⓔ
107 Ⓐ Ⓑ Ⓒ Ⓓ Ⓔ
108 Ⓐ Ⓑ Ⓒ Ⓓ Ⓔ
109 Ⓐ Ⓑ Ⓒ Ⓓ Ⓔ
110 Ⓐ Ⓑ Ⓒ Ⓓ Ⓔ

111 Ⓐ Ⓑ Ⓒ Ⓓ Ⓔ
112 Ⓐ Ⓑ Ⓒ Ⓓ Ⓔ
113 Ⓐ Ⓑ Ⓒ Ⓓ Ⓔ
114 Ⓐ Ⓑ Ⓒ Ⓓ Ⓔ
115 Ⓐ Ⓑ Ⓒ Ⓓ Ⓔ

116 Ⓐ Ⓑ Ⓒ Ⓓ Ⓔ
117 Ⓐ Ⓑ Ⓒ Ⓓ Ⓔ
118 Ⓐ Ⓑ Ⓒ Ⓓ Ⓔ
119 Ⓐ Ⓑ Ⓒ Ⓓ Ⓔ
120 Ⓐ Ⓑ Ⓒ Ⓓ Ⓔ

121 Ⓐ Ⓑ Ⓒ Ⓓ Ⓔ
122 Ⓐ Ⓑ Ⓒ Ⓓ Ⓔ
123 Ⓐ Ⓑ Ⓒ Ⓓ Ⓔ
124 Ⓐ Ⓑ Ⓒ Ⓓ Ⓔ
125 Ⓐ Ⓑ Ⓒ Ⓓ Ⓔ

126 Ⓐ Ⓑ Ⓒ Ⓓ Ⓔ
127 Ⓐ Ⓑ Ⓒ Ⓓ Ⓔ
128 Ⓐ Ⓑ Ⓒ Ⓓ Ⓔ
129 Ⓐ Ⓑ Ⓒ Ⓓ Ⓔ
130 Ⓐ Ⓑ Ⓒ Ⓓ Ⓔ

131 Ⓐ Ⓑ Ⓒ Ⓓ Ⓔ
132 Ⓐ Ⓑ Ⓒ Ⓓ Ⓔ
133 Ⓐ Ⓑ Ⓒ Ⓓ Ⓔ
134 Ⓐ Ⓑ Ⓒ Ⓓ Ⓔ
135 Ⓐ Ⓑ Ⓒ Ⓓ Ⓔ

136 Ⓐ Ⓑ Ⓒ Ⓓ Ⓔ
137 Ⓐ Ⓑ Ⓒ Ⓓ Ⓔ
138 Ⓐ Ⓑ Ⓒ Ⓓ Ⓔ
139 Ⓐ Ⓑ Ⓒ Ⓓ Ⓔ
140 Ⓐ Ⓑ Ⓒ Ⓓ Ⓔ

141 Ⓐ Ⓑ Ⓒ Ⓓ Ⓔ
142 Ⓐ Ⓑ Ⓒ Ⓓ Ⓔ
143 Ⓐ Ⓑ Ⓒ Ⓓ Ⓔ
144 Ⓐ Ⓑ Ⓒ Ⓓ Ⓔ
145 Ⓐ Ⓑ Ⓒ Ⓓ Ⓔ

146 Ⓐ Ⓑ Ⓒ Ⓓ Ⓔ
147 Ⓐ Ⓑ Ⓒ Ⓓ Ⓔ
148 Ⓐ Ⓑ Ⓒ Ⓓ Ⓔ
149 Ⓐ Ⓑ Ⓒ Ⓓ Ⓔ
150 Ⓐ Ⓑ Ⓒ Ⓓ Ⓔ

151 Ⓐ Ⓑ Ⓒ Ⓓ Ⓔ
152 Ⓐ Ⓑ Ⓒ Ⓓ Ⓔ
153 Ⓐ Ⓑ Ⓒ Ⓓ Ⓔ
154 Ⓐ Ⓑ Ⓒ Ⓓ Ⓔ
155 Ⓐ Ⓑ Ⓒ Ⓓ Ⓔ

156 Ⓐ Ⓑ Ⓒ Ⓓ Ⓔ
157 Ⓐ Ⓑ Ⓒ Ⓓ Ⓔ
158 Ⓐ Ⓑ Ⓒ Ⓓ Ⓔ
159 Ⓐ Ⓑ Ⓒ Ⓓ Ⓔ
160 Ⓐ Ⓑ Ⓒ Ⓓ Ⓔ

161 Ⓐ Ⓑ Ⓒ Ⓓ Ⓔ
162 Ⓐ Ⓑ Ⓒ Ⓓ Ⓔ
163 Ⓐ Ⓑ Ⓒ Ⓓ Ⓔ
164 Ⓐ Ⓑ Ⓒ Ⓓ Ⓔ
165 Ⓐ Ⓑ Ⓒ Ⓓ Ⓔ

166 Ⓐ Ⓑ Ⓒ Ⓓ Ⓔ
167 Ⓐ Ⓑ Ⓒ Ⓓ Ⓔ
168 Ⓐ Ⓑ Ⓒ Ⓓ Ⓔ
169 Ⓐ Ⓑ Ⓒ Ⓓ Ⓔ
170 Ⓐ Ⓑ Ⓒ Ⓓ Ⓔ

171 Ⓐ Ⓑ Ⓒ Ⓓ Ⓔ
172 Ⓐ Ⓑ Ⓒ Ⓓ Ⓔ
173 Ⓐ Ⓑ Ⓒ Ⓓ Ⓔ
174 Ⓐ Ⓑ Ⓒ Ⓓ Ⓔ
175 Ⓐ Ⓑ Ⓒ Ⓓ Ⓔ

176 Ⓐ Ⓑ Ⓒ Ⓓ Ⓔ
177 Ⓐ Ⓑ Ⓒ Ⓓ Ⓔ
178 Ⓐ Ⓑ Ⓒ Ⓓ Ⓔ
179 Ⓐ Ⓑ Ⓒ Ⓓ Ⓔ
180 Ⓐ Ⓑ Ⓒ Ⓓ Ⓔ